Essentials of Clinical Geriatrics

Fourth Edition

Robert L. Kane, M.D.

*Professor and Minnesota Endowed Chair
in Long-Term Care and Aging
School of Public Health
University of Minnesota
Minneapolis, Minnesota*

Joseph G. Ouslander, M.D.

*Professor of Medicine
Director, Division of Geriatric Medicine
and Gerontology
Vice President for Professional Affairs
Wesley Woods Center of Emory University
Director, Atlanta VA Rehabilitation
Research & Development Center
Atlanta, Georgia*

Itamar B. Abrass, M.D.

*Professor and Head, Division of Gerontology
and Geriatric Medicine
University of Washington
Seattle, Washington*

McGraw-Hill
HEALTH PROFESSIONS DIVISION

New York   St. Louis   San Francisco   Auckland
Bogotá   Caracas   Lisbon   London
Mexico City   Milan   Montreal   New Delhi   Paris
San Juan   Singapore   Sydney   Tokyo   Toronto

McGraw-Hill

A Division of The McGraw-Hill Companies

ESSENTIALS OF CLINICAL GERIATRICS
Fourth Edition

1234567890 DOCDOC 99

ISBN 0-07-034458-2

This book was set in Times Roman by The PRD Group
The editors were Stephen Zollo and Muza Navrozov.
The production supervisor was Richard Ruzycka.
The cover was designed by José Fonfrias.
The index was prepared by Tony Greenberg, M.D.
R. R. Donnelley & Sons was printer and binder.

This book is printed on recycled, acid-free paper.

Library of Congress Cataloging-in-Publication Data

Kane, Robert L., date
    Essentials of clinical geriatrics / Robert L. Kane, Joseph G.
Ouslander, Itamar B. Abrass.—4th ed.
        p.   cm.
    Includes bibliographical references and index.
    ISBN 0-07-034458-2
    1. Geriatrics. 2. Aging. 3. Aged—Health and hygiene.
I. Ouslander, Joseph G. II. Abrass, Itamar B. III. Title.
    [DNLM: 1. Geriatrics. 2. Aging. WT 100 K16e 1999]
RC952.K36   1999
618.97—dc21
DNLM/DLC
for Library of Congress

Essentials of Clinical Geriatrics

NOTICE

Medicine is an ever-changing science. As new research and clinical experience broaden our knowledge, changes in treatment and drug therapy are required. The authors and the publisher of this work have checked with sources believed to be reliable in their efforts to provide information that is complete and generally in accord with the standards accepted at the time of publication. However, in view of the possibility of human error or changes in medical sciences, neither the authors nor the publisher nor any other party who has been involved in the preparation or publication of this work warrants that the information contained herein is in every respect accurate or complete, and they are not responsible for any errors or omissions or for the results obtained from use of such information. Readers are encouraged to confirm the information contained herein with other sources. For example and in particular, readers are advised to check the product information sheet included in the package of each drug they plan to administer to be certain that the information contained in this book is accurate and that changes have not been made in the recommended dose or in the contraindications for administration. This recommendation is of particular importance in connection with new or infrequently used drugs.

CONTENTS

APPENDIX   SUGGESTED GERIATRIC MEDICAL FORMS

LIST OF TABLES AND FIGURES

CHAPTER THREE

CHAPTER FOUR

CHAPTER FIVE

CHAPTER SIX

CHAPTER SEVEN

CHAPTER EIGHT

CHAPTER NINE

CHAPTER TEN

CHAPTER TWELVE

CHAPTER THIRTEEN

CHAPTER FOURTEEN

CHAPTER FIFTEEN

CHAPTER SIXTEEN

PREFACE

The world of geriatrics has changed substantially since we wrote the first edition of this book, but the same goals still pertain. This book is intended to provide an overview and an introduction to the elements of the care of older persons. It is not intended to supplant a textbook in medicine. Rather, it emphasizes those aspects of care that are not usually well addressed in such books. This book is designed to be useful to practitioners at various levels of training. We continue to rely heavily on tables and figures to summarize information. We are proud that many educators have told us that they use these illustrations for their own presentations.

We have reorganized this edition of the book to reflect the changes in emphasis. The material on iatrogenesis has been combined with the expanded and substantially revised work on clinical expectations. Long-term care has been expanded to become health services. The chapter on temperature regulation has been combined with vitality. The chapter on ethical issues has been restored and expanded.

We have updated almost all areas. While there have been notable clinical advances in areas such as osteoporosis, the treatment of dementia and cardiac care, the greatest changes continue to occur in the way services are organized. Managed care has become a significant force on the aging scene. It is not yet clear whether it will achieve

anything close to its potential to support the establishment of a chronic care approach. Long-term care has diversified. We are beginning to recognize the need for a more fundamental revolution in the way we practice medicine. The dominant model, which has been based on an acute care paradigm, must yield to a new model that responds to the overwhelming prevalence of chronic disease. This transition implies a need to develop models of care that address extended episodes rather than discrete events. We need to think in terms of investments in care that will prevent or delay exacerbations. Management and function gain take precedence over eliminating disease or avoiding death. The medical and social aspects of care must be synergized.

Essentials of Clinical Geriatrics

PART
ONE

THE AGING PATIENT AND GERIATRIC ASSESSMENT

CHAPTER ONE

CLINICAL IMPLICATIONS
OF THE AGING PROCESS

The care of older patients differs from that of younger patients for a number of reasons. Some of these can be traced to the changes that occur in the process of aging, some are caused by the plethora of diseases and disruptions that accompany seniority, and still others result from the way old people are treated.

Perhaps one of the most intriguing challenges in medicine is to unravel the process of aging. Although we may be able to see pure aging in a cellular culture, it is very hard to visualize in the intact organism. Discussions about aging seem to imply accumulation of chronic diseases. How then does one separate the changes caused solely by aging from the sequelae of disease? Would a group of disease-free older persons be the appropriate models to help us understand the aging process? The prospect sounds uncomfortably like describing life on the basis of a colony of germ-free mice.

Nonetheless, the distinction between so-called normal aging and pathologic changes is critical to the care of older people. We wish to avoid both dismissing treatable pathology as simply a concomitant of old age and treating natural aging processes as though they were diseases. The latter is particularly dangerous because older adults are so vulnerable to iatrogenic effects.

There is growing appreciation that everyone does not age in the same way or at the same rate. The changing composition of today's older adults compared with that of a generation ago may actually reflect a bimodal shift wherein there are both more disabled people and more healthy older people. Attention has become focused on the variations in aging, with great interest directed toward those described as aging successfully—that is, showing the least decline in function with time (Rowe and Kahn, 1987).

CHANGES ASSOCIATED WITH "NORMAL" AGING

We have already noted the critical and difficult distinction a clinician must make to attribute a finding to either the expected course of aging or the result of pathologic changes. This distinction perplexes the researcher as well. We currently lack precise knowledge of what constitutes normal aging. Much of our information comes from cross-sectional studies, which compare findings from a group of younger persons with those from a group of older individuals. Such data may reflect differences other than simply the effects of age. The older group grew up in a different environment, perhaps with different diet and activities. They represent a cohort of survivors. We have come to appreciate that what we see in the older patient is largely a result of what is brought to old age. For example, the decrease in the frequency of osteoporosis today has been related to the observation that women entering the high-risk period (postmenopause) have stronger bones with thicker cortices.

Many of the changes associated with aging result from gradual loss. These losses may often begin in early adulthood, but—thanks to the redundancy of most organ systems—the decrement does not become functionally significant until the loss is fairly extensive.

Based on cross-sectional comparisons of groups at different ages (Andres and Tobin, 1977), most organ systems seem to lose function at about 1 percent a year beginning around age 30. More recent data (Svanborg et al., 1982) suggest that the changes in people followed longitudinally are much less dramatic and certainly begin well after age 70.

In some organ systems, such as the kidney, a subgroup of persons appear to experience gradually declining function over time, whereas others' function remains constant (Lindeman et al., 1985). If these

newer findings are substantiated, the earlier theory of gradual loss must be reassessed as reflecting disease rather than aging.

Given a pattern of gradual deterioration—whether from aging, disease, or both—we are best advised to think in terms of thresholds. The loss of function does not become significant until it crosses a given level. Thus the functional performance of an organ in an older person depends on two principal factors: (1) the rate of deterioration and (2) the level of performance needed. It is not surprising then to learn that most older persons will have normal laboratory values. The critical difference—in fact, the hallmark of aging—lies not in the resting level of performance but in how the organ (or organism) adapts to external stress. For example, an older person may show a normal blood sugar at rest but be unable to handle a glucose load within the normal parameters for younger subjects. The glucose tolerance test thus must be reinterpreted for older subjects, and 2-h postprandial glucose levels are less helpful than fasting blood sugars to detect diabetes.

The same pattern of decreased response to stress can be seen in the performance of other endocrine systems or the cardiovascular system. An older individual may have a normal resting pulse and cardiac output but be unable to achieve an adequate increase in either with exercise.

Sometimes the changes of aging work together to produce apparently normal resting values in other ways. For example, although both glomerular filtration and renal blood flow decrease with age, many elderly persons have normal serum creatinine levels because of the concomitant decreases in lean muscle mass and creatinine production. Thus serum creatinine is not as good an indicator of renal function in the elderly as in younger persons. Because knowledge of kidney function is so critical in drug therapy, it is important to get some measure of this parameter. A useful formula for estimating creatinine clearance on the basis of serum creatinine values in the elderly has been developed (Cockcroft and Gault, 1976). (The actual formula is provided in Chap. 14.)

Table 1-1 summarizes some of the pertinent changes that occur with aging. For many items, the changes begin in adulthood and proceed gradually; others may not manifest themselves until well into seniority. Readers interested in a more detailed discussion of the changes associated with aging should consult the several excellent reviews on the subject from which this table was derived (Birren and Schaie, 1985; Finch and Schneider, 1985).

Table 1-1 Changes associated with aging

Item	Morphology	Function
Overall	Decreased height (vertebral compression and stooped posture secondary to increased kyphosis) Decreased weight (after age 80 in longitudinal studies) Increased fat-to-lean body mass ratio Decreased total body water Increased wrinkling	
Skin	Atrophy of sweat glands	
Cardiovascular system	Elongation and tortuosity of arteries, including aorta Increased intimal thickening of arteries Increased fibrosis of media of arteries Sclerosis of heart valves	Decreased cardiac output Decreased heart rate response to stress Decreased compliance of peripheral blood vessels
Kidney	Increased number of abnormal glomeruli	Decreased creatinine clearance Decreased renal blood flow Decreased maximum urine osmolality
Lung	Decreased elasticity Decreased activity of cilia	Decreased forced vital capacity and forced expiratory volume Decreased maximal oxygen uptake Decreased cough reflex
Gastrointestinal tract	Decreased hydrochloric acid Fewer taste buds	Slowed intestinal motility
Skeleton	Osteoarthritis Loss of bone substance	
Eyes	Arcus senilis Decreased pupil size Growth of lens	Decreased accommodation Hyperopia Decreased acuity Decreased color sensitivity Decreased depth perception

Table 1-1 Changes associated with aging *(Continued)*

Item	Morphology	Function
Hearing	Degenerative changes of ossicles Increased obstruction of eustachian tube Atrophy of external auditory meatus Atrophy of cochlear hair cells Loss of auditory neurons	Decreased perception in high frequencies Decreased pitch discrimination
Immune system		Decreased T-cell activity
Nervous system	Decreased brain weight Decreased cortical cell count	Increased motor response time Slower psychomotor performance Decreased intellectual performance Decreased complex learning Decreased hours of sleep Decreased hours of REM sleep
Endocrine	Decreased triiodothyronine (T$_3$) Decreased free (unbound) testosterone Increased insulin Increased norepinephrine Increased parathoromone Increased vasopressin	

BIOLOGICAL AGING

It is now a commonly accepted notion that aging is a multifactorial process. Extended longevity is frequently associated with enhanced metabolic capacity and response to stress. The importance of genetics in the regulation of biological aging is demonstrated by the characteristic longevity of each animal species. However, heritability of life-span accounts for ≤35 percent of its variance, whereas environmental factors account for >65 percent of the variance (Finch and Tanzi, 1997).

Several theories of aging have been promulgated and recently reviewed (Goldstein, 1989; Abrass, 1991; Vijg and Wei, 1995). These theories fall into two general categories: accumulation of damage to informational molecules or the regulation of specific genes (Table 1-2).

DNA undergoes continuous change both in response to exogenous agents and intrinsic processes. Stability is maintained by the double-strandedness of DNA and by specific repair enzymes. It has been proposed that somatic mutagenesis, either owing to greater susceptibility to mutagenesis or deficits in repair mechanisms, is a factor in biological aging. In fact, there is a positive correlation of species longevity with DNA repair enzymes. However, in humans, the spontaneous mutagenesis rate is not adequate to account for the number of changes that would be necessary, and there is no evidence that a failure in repair systems causes aging.

A related theory, the error catastrophe theory, proposes that errors occur in DNA, RNA, and protein synthesis, each augmenting the other and finally culminating in an error catastrophe. Translation was considered the most likely source for age-dependent errors, since it was the final common pathway. However, increased translational errors have not been found in either in vivo or in vitro aging. Amino acid substitutions do not increase with age, although some enzyme activities may be altered by changes in posttranslational modification, such as glycosylation.

The major by-products of oxidative metabolism include superoxide radicals that can react with DNA, RNA, proteins, and lipids,

Table 1-2 Major theories on aging

Theory	Mechanisms	Manifestations
Accumulation of damage to informational molecules	Spontaneous mutagenesis	Copying errors
	Failure in DNA repair systems	
	Errors in DNA, RNA, and protein synthesis	Error catastrophe
	Superoxide radicals and loss of scavenging enzymes	Oxidative cellular damage
Regulation of specific genes	Appearance of specific protein(s)	Genetically programmed senescence

leading to cellular damage and aging. There are several scavenging enzymes and some small molecules, such as vitamins C and E, that protect the cell from oxidative damage. There is no significant loss of scavenging enzymes in aging, and vitamins C and E do not increase longevity in experimental animals. However, interest in this hypothesis persists, since overexpression of antioxidative enzymes retards the age-related accrual of oxidative damage and extends the maximum life span of transgenic fruit flies; moreover, caloric restriction lowers levels of oxidative stress and damage and extends the maximum life span of rodents (Sohal and Weindruch, 1996).

One concept of aging is that it is regulated by specific genes. Support for such a hypothesis has been gained mainly from yeast, nematodes, fruit flies, and models of in vitro aging. Several genes in yeast, nematodes, and fruit flies have been found to extend the species life span. They appear to reinforce the importance of metabolic capacity and stress responses in aging.

In adulthood, cells can be placed into one of three categories based on their replicative capacity: continuously replicating, replicating in response to a challenge, and nonreplicating. Epidermal, gastrointestinal, and hematopoietic cells are continuously renewed; liver can regenerate in response to injury; while neurons and cardiac and skeletal muscle do not regenerate.

In vitro replication is closely related to in vivo proliferation. Neurons and cardiac myocytes from adults can be maintained in culture but do not divide, whereas hepatocytes, marrow cells, endothelial cells, and fibroblasts replicate in vitro. Since they are easily obtained from skin, fibroblasts have been the most extensively studied. Although some cells continuously replicate in vivo, they have a finite replicative life. For fibroblasts in vitro, this is about 50 doublings (Hayflick, 1979). Replicative life in vitro correlates with the age of the donor, such that the older the donor, the fewer the doublings in vitro. With time in culture, doubling time decreases and ultimately stops.

When fibroblasts from younger donors are fused with nonreplicating senescent cells, DNA synthesis is inhibited in both nuclei. Transient inhibition of protein synthesis immediately following fusion increased DNA synthesis in both nuclei, suggesting that a protein factor may be involved in the inhibition of replication and should exist in the cytoplasm. When senescent cytoplasts (cells without nuclei) are fused with young, dividing cells, DNA synthesis is depressed. Growth

arrest both in vivo and in vitro has now been associated with the appearance of a specific protein. This is a nuclear protein that may be involved in DNA replication.

With each cell division, a portion of the terminal end of chromosomes (the telomere) is not replicated and therefore shortens. It is proposed that telomere shortening is the clock that results in the shift to a senescent pattern of gene expression and ultimately cell senescence (Fossel, 1998). Telomerase is an enzyme that acts by adding DNA bases to telomeres. Transfection of the catalytic component of this enzyme into senescent cells extends their telomeres as well as the replicative life span of the cells and induces a pattern of gene expression typical of young cells. It is now possible to explore the role of replicative senescence in aging and associated chronic disease processes.

These experiments help define the finite life span of cells in vitro but do not themselves explain in vivo aging, since organisms do not suddenly die because all their cells stop replicating and die. However, factors associated with finite cell replication may more directly influence in vivo aging. Fibroblasts aged in vitro or obtained from older adult donors are less sensitive to a host of growth factors. Such changes occur at both the receptor and postreceptor levels. A decrease in such growth factors, a change in sensitivity to growth factors, and/or a slowing of the cell cycle may slow wound healing and thus place the older individual at greater risk for infection.

For tissues with nonreplicating cells, cell loss may lead to a permanent deficit. With aging, dopaminergic neurons are lost, thus influencing gait and balance and the susceptibility to drug side effects. With further decrements such as ischemia or viral infection, Parkinson's disease may develop. Similar cell loss and/or functional deficits may occur in other neurotransmitter systems and lead to autonomic dysfunction as well as alteration in mental function and neuroendocrine control.

The immune system demonstrates similar phenomena. Lymphocytes from older adults have a diminished proliferative response to a host of mitogens. This appears to be due to both a decrease in lymphokines and a decreased response to extracellular signals. As the thymus involutes after puberty, levels of thymic hormones (thymosins) decrease. Basal and stimulated interleukin-2 (IL-2) production and IL-2 responsiveness also diminish with age. The latter appears to be due, at least in part, to a decreased expression of IL-2 receptors. Some

immune functions can be restored by the addition of these hormones to lymphocytes in vitro, or, in vivo, by their administration to aged animals. The proliferative defect can also be reversed in vitro by calcium ionophores and activators of protein kinase C, suggesting that the T-cell defect may be in transduction of extracellular signals to intracellular function.

In vivo, molecular mechanisms such as those described above contribute to physiologic deficits and altered homeostatic mechanisms that predispose older individuals to dysfunction in the face of stress and disease.

The gene for Werner's syndrome, a progeric syndrome associated with early onset of age-related changes—such as gray hair, balding, atherosclerosis, insulin resistance, and cataracts but not Alzheimer's disease—has recently been cloned. The gene codes for a helicase involved in DNA replication. There is great interest in understanding how a defect in just this one gene leads to the multiple abnormalities of this syndrome.

Molecular geneticists have also recently cloned several genes related to early-onset familial Alzheimer's disease and identified susceptibility genes for the late-onset form of the disease (Tanzi et al., 1996). A small number of families have mutations in the amyloid precursor protein located on chromosome 21. The largest number of families with early-onset familial Alzheimer's disease have a mutation in a gene on chromosome 14. This gene has been named presenilin 1. A similar gene has been identified on chromosome 1 and labeled presenilin 2. The role of the presenilins in Alzheimer's disease pathology is not yet known, but the identification of the three loci mentioned above has led to much excitement for the potential understanding of pathophysiologic mechanisms in this devastating disease. Similarly, the identification of apo E alleles as risk factors for late-onset Alzheimer's disease has raised interest in both the diagnosis and pathology of this disease.

CLINICAL IMPLICATIONS

As we try to understand aging, we appreciate the limitations of available information. As noted earlier, most of the data cited to document changes with age come from cross-sectional studies in which individuals of different ages are compared in terms of group averages. Such

an approach generally reveals a gradual decline in organ function with age, beginning in early middle life. A few studies have followed cohorts of people longitudinally as they age. Their conclusions are quite different. In several parameters, performance actually increases with age. For example, cognitive function can improve over time among older persons (Schaie, 1970). Similarly, cardiac function in subjects free of heart disease does not show inevitable decline with age (Gerstenblith et al., 1985).

The physician must be able to take data derived from group studies and apply them to the individual. It is essential to keep in mind the principle of individual variation. The best predictor of a given patient's performance now is that person's earlier performance rather than an average age-related decline documented in cross-sectional studies. Thus, an 80-year-old runner may well have better cardiovascular function than a 50-year-old sedentary doctor.

Aging is not simply a series of biological changes. That is, when one looks in the mirror and confronts an old person, the noted changes are associated with a variety of alterations in life. Aging is a time of losses: loss of social role (usually through retirement), loss of income, loss of friends and relatives (through death and mobility). It can also be a time of fear: fear for personal safety, fear of financial insecurity, fear of dependency.

In the face of these enormous threats, we should pause to rethink our views about older adults. Rather than being victims, they are the survivors. Most elderly persons have developed mechanisms to cope with multiple limitations. Most nevertheless continue to function. The physician's role is to enhance this coping ability by identifying and treating remediable problems and facilitating changes in the environment to maximize function in the face of those problems that remain.

In some instances, the patient's coping skills may make the physician's task more difficult. The elderly patient has often adapted to problems by denying or ignoring them. In such cases, it will be difficult to obtain a good history. Other patients cope with their disabilities by employing adaptive techniques. For example, a person who is hard of hearing may talk a great deal to hide a hearing deficit. A particularly troublesome problem is the skillful compensation for cognitive losses. At least once in every physician's career, he or she will encounter a patient who carries on a perfectly lucid conversation, only to discover on closer examination that the patient is completely disoriented to time, place, and person. Because it is easy to miss these cognitive

deficits, we recommend that an evaluation of older persons include a formal screening for mental status. A simple method for doing this is described in Chap. 5.

The physician's role is thus a delicate one. The physician must remove barriers erected by coping mechanisms but be equally attentive to restoring and reinforcing those coping skills that enhance functioning.

Coping is not the only factor that complicates getting reliable information from geriatric patients. At the most tangible level, we must first be sure that communication has truly been established. Patients with hearing impairments or severe vision problems may not be receiving the questions and messages we are sending. If they are accustomed to dealing with this deficit by giving ready answers that do not necessarily respond to the questions posed, no useful information is exchanged. It is often helpful to check communication early in the interview by asking the patient to repeat what you have said.

The problems of the geriatric patient may present quite differently from those of younger patients. Because of the increased prevalence of chronic disease, the presenting problem may not be as distinct as with a younger patient, who is typically well until the onset of a new symptom complex. With an elderly patient, the new problem is generally superimposed on a background of already existing signs and symptoms. The onset may be less clear and the manifestations less precise. In addition, we need to recall that many symptoms and signs are not produced by the disease itself but by the body's response to that insult. One of the hallmarks of aging is the reduced response to stress, including the stress of disease. Thus, the symptom intensity may be dampened by the aged body's decreased responsiveness. The presentation of illness in the geriatric patient can be thought of as a combination of dampened primary sound in the presence of background noise.

In treating an older adult, it is useful to keep in mind that an individual's ability to function depends on a combination of his or her characteristics (e.g., innate capacity, motivation, pain tolerance) and the setting in which that person is expected to function. The same individual may be functional in one setting and dependent in another. The physician's first responsibility is to treat the patient, to remedy the remediable by searching for and dealing with those conditions that are treatable. Having improved the patient's ability (physiologically and psychologically) as much as possible, the physician's next

task is to structure an environment that will facilitate the patient's functioning with maximum autonomy. This latter mandate should not rest exclusively on the doctor's shoulders. A variety of health-related professionals are available in most situations to play major roles in locating and utilizing supportive environments. But the physician must not abrogate this task. To ignore the environment of a disabled individual is tantamount to prescribing drugs and ignoring the patient's compliance with the treatment regimen.

Conversely, the environment can produce dysfunction. At the simplest level, it may produce hazards that lead to falls (see Chap. 8). At a more subtle level, it may necessitate a level of effort that produces decompensation. For example, an elderly person with dyspnea on exertion may get along reasonably well in a ground-floor apartment but become unmanageable in an apartment on the second floor of a building with no elevator. Similarly, patients with compromised pulmonary or cardiac function will show increased morbidity and mortality as air pollution levels increase. Finally, the environment may create disability by fostering dependency.

At a somewhat more subtle level, physicians must be aware of the forces among caregivers that foster dependency. Patients may be immobile because of the care they get. One important factor is risk aversion. Nursing personnel may be reluctant to mobilize patients for fear that they will fall and sustain injuries. We must provide assurance to staff that they will not be penalized for activating patients appropriately. Nor is risk aversion confined to professionals. Families may be equally protective, insisting on limiting an older relative's activities or moving him or her to a more closely supervised situation. Such fears are often infused with guilt and may manifest as anger. Families can be helped to see the dangers of such restricted activity.

CLASSIFYING GERIATRIC PROBLEMS

Because diagnoses often do not tell the whole story in geriatrics, it is more helpful to think in terms of presenting problems. One aid to recalling some of the common problems of geriatrics uses a series of I's:

- Immobility
- Instability

- Incontinence
- Intellectual impairment
- Infection
- Impairment of vision and hearing
- Irritable colon
- Isolation (depression)
- Inanition (malnutrition)
- Impecunity
- Iatrogenesis
- Insomnia
- Immune deficiency
- Impotence

The list is important for several reasons. Especially with older patients, the expression of the problem may not be a good clue to the etiology. Conversely, a problem may occur for a variety of reasons. For example, an individual may be immobilized by a broken hip, by severe angina, or by arthritis. But the patient may also be immobilized by fear. The elderly patient with a successfully repaired hip fracture may be unwilling to walk again for fear of falling and sustaining another fracture. An elderly person living in a deteriorated neighborhood may be confined to the home not by physical limitations but because of a fear of being molested. Such an individual may decide to enter a long-term-care institution to seek a safer environment. In each instance, the physician and coworkers must obtain a sufficient history to understand the true etiology of the problem if they are to develop a successful approach to remedying the condition.

Another factor in generating dependency is cost. It is often much easier and cheaper to do things *for* people with functional limitations than to invest the effort needed to encourage them to do for themselves. Unfortunately such savings are short-ranged; they will increase the level of dependency and ultimately the amount of care needed.

Among the list of I's, we have included iatrogenesis. The least desirable outcome of medical care is a decrease in the patient's health as a result of contact with the care system. In some cases, there is a real risk that untoward consequences of treatment may worsen a patient's health. The risk-benefit calculation as a basis for urging intervention must be performed carefully for each elderly patient in the context of his or her condition. Many risks are within the ordinary bounds of medicine.

We are concerned here with those events that result from indifferent or superficial care. The physician who casually adds another drug to the patient's polypharmacy portfolio is playing with a living chemistry set. The reduced rate of drug metabolism and excretion in many elderly persons exacerbates the problem of drug interactions (Chap. 4). Even more dangerous is the careless, hasty application of clinical labels. The patient who becomes confused and disoriented in the hospital may not be suffering from dementia. The individual who has an occasional urinary accident is not necessarily incontinent. Labeling patients as demented or incontinent is too often the first step toward their placement in a nursing home, a setting that can make such labels self-fulfilling prophecies. We must exercise great caution in applying these potent labels. They should be reserved for patients who have been carefully evaluated, lest we unnecessarily condemn countless persons to lifetimes of institutionalization.

DIAGNOSIS VERSUS FUNCTIONAL STATUS

One of the persistent problems surrounding growing discussions about care of the elderly has arisen from the emphasis on functioning. This emphasis on the need to direct clinical attention to the patient's functional status as well as to specific medical conditions has occasionally been misinterpreted. The point is not that functional status is more important or more useful than diagnosis but that both are needed. One is incomplete without the other. Functioning is the result of the innate abilities of the patient and the environment that supports those abilities.

Clearly the optimal management of an elderly patient involves identifying a correctable problem and correcting it. The first and principal task of the physician is to do precisely that. No amount of rehabilitation, compassionate care, or environmental manipulation will compensate for missing a remediable diagnosis. However, diagnoses alone are usually insufficient. The elderly are the repositories of chronic disease more often cared for than cured.

The process of geriatrics is thus twofold: (1) careful clinical assessment and management to identify remediable problems and (2) equally careful and competent functional assessment to ascertain how the patient's autonomy can be maximized by appropriate human and mechanical assistance and environmental manipulations.

Our goal in orienting primary care providers is to raise their consciousness about the need to consider the whole patient and his or her environment, but never at the cost of neglecting the search for correctable causes for the patient's problems. In that search for causes, the a priori probabilities will often differ substantially from those of younger patients. For this reason, a problem-focused approach, like that of the I's, outlined above, may prove useful.

REFERENCES

Abrass IB: Biology of aging, in Wilson JD, Braunwald E, Isselbacher KJ, et al (eds): *Principles of Internal Medicine,* 12th ed. New York, McGraw-Hill, 1991.

Andres R, Tobin JD: Endocrine systems, in Finch CE, Hayflick L (eds): *Handbook of the Biology of Aging.* New York, Van Nostrand Reinhold, 1977.

Birren J, Schaie W (eds): *Handbook of the Psychology of Aging,* 2d ed. New York, Van Nostrand Reinhold, 1985.

Cockcroft DW, Gault MH: Prediction of creatinine clearance from serum creatinine. *Nephron* 16:31–41, 1976.

Finch C, Schneider E (eds): *Handbook of the Biology of Aging,* 2d ed. New York, Van Nostrand Reinhold, 1985.

Finch CE, Tanzi RE: Genetics of aging. *Science* 278:407–411, 1997.

Fossel M: Telomerase and the aging cell. *JAMA* 279:1732–1735, 1998.

Gerstenblith G, Weisfeldt ML, Lakatta EG: Disorders of the heart, in Andres R, Bierman EL, Hazzard WR (eds): *Principles of Geriatric Medicine.* New York, McGraw-Hill, 1985.

Goldstein S: The biology of aging, in Kelley WN, DeVita VT, DuPont HL, et al (eds): *Textbook of Internal Medicine.* Philadelphia, Lippincott, 1989.

Hayflick L: Cell biology of aging. *Fed Proc* 38:1847–1850, 1979.

Lindeman RD, Tobin J, Shock NW: Longitudinal studies on the rate of decline in renal function with age. *J Am Geriatr Soc* 33:278–285, 1985.

Rowe JW, Kahn RL: Human aging: Usual and successful. *Science* 237:143–149, 1987.

Schaie KW: A reinterpretation of age-related changes in cognitive structure and functioning, in Goulet LR, Baltes PB (eds): *Life-Span Developmental Psychology: Research and Theory.* New York, Academic Press, 1970.

Shock NW: System integration, in Finch CE, Hayflick L (eds): *Handbook of the Biology of Aging.* New York, Van Nostrand Reinhold, 1977.

Sohal RS, Weindruch R: Oxidative stress, caloric restriction, and aging. *Science* 273:59–63, 1996.

Svanborg A, Bergstrom G, Mellstrom D: *Epidemiological Studies on Social and Medical Conditions of the Elderly.* Copenhagen, World Health Organization, 1982.

Tanzi RE, Kovacs DM, Kim T-W, et al: The gene defects responsible for familial Alzheimer's disease. *Neurobiol Dis* 3(0016):159–168, 1996.

Vijg J, Wei JY: Understanding the biology of aging: the key to prevention and therapy. *J Am Geriatr Soc* 43:426–434, 1995.

SUGGESTED READINGS

Binstock RH, Shanas E (eds): *Handbook of Aging and the Social Sciences,* 2d ed. New York, Van Nostrand Reinhold, 1985.

Finch CE: The regulation of physiological changes during mammalian aging. *Q Rev Biol* 51:49–83, 1976.

Fries JF, Crapo LM: *Vitality and Aging.* San Francisco, Freeman, 1981.

Haynes SG, Feinleib M: *Second Conference on the Epidemiology of Aging.* Washington, DC, U.S. Government Printing Office, 1980.

Jazwinski SM: Longevity, genes, and aging. *Science* 273:54–59, 1996.

Levy-Lahad E, Bird TD: Genetic factors in Alzheimer's Disease: A review of recent advances. *Ann Neurol* 40:829–840, 1996.

Portnoi VA: Diagnostic dilemma of the aged. *Arch Intern Med* 141:734–737, 1981.

Rowe JW: Clinical research on aging: Strategies and directions. *N Engl J Med* 297:1332–1336, 1977.

Scoggin GH: The cellular biochemical and genetic basis of aging, in Schrier RW (ed): *Clinical Internal Medicine in the Aged.* Philadelphia, Saunders, 1982.

Shock NW: The physiology of aging. *Sci Am* 206:100–110, 1962.

Shock NW, Greulich RC, Andres R, et al: *Normal Human Aging: The Baltimore Longitudinal Study of Aging.* NIH Publ. No. 84-2450. Washington, DC: U.S. Government Printing Office, 1984.

Weindruch RH, Kristie JW, Cheney KE, et al: Influence of controlled dietary restriction on immunologic function and aging. *Fed Proc* 38:2007–2016, 1979.

Williams TF, Hill JG, Fairbank ME, Knox KG: Appropriate placement of the chronically ill and aged: A successful approach by evaluation. *JAMA* 226:1332–1335, 1973.

CHAPTER TWO

THE GERIATRIC PATIENT: DEMOGRAPHY AND EPIDEMIOLOGY

From the physician's perspective, the demographic curve strongly argues that medical practice in the future will entail a great deal of geriatrics. Persons aged 65 and older currently represent a little over one-third of the patients seen by a primary care physician. In the next century, we can safely predict that at least every other adult patient will be an older person.

The concern so often heard about the epidemic of aging stems primarily from two factors: numbers and dollars. We hear a great deal of talk about the incipient demise of Social Security, the bankrupt status of Medicare, the death of the family, and dire predictions of demographic cataclysms. There is indeed cause for concern but not necessarily for alarm. The message of the numbers is straightforward: we cannot go on as we have; new approaches are needed. The shape of those approaches to meeting the needs of growing numbers of elderly persons in this society will reflect societal values. We are already witnessing major changes in the way we provide care that have been stimulated by the costs associated with an aging society. However, aging alone is not the major contributor to the rapidly

escalating costs of care. Although older people use a disproportionately large amount of medical care, most of the growth in costs is traceable to tremendous expansion in medical technology, both diagnostic and therapeutic. We have potent but often expensive tools at our disposal. In some ways, we can be said to be reaping the fruits of our success. While a substantial number of older people live to enjoy many active years, some persons who might not have survived in earlier times are now living into old age and bringing with them the chronic disease burden that would have been avoided by death. Indeed, one of the great demographic ironies is the observation that preventing most of the common diseases would actually increase the numbers of disabled persons rather than reducing them. (Of course, we would have more healthy people as well, but some would now survive to develop other chronic problems.)

The press for dramatic responses to the growth in the older population and its concurrent medical costs has led in two directions. Programs like managed care have been launched to serve Medicare beneficiaries in the hopes that such approaches might constrain costs. To date, this promise has not been achieved; most analyses suggest that the managed care programs have benefited from favorable selection, which has undermined any potential savings, but the hope persists that some variant of risk-based care will create incentives for greater efficiencies. The second strategy has promoted rationing through the back door, by emphasizing the avoidance of futile care at the end of life. The technique for implementing this objective has been the use of advance directives. Rather than overtly limiting the availability of treatment, advance directives empower patients to authorize less care. However, as discussed in Chap. 16, advance directives may not appeal to many older persons. If such directives fail to stem the tide of end-of-life care, will more draconian strategies be employed?

GROWTH IN NUMBERS

A look at a few trends will help to focus the problem. The numbers of older people in this country (and in the world) have been growing in both absolute and relative terms. The growth in numbers can be traced to two phenomena: (1) the advances in medical science that have improved survival rates from specific diseases and (2) the birth rate. The relative numbers of older persons is primarily the result of

two birth rates: (1) the one that occurred 65 or more years ago and the current one. The first one provides the people, most of whom will survive to become old. The second means that the proportion of those who are old depends on how many were born subsequently. This ratio is critical in estimating the size of the work force available to support an elderly population. The looming demographic crisis is based on the forecast of a large number of older persons increasing through the first half of the next century as a result of the post–World War II baby boom. That group of people, born in the late forties and early fifties, will begin to reach seniority by 2010. Figure 2-1 describes the growth in the older sector of the population. Not only is this group increasing, but the relative rate of growth increases with each decade over age 75. Indeed, many older persons are now surviving longer. It is no longer rare to encounter a centenarian. Hallmark even makes "Happy 100th Birthday" greeting cards. The impact of this projection can be better appreciated by looking at Table 2-1, which expresses the growth as a percentage of the total population. Although these forecasts can vary with the future birth and death rates, they are likely to be reasonably accurate. Thus, since the turn of the century, we

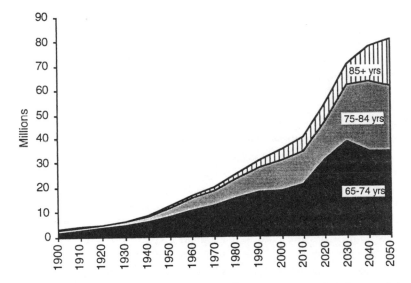

Figure 2-1 Growth in the U.S. population, age 65 and over. *(From U.S. Bureau of the Census, 1996.)*

Table 2-1 The elderly population of the United States: Trends 1900–2050

	Percent of the total population						
Age	1900	1940	1960	1990	2010	2030	2050
65–74	2.9	4.8	6.1	7.3	7.4	12.0	10.5
75–84	1.0	1.7	2.6	4.0	4.3	7.1	7.2
85+	0.2	0.3	0.5	1.3	2.2	2.7	5.1
65+	4.0	6.8	9.2	12.6	13.9	21.8	22.9

Source: U.S. Senate, 1991.

have gone from a situation in which 4 percent of the population was 65 or older to a time when more than 12 percent has reached seniority. By the year 2030, that older population will have almost doubled. Put another way, in 2030 there will be as many people over 75 as there are today over 65. When that observation is combined with the reduction in births in the cohort behind the baby boomers, then social implications become more obvious. There will be many fewer workers to support the larger older population. This demographic observation has led to several urgent recommendations: (1) redefine retirement age to recognize the increase in life expectancy and thereby reduce the ratio of retirees to workers, (2) encourage younger persons to personally save more for their retirement to avoid excessive dependency on public funds, and (3) change public programs to accrue surpluses to meet these projected drains.

We recognize that older people use more health care services than do younger people. The result is an even greater demand on the health care system and a concomitant rise in total health care costs. Because Medicare beneficiaries use more institutional services (i.e., hospital and nursing home care), their health care costs are higher than those for younger groups. Only 12 percent of the population, those age 65 and over, account for over one-third of health expenditures. Data from the National Medical Expenditure Survey indicate that the per capita cost of health care for older persons was over $7039 in 1995, compared with $2471 for the population as a whole.

The increased number of older persons has been accompanied by a number of changes in the way medical care is financed. Although

these programs are discussed in more detail in Chap. 14, we note here that the appearance of programs like Medicare and Medicaid, with all their shortcomings, has been associated with a growing expenditure on health care for older people and an increasing role in this area for public dollars. It is important to bear in mind that even in the face of greatly increased public financing, the elderly person still must bear a considerable share of the financial burden. In fact, in 1995, elderly persons' out-of-pocket costs for health care represented about 21 percent of their income, a figure comparable to before the passage of Medicare (Moon, 1996).

The growing number of older persons has created great consternation among forecasters. There is a sense of doom about a future in which all resources will go to support the elderly members of our society. To counter this ageist misimpression, two projections should be borne in mind: (1) The Office of the Actuary in the Health Care Financing Administration estimates that aging of the population alone would increase the proportion of the Gross National Product (GNP) spent on health from 12 percent in 1990 to only 13.4 percent in 2020; however, if the current rate of annual increase attributed to intensity of care or technology continues, we will be devoting 36 percent of the GNP to health. Thus, the aging of the population serves as a convenient scapegoat to deflect attention from the major role of technology in raising health care costs. (2) The increasing numbers of older persons will be accompanied by a decrease in the proportion of those under age 18. It is important to consider the overall dependency ratio. This index compares the proportion of the population under 18 and over 65 with that between 18 and 64 (the group presumed to be working to support the rest). Figure 2-2 traces the changes in the index and its principal components from 1900 through projections to the year 2050. It is important to note that while the relative contribution of the older population will increase impressively, the total will never be as high as it was in the mid-1960s.

The growth in the number of aged persons results from improvements in both social living conditions and medical care. Over the course of this century, we have moved from a preponderance of acute diseases (especially infections) to an era of chronic illnesses. Today at least two-thirds of all the money spent on health care goes toward chronic disease. Medical care can be criticized for continuing to practice in a mode more suited to acute illness than chronic care. Information systems have not yet arisen in common practice to channel clinicians' attention to the problems associated with chronic care.

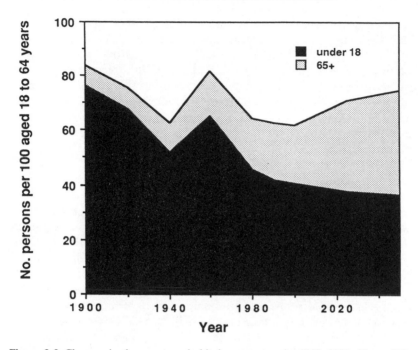

Figure 2-2 Changes in the young and elderly support ratio, 1900–2050. *(From U.S. Senate, 1991.)*

Table 2-2 reflects the changes in the common causes of death from 1900 to the present. Many of those common at the turn of the century are no longer even listed. Today the pattern of death in old age is generally similar to that of the population as a whole (with a few dramatic exceptions, such as AIDS). The leading causes are basically the same, but there are some differences in the rankings. The leading causes of death are heart disease, cancer, stroke, chronic obstructive pulmonary disease (COPD), and influenza/pneumonia. Although the most dramatic reduction of mortality has occurred in infants and mothers, there has been a perceptible increase in survival even after age 65. This increased survival is plotted in Fig. 2-3. Our stereotypes of what to expect from older people may therefore need reexamination. The average 65-year-old woman can expect to live another 19 years, and a 65-year-old man another 15 years. As shown in Fig. 2-4, even at age 85, there is an expectation of over 5 years.

Table 2-2   Changes in the commonest causes of death, 1900–1995, all ages and for those over 65

| | All ages | | | | 65+ | |
| | 1900 | | 1995 | | 1995 | |
	Rate*	Rank	Rate	Rank	Rate	Rank
Diseases of the heart	13.8	4	28.1	1	183.5	1
Malignant neoplasms	6.4	8	20.5	2	113.7	2
Cerebrovascular diseases	10.7	5	6.0	3	41.4	3
COPD and allied conditions	4.5	9	3.9	4	26.4	4
Accidents and adverse effects	7.2	7	3.6	5	8.7	7
Pneumonia and influenza	22.9	1	3.2	6	22.2	5
Diabetes mellitus	1.1		2.3	7	13.3	6
HIV infection	NR		1.6	8		
Suicide	1.0		1.2	9		
Chronic liver disease/cirrhosis	1.2		1.0	10		
Nephritis and neophrosis	8.9	6			6.0	9
Tuberculosis	19.4	2				
Diarrhea and enteritis	14.3	3				
Senility	5.0	10				
Alzheimer's disease					6.0	8
Septicemia					5.0	10

* Rate per 10,000 population.

Key: NR, not reported; COPD, chronic obstructive pulmonary disease; HIV, human immunodeficiency virus.

Sources: Data for 1900 from Linder and Grove, 1947; data for 1995 from Anderson et al., 1997; with permission.

However, this gain in survival includes both active and dependent years. Indeed, one of the great controversies of modern gerontologic epidemiology is whether the gain in life expectancy brings with it equivalent gains in years free of dependency. Although the concept of compression of morbidity has been popularized (Fries, 1980), the debate still rages about whether disability rates are rising or falling. Katz and his colleagues (Katz et al., 1983) have introduced the concept of active life expectancy to distinguish the years spent free of disability. As shown in Fig. 2-5, much of the advantage enjoyed by females comes in the form of dependent years. However, the concept of active life expectancy is more dynamic than it first appears. More recent work has shown that disability need not be a permanent state.

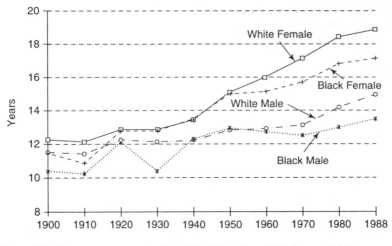

Figure 2-3 Life expectancy at age 65, 1900–1988. *(From U.S. Senate, 1991.)*

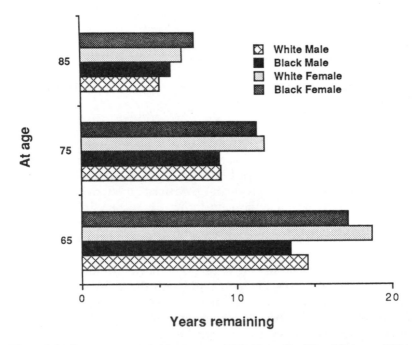

Figure 2-4 Life expectancy of older persons, 1984. *(From Havlik and Suzman, 1987.)*

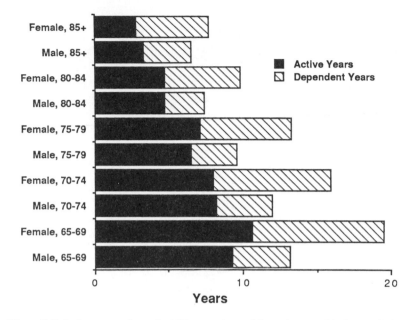

Figure 2-5 Active versus dependent life expectancy, Massachusetts elderly population, 1974. *(From Katz et al., 1983.)*

Some people become less disabled over time and some even move completely out of a disabled state. More recent population studies that compare current and past cohorts suggest that the overall rate of disability may actually be decreasing (Manton et al., 1995; Vita et al., 1998).

Some analysts have used disability as the basis for defining quality of life. They have then seized on the concept of active life expectancy to create a concept of quality-adjusted life years (QALYs). Under this formulation, which is especially popular with economists who are seeking a common denominator against which to weigh all interventions, the goal of health care is to maximize individuals' periods of disability-free time. However, such a formulation immediately raises concerns about the care of all those who are already frail; they would derive no benefit from any actions on their behalf unless they could convert them to a disability-free state.

DISABILITY

The World Health Organization distinguishes between impairments, disabilities, and handicaps. A disease may create an impairment in organ function. That failure can eventually lead to a reduced ability to perform certain tasks. This inability to perform may become a handicap when those tasks are necessary to carry out social activities. Hence, a handicap is the result of external demands and may be mitigated by environmental alterations. The distinction can provide a useful framework within which to consider the care of older persons. As shown in Fig. 2-6, there is a general pattern of increased impairment in the senses and in orthopedic problems with age. Indeed, not surprisingly, the prevalence of chronic conditions increases with age. However, the nature of survivorship produces the occasional twist. The association between prevalence and age is not absolute. Those afflicted with diabetes and those with chronic lung disease, for example, do not survive as readily to age 85 and above. Despite having more chronic conditions and impairments, older people tend to report their health as generally good; 40 percent of those aged 65 and older rate their health as very good or excellent, and another 32 percent rate it as good. This contrast highlights the coping abilities of elderly persons discussed in Chap. 1.

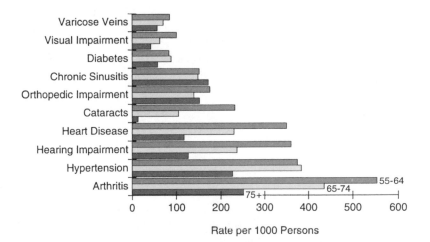

Figure 2-6 Top-10 chronic conditions for people 55+, 1989. *(From U.S. Senate, 1991.)*

Because physicians tend to see the sick, they may form a distorted picture of the senior citizens. Most older persons are indeed self-sufficient and able to function on their own or with minimal assistance. Those who need help are likely to be the very old. Functioning can be measured in a variety of ways. Commonly we use the ability to perform specific tasks as a reflection of independence. These are grouped into two classes of measures. The term *instrumental activities of daily living* (IADLs) refers to tasks required to maintain an independent household. IADLs include such tasks as using the telephone, managing money, shopping, preparing meals, doing light housework, and getting around the community. They generally demand a combination of both physical and cognitive performance. Even among those at age 85 and above, over half the population living in the community can still perform these tasks independently.

The ability to carry out basic self-care activities is reflected in the so-called *activities of daily living* (ADLs). Dependencies in terms of ADLs—which include such tasks as eating, using the toilet, dressing, transferring, walking, and bathing—are less common than IADL losses. As shown in Fig. 2-7, even among the oldest groups, the prevalence of ADL dependency is quite low. Forty percent of females aged 85 or more living in the community needed no assistance with any

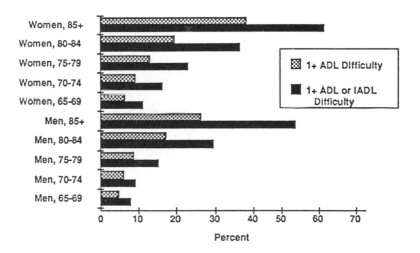

Figure 2-7 Prevalence of ADL and IADL difficulties among community living older persons, 1985. *(From U.S. Senate, 1991.)*

IADL, and more than 60 percent needed no help with ADLs. Overall, among those aged 85 or more of both sexes living in the community, 16 percent needed help with one ADL, 10 percent with two or three ADLs, and 9 percent with four or more ADLs.

SOCIAL SUPPORT

An important feature in determining an older person's ability to live in the community is the extent of support available. The family is the heart of long-term care (LTC). Family and friends provide the bulk of services in each category with, or more often without, the help of formal caregivers. Informal care is largely provided by women. Women are both the major givers and receivers of long-term care. Hence, a natural coalition has formed between those advocating for improved LTC and women's organizations. Even as women are entering the work force in large numbers, they continue to bear the majority of the caregiving load. Largely because they outlive men, over twice as many older women, compared with men, live alone (Fig. 2-8), but

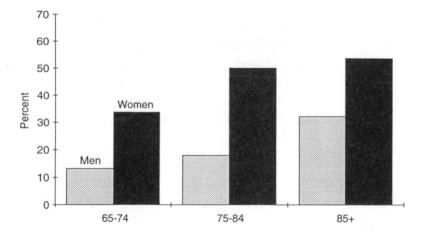

Figure 2-8 Percent of older persons living alone in the community, 1989. *(From U.S. Senate, 1991.)*

the gap narrows by age 85. As shown in Fig. 2-9, wives and daughters are the most important source of family support for older persons. Survey data suggest that over 70 percent of persons aged 65 and older have surviving children. (Remember that the children of persons age 85 and older may themselves be aged 65 or older.) These "children" provide over a third of the informal care.

The difference between needing and not needing a nursing home can depend on the availability of such support. Extrapolating from available data, we estimate that for every person over age 65 in a nursing home, there are from one to three people equally disabled living in the community. The importance of social support must be kept continuously in mind. Formal community supports will continue to rely heavily on family and friends to see that adequate amounts of care are provided to maintain an elderly individual in the community. The physician must work diligently to maintain and bolster such support so as to avoid nursing home placement.

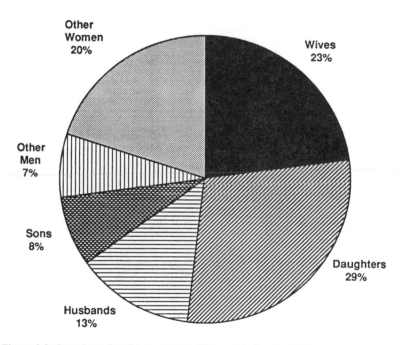

Figure 2-9 Caregivers for older persons. *(From U.S. Senate, 1991.)*

USE OF SERVICES

In general, there is an increase in the utilization of health care with age. Table 2-3 summarizes some of these differences. The exception to the pattern of age-related increase is seen with dental care; it is not clear whether this reflects the lack of coverage under Medicare or a loss of teeth but probably is at least greatly influenced by the former. With the introduction of the new prospective payment system (PPS) for hospitals under Medicare in 1984, some changes in length of stay and admission rates had been expected. The use of the diagnosis-related group (DRG) as a basis for determining flat rates per admission means that hospitals can vary either the intensity of care per day or the number of days per admission. Figures 2-10 and 2-11 trace the patterns of care before and after PPS. As expected, length of stay decreased, although it had already been declining. After a plateau, it has begun to fall again in recent years. To the surprise of many, admission rates fell rather than increased. Their pattern is similar to length of stay, with a plateau after the initial decrease, but here the recent findings suggest an increase in use, the mirror image of the length-of-stay data. Table 2-4 shows the most common discharge diag-

(Text continues on page 36.)

Table 2-3 Health services utilization by various age groups

	Age groups		
	45–64	65–74	75+
Annual hospital discharges/100	14.2	23.7	33.7
Average length of stay	6.8	8.7	8.3
Short-stay hospital days in past year	9.6	12.5	12.1
Percent of persons with no hospital days	90.3	84.6	79.7
No. of procedures/100*	19.7	38.7[†]	
Percent seeing a physician in past year	75.0	82.2	87.2
Average number of physician contacts per year	6.6	8.1	10.6
Percent seeing a dentist in past year	55.9	42.6[†]	

* The term *procedures* refers to a broader category of activities in short-stay hospitals than just operations; it includes such things as arteriography, angiocardiography, CT scans, diagnostic ultrasound, and endoscopies.

[†] 65 years and over.

Source: From Dawson, 1987, with permission.

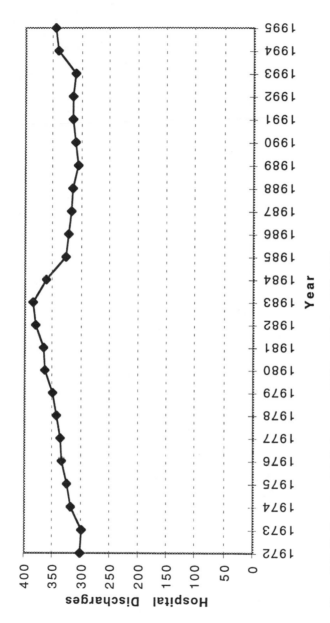

Figure 2-10 Medicare hospital discharges per 1000 beneficiaries, 1972–1995.

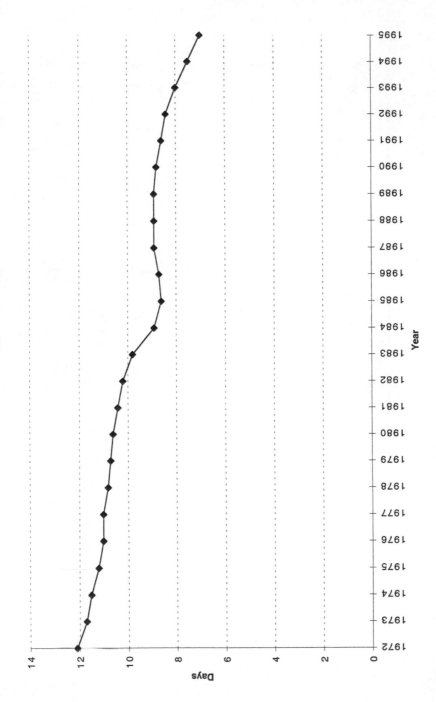

Figure 2-11 Medicare hospital length of stay, 1972–1995.

Table 2-4 Most common hospital discharges for patients over age 65, 1995

Diagnostic category	No. of discharges (1000s)	Percent of discharges
All conditions	11,556	100
Heart disease	2,618	22.7
Acute myocardial infarction	471	4.1
Coronary atherosclerosis	501	4.3
Other ischemic heart disease	265	2.3
Cardiac dysrhythmias	400	3.5
Congestive heart failure	698	6.0
Malignant neoplasms	774	6.7
Malignant neoplasm of large intestine and rectum	105	0.9
Malignant neoplasm of trachea, bronchus, and lung	109	0.9
Cerebrovascular disease	704	6.1
Pneumonia	687	5.9
Fractures	489	4.2
Fracture of neck of femur	274	2.4
Arthropathies and related disorders	322	2.8
Psychosis	256	2.2
Chronic bronchitis	244	2.1
Urinary tract infection, not specified	223	1.9
Volume depletion	210	1.8
Septicemia	210	1.8
Diabetes mellitus	188	1.6

Procedure category		
Total surgical procedures	7,410	100
Cardiac catheterization	530	7.2
Coronary artery bypass graft	320	4.3
Insertion, replacement, removal, and repair of pacemaker leads or device	256	3.5
Esophagogastroduodenoscopy with closed biopsy	256	3.5
Removal of coronary artery obstruction	209	2.8
Prostatectomy	184	2.5

(continued)

Table 2-4 Most common hospital discharges for patients over age 65, 1995 *(Continued)*

Diagnostic category	No. of discharges (1000s)	Percent of discharges
Procedure category		
Open reduction and internal fixation of fracture	178	2.4
Cholecystectomy	165	2.2
Total knee replacement	157	2.1
Debridement of wound, infection, or burn	133	1.8

Source: From Gillum et al., 1998, with permission.

noses and surgical procedures in 1995. Heart disease, cancer, stroke and pneumonia continue to dominate the scene. The growth of technology can be seen in the frequent use of procedures, especially catheterization and endoscopy.

The introduction of PPS greatly spurred the use of post–acute care. Patients discharged earlier from hospitals often needed someplace to recuperate. As a result, Medicare began paying twice for hospital care. It paid a fixed amount for shorter stays and then often paid for the post–hospital care. In fiscal year 1997, 14.5 percent of Medicare patients discharged from an acute care hospital went to a skilled nursing facility, 7.5 percent went home with home health care, and another 3.3 percent went to specialty hospitals (e.g., for rehabilitation).

Table 2-5 describes the patterns for ambulatory visits at various ages. Despite the general principle that bad things are more common with increasing age after 75, not all diagnoses increase with age.

NURSING HOME USE

The nursing home has traditionally been used as the touchstone for long-term care, but its role has changed with the changes in hospital payment under Medicare. The fixed-payment approach and the consequent shortening of hospital stays have spawned a new industry of post–hospital care, sometimes called subacute care. In effect, care

Table 2-5 Percent of office visits by selected medical conditions, 1996

	45–64 years	65–74 years	75+ years
Arthritis	11.9	23.6	33.4
Atherosclerosis	3.4	9.9	15.1
Chronic obstructive pulmonary disease	3.4	7.5	8.5
Depression	8.9	5.2	5.2
Diabetes	9.8	13.9	11.6
Hypertension	24.5	35.9	36.9
Obesity	11.4	7.3	4.7

Source: From Woodwell, 1997, with permission.

that was formerly rendered in a hospital is now provided in other settings, including the nursing home and the home of the patient. Some nursing homes have sought to increase their capacity to support such care by upgrading their nursing staffs, but others have adopted the new title without changing their modus operandi. Thus, the typical distinction between long-stay and short-stay nursing home residents has become more exaggerated. Some residents are there for chronic care, whereas others are just visiting for a brief spell of recuperation and rehabilitation.

We are prone to cite a figure of 5 percent for the proportion of those aged 65 and older in nursing homes at any moment. Such a figure is a potentially misleading generalization. As Fig. 2-12 suggests, age is a very important factor. Among those 65 to 74 years old, the rate is less than 2 percent. It rises to about 7 percent for those aged 75 to 84, and then jumps to 20 percent for those 85 and older. It is also helpful to distinguish between these prevalence rates and the lifetime probability of entering a nursing home. Longitudinal studies suggest that persons aged 65 have better than a 40 percent chance of spending some time in a nursing home before they die. Of those who enter a nursing home, 55 percent will spend at least 1 year there and 21 percent will spend 5 years or more (Kemper and Murtaugh, 1991). The proportion of persons spending at least some time in a nursing home is likely to increase if nursing homes continue to play a role in subacute care.

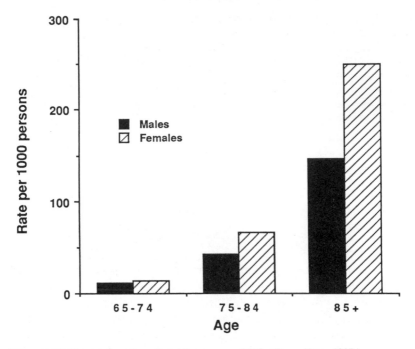

Figure 2-12 Nursing home use by older persons, 1985. *(From Hing, 1987.)*

Nursing homes are needed not only because of the presence of diseases or even functional disabilities. It is also a result of a lack of social support. Often the family becomes exhausted after caring for an elderly patient for a long period. Family fatigue is especially a problem when the patient has symptoms that are very disruptive. Among the most disturbing are incontinence and behavior problems that involve wandering or disruptive behavior. Table 2-6 summarizes the factors associated with increased likelihood of nursing home placement.

About three-fourths of nursing home admissions come from hospitals. A 3-day hospital stay is a prerequisite for nursing home coverage available under Medicare. Often the hospitalization represents the last step in a series of steps involving the deterioration of the patient and the patient's social supports. For others, the hospitalization results from an acute event, e.g., a broken hip or a stroke, which then necessitates long-term care.

Table 2-6 Factors affecting the need for nursing home admission

Characteristics of the individual
  Age, sex, race
  Marital status
  Living arrangements
  Degree of mobility
  Activities of daily living
  Instrumental activities of daily living
  Clinical prognosis
  Level of function prior to hospitalization
  Urinary continence
  Behavior problems
  Mental status/memory impairment
  Mood disturbance
  Ability to distinguish both sides of body
  Vertigo and falls
  Ability to manage medication
  Income
  Payment eligibility
  Need for special services

Characteristics of the support system
  Family capability
    For married respondents, age of spouse
    Presence of responsible relative (usually adult
      child)
    Family structure of responsible relative
    Employment status of responsible relative
  Physician availability
  Amount of care currently received from family
    and others

Community resources
  Formal community resources
  Informal support systems
  Presence of long-term-care institutions
  Characteristics of long-term-care institutions

In 1997 almost 15 percent of hospital patients age 65 and older were discharged to nursing homes. As with those from the community, the rate of nursing home placement increases with age and is greater for females than for males. Table 2-6 summarizes some of the factors that can identify those older patients in hospitals at risk of nursing

home placement. The most significant single factor predicting discharge to a nursing home is being admitted from one. Effectively all of the nursing home residents who survive their hospital stay will be returned to a nursing home. For those patients originating from the community, the most important factors are associated with dependency and cognitive status. Compared with those going home or to a rehabilitation unit, nursing home admissions are likely to have worse functional status and more confusion (Kane et al., 1996). Models have been developed to predict the time to nursing home admission for persons with Alzheimer's disease (Stern et al., 1997).

Talk about nursing home patients must carefully distinguish between data based on a study of those resident in a facility at a given time and those entering or leaving the facility. The conclusions reached about nursing home patients may be quite different depending on which groups are examined. Researchers have identified two streams of patients entering the nursing home—one group will leave fairly quickly (within 3 to 6 months); the other will stay several years (Keeler et al., 1981). These two groups have distinct characteristics. The short-term patients tend to be younger, have more physical problems, and enter from the hospital. The long-term patients are more likely to be older, confused, and incontinent. At admission, the patients are about equally distributed between short-term and long-term patients, but a study of residents will find about nine times as many long-term patients.

Nursing home data can be very confusing. Not only must one distinguish between admissions and residents but one must also look at the time course of former residents to appreciate the true nature of such long-term care. On the one hand, the picture is much more dynamic than is usually suspected. Over half the persons admitted at a nursing home are discharged within 3 months. On the other hand, many of these people die in the nursing home, and many of the discharges are really transfers to hospitals. From there a majority of patients either return to the nursing home or die in a hospital. About a third of nursing home discharges do go back to the community, but even then many return to a nursing home in time. Figure 2-13 offers a simplified portrayal of the true dynamics of nursing home discharges and the transitions involved. It is more accurate to talk about long-term care "careers" than to think in terms of discrete episodes.

As we enter an era of more aged persons with chronic disease, physicians will find themselves working increasingly in institutions such as nursing homes. They will be challenged to provide leadership

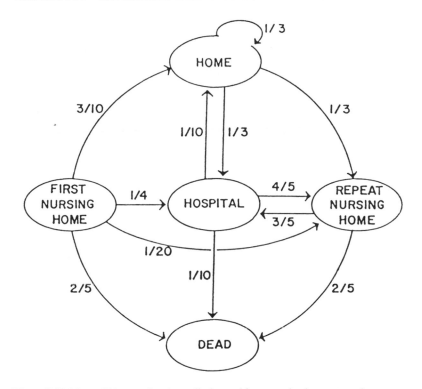

Figure 2-13 Natural history of patients discharged from nursing homes transfer patterns of nursing home patients. The fractions indicate the approximate proportion of patients moving from one status to another. For example, about three-tenths of first admissions went home on discharge, a fourth went to the hospital, a twentieth went to another nursing home, and two-fifths died. Of those going home, a third stayed at home a third went to the hospital, and a third went back to a nursing home. *(From Lewis et al., 1985.)*

in upgrading the care available in such settings. They will need to be familiar with the array of resources available to meet the needs of their patients and the factors determining access to these resources. A guide to long-term-care resources is presented in Chap. 14.

REFERENCES

Anderson RN, Kochanek KD, Murphy SL: *Report of Final Mortality Statistics, 1995* (Monthly vital statistics report: vol. 45, no. 11, suppl. 2, Table 7). Hyattsville, MD, National Center for Health Statistics, 1997.

Dawson DA: *Current Estimates from National Health Interview Survey, United States, 1986.* Washington, DC, U.S. Government Printing Office, 1987.

Fries JF: Aging, natural death, and the compression of morbidity. *N Engl J Med* 303:130–136, 1980.

Gillum BS, Graves EJ, Wood E: National hospital discharge survey: Annual summary, 1995. *Vital Health Statistics* 13(133): 1998.

Havlik RJ, Suzman R: Health status—Mortality, in Havilk RJ, Liu MG, Kovar MG, et al (eds): *Health Statistics on Older Persons, United States, 1986. Vital and Health Statistics,* Series 3, No. 25. DHHS Publ. No (PHS)87-1409. Public Health Service, U.S. Government Printing Office, June 1987.

Hing E: Use of nursing homes by the elderly: Preliminary data from the 1985 National Nursing Home Survey, in *Advance Data from Vital and Health Statistics,* No. 135. DHHS Publ. No. (PHS)87-1250. Hyattsville, MD, Public Health Service, May 14, 1987.

Kane RL, Finch M, Blewett L, et al: Use of post-hospital care by Medicare patients. *J Am Geriatr Soc* 44:242–250, 1996.

Katz K, Branch LG, Branson MH, et al: Active life expectancy. *N Engl J Med* 309:1218–1224, 1983.

Keeler EB, Kane RL, Solomon DH: Short- and long-term residents of nursing homes. *Med Care* 19:363–369, 1981.

Kemper P, Murtaugh CM: Lifetime use of nursing home care. *N Engl J Med* 324:595–600, 1991.

Lewis MA, Cretin S, Kane RL: The natural history of nursing home patients. *Gerontologist* 25:382–388, 1985.

Linder FE, Grove RD: *Vital Statistics Rates in the United States 1900–1940.* Washington, DC, U.S. Government Printing Office, 1947.

Manton KG, Stallard E, Corder L: Changes in morbidity and chronic disability in the U.S. elderly population: Evidence from the 1982, 1984, and 1989 National Long-Term Care Surveys. *J Gerontol Ser B* 50(4):S194–S204, 1995.

Moon M: What Medicare has meant to older Americans. *Health Care Fin Rev* 18(2):49–59, 1996.

Stern Y, Tang M-X, Albert MS, et al: Predicting time to nursing home care and death in individuals with Alzheimer disease. *JAMA* 277:806–812, 1997.

U.S. Bureau of the Census: *Current Population Reports, Special Studies, 65+ in the United States,* Washington, DC, U.S. Government Printing Office, 1996, pp. 23–90.

U.S. Senate Subcommittee on Aging, American Association of Retired Persons, Federal Council on Aging, and U.S. Administration on Aging. *Aging America: Trends and Projections* [DHHS Publ No. (FCoA)91-28001]. Washington, DC, U.S. Department of Health and Human Services, 1991.

Vita AJ, Terry RB, Hubert HB, et al: Aging, health risks, and cumulative disability. *N Engl J Med* 338:1035–1041, 1998.

Woodwell DA: *National Ambulatory Medical Care Survey: 1996 Summary. Advance Data from Vital and Health Statistics* (295). Hyattsville, MD, National Center for Health Statistics, 1997.

THREE

EVALUATING THE GERIATRIC PATIENT

Comprehensive evaluation of an older individual's health status is one of the most challenging aspects of clinical geriatrics. It requires a sensitivity to the concerns of older people, an awareness of the many unique aspects of their medical problems, an ability to interact effectively with a variety of health professionals, and often a great deal of patience. Most importantly, it requires a perspective different from that used in the evaluation of younger individuals. Not only are the a priori probabilities of diagnoses different, but one must be attuned to more subtle findings. Progress may be measured on a finer scale. Special tools are needed to ascertain relatively small improvements in chronic conditions and overall function compared with the more dramatic cures of acute illnesses often possible in younger patients. Creativity is essential in order to incorporate these tools efficiently in a busy clinical practice.

The purposes of the evaluation and the setting in which it takes place will determine its focus and extent. Considerations important in admitting a geriatric patient with a fractured hip and pneumonia to an acute care hospital during the middle of the night are obviously different from those in the evaluation of an older demented patient exhibiting disruptive behavior in a nursing home. Elements included in

screening for treatable conditions in an ambulatory clinic are different from those in assessment of older individuals in their own homes or in long-term-care facilities.

Despite the differences dictated by the purpose and setting of the evaluation, several essential aspects of evaluating older patients are common to all purposes and settings. Figure 3-1 depicts these aspects; they can be summarized as follows:

1. Physical, psychological, and socioeconomic factors interact in complex ways to influence the health and functional status of the geriatric population.
2. Comprehensive evaluation of an older individual's health status requires an assessment of each of these domains. The coordinated efforts of several different health care professionals functioning as an interdisciplinary team are needed.
3. Functional abilities should be a central focus of the comprehensive evaluation of geriatric patients. Other more traditional measures of health status (such as diagnoses and physical and laboratory findings) are useful in dealing with underlying etiologies and detecting treatable conditions, but in the geriatric population, measures of function are often essential in determining overall health, well-being, and the need for health and social services.

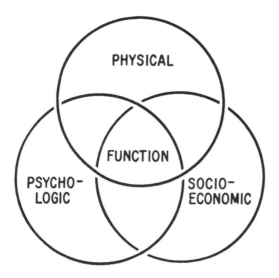

Figure 3-1 Components of assessment of older patients.

Just as function is the common language of geriatrics, assessment lies at the heart of its practice. Special techniques that address multiple problems and their functional consequences offer a way to structure the approach to complicated geriatric patients. Geriatric assessment has been tested in a variety of forms. The findings from a number of randomized, controlled trials of different approaches to geriatric assessment are summarized in Table 3-1 (Rubenstein, 1991). A recent randomized trial demonstrated the potential for annual in-home comprehensive geriatric assessment to delay the development of disability and reduce permanent nursing home stays (Stuck et al., 1995). More recent controlled trials of approaches to hospitalized geriatric patients suggest comprehensive geriatric assessment by a consultation team with limited follow-up does not improve health or survival of selected geriatric patients (Reuben et al., 1995), but that a special acute geriat-

Table 3-1 Examples of randomized controlled trials of geriatric assessment

Setting	Examples of assessment strategies	Selected outcomes*
Community/outpatients	Social worker assessment and referral Nursing assessment and referral Annual in-home assessment by nurse practitioner Multidisciplinary clinic assessment	Reduced mortality Reduced hospital use Reduced permanent nursing home use Delayed development of disability
Hospital inpatient (specialized units)	Interdisciplinary teams with focus on function, geriatric syndromes, rehabilitation	Reduced mortality Improved function Reduced acute hospital and nursing home use
Hospital inpatient consultation	Geriatric consultation teams	Mixed results Some studies improved function and lower short-term mortality Other studies show no effects

* Not all studies show improvements in all outcomes. See text and Rubenstein et al., 1991.

ric unit can improve function and reduce discharges to institutional care (Landefeld et al., 1995).

There is considerable variation in approaches to the comprehensive assessment of geriatric patients. Various screening and targeting strategies have been used to identify appropriate patients for more comprehensive assessment. These strategies range from selection based on age to targeting patients with a certain number of impairments or specific conditions. Sites of assessment vary as well, and include the clinic, the home, the hospital, and different levels of long term care. Geriatric assessment also varies in terms of which discipline carries out the different components of the assessment as well as in the specific assessment tools used. Despite the dramatic variation in approach to targeting, personnel used, and measures employed, a clear pattern of effectiveness has emerged. Taken together, these results are both heartening and cautioning. Systematic approaches to patient care are obviously desirable. The issue is more how formalized these assessments should be. Research data suggest that the specifics of the assessment process seem to be less important than the very act of systematically approaching older people with the belief that improvement is possible.

Because of the multidimensional nature of geriatric patients' problems and the frequent presence of multiple interacting medical conditions, comprehensive evaluation of the geriatric patient can be time-consuming and thus costly. Strategies that can make the evaluation process more efficient include the following:

1. The development of a close-knit interdisciplinary team with minimal redundancy in the assessments performed.
2. Use of carefully designed questionnaires that reliable patients and/or caregivers can complete before an appointment.
3. Incorporation of screening tools that target the need for further, more in-depth assessment.
4. Use of assessment forms that can be readily incorporated into a computerized relational data base.
5. Integration of the evaluation process with case management activities that target services based on the results of the assessment.

This chapter focuses on the general aspects of assessing geriatric patients. Sections on geriatric consultation, preoperative evaluation, and environmental assessments are included at the end of the chapter.

Chapter 14 includes information on case management and other health services, and Chap. 15 is devoted to the assessment and management of geriatric patients in the nursing home setting.

THE HISTORY

Sir William Osler's aphorism "Listen to the patient, he'll give you the diagnosis" is as true in the older patients as it is in the young. In the geriatric population, however, several factors make taking histories more challenging, difficult, and time-consuming.

Table 3-2 lists difficulties commonly encountered in taking histories from geriatric patients, the factors involved, and some suggestions for overcoming these difficulties. Impaired hearing and vision (despite corrective devices) are common and can interfere with effective communication. Techniques such as eliminating extraneous noises, speaking slowly and in deep tones while facing the patient, and providing adequate lighting can be helpful. The use of simple, inexpensive amplification devices with "Walkman"-style earphones can be especially effective, even among the severely hearing impaired. Patience is truly a virtue in obtaining a history; because thought and verbal processes are often slower in older than in younger individuals, patients should be allowed adequate time to answer in order not to miss potentially important information.

Many older individuals underreport potentially important symptoms because of their cultural and educational backgrounds as well as their expectations of illness as a normal concomitant of aging (Brody et al., 1983). Fear of illness and disability or depression accompanied by a lack of self-concern may also render the reporting of symptoms less frequent. Altered physical and physiologic responses to disease processes (see Chap. 1) can result in the absence of symptoms (such as painless myocardial infarction or ulcer and pneumonia without cough). Symptoms of many diseases can be vague and nonspecific because of these age-related changes. Impairments of memory and other cognitive functions can result in an imprecise or inadequate history and compound these difficulties. Asking specifically about potentially important symptoms (such as those listed in Table 3-3) and using other sources of information (such as relatives, friends, and other caregivers) can be very helpful in collecting more precise and useful information in these situations.

Table 3-2 Potential difficulties in taking geriatric histories

Difficulty	Factors involved	Suggestions
Communication	Diminished vision Diminished hearing	Use well-lit room Eliminate extraneous noise Speak slowly in a deep tone Face patient, allowing patient to see your lips Use simple amplification device for severely hearing impaired If necessary, write questions in large print
	Slowed psychomotor performance	Leave enough time for the patient to answer
Underreporting of symptoms	Health beliefs Fear Depression Altered physical and physiologic responses to disease process Cognitive impairment	Ask specific questions about potentially important symptoms (see Table 3-3) Use other sources of information (relatives, friends, other caregivers) to complete the history
Vague or nonspecific symptoms	Altered physical and physiologic responses to disease process Altered presentation of specific diseases Cognitive impairment	Rule out treatable diseases, even if the symptoms (or signs) are not typical or specific when there has been a rapid change in funtion Use other sources of information to complete history
Multiple complaints	Prevalence of multiple coexisting diseases Somatization of emotions—"masked depressed" (see Chap. 5)	Attend to all somatic symptoms, ruling out treatable conditions Get to know the patient's complaints; pay special attention to new or changing symptoms Interview the patient on several occasions to complete the history

Table 3-3 Important aspects of the geriatric history

Social history

Living arrangements
Relationships with family and friends
Expectations of family or other caregivers
Economic status
Abilities to perform activities of daily living (Table 3-8)
Social activities and hobbies
Mode of transportation
Advance directives (Chap. 16)

Past medical history

Previous surgical procedures
Major illnesses and hospitalizations
Immunization status
  Influenza, pneumococcal, tetanus

Preventive health measures
  Mammography
  Pap smear
  Flexible sigmoidoscopy
  Antimicrobial prophylaxis
  Estrogen replacement

Tuberculosis history and testing

Medications (use the "brown bag" technique; see text)
  Previous allergies
  Knowledge of current medication regimen
  Compliance

Perceived beneficial or adverse drug effects

Systems review

Ask questions about general symptoms that may indicate treatable underlying
  disease such as fatigue, anorexia, weight loss, insomnia, recent change in
  functional status
Attempt to elicit key symptoms in each organ system, including the following:

System	Key symptoms
Respiratory	Increasing dyspnea
	Persistent cough
Cardiovascular	Orthopnea
	Edema

(continued)

Table 3-3 Important aspects of the geriatric history *(Continued)*

System	Key symptoms
	Angina
	Claudication
	Palpitations
	Dizziness
	Syncope
Gastrointestinal	Difficulty chewing
	Dysphagia
	Abdominal pain
	Change in bowel habit
Genitourinary	Frequency
	Urgency
	Nocturia
	Hesitancy, intermittent stream, straining to void
	Incontinence
	Hematuria
	Vaginal bleeding
Musculoskeletal	Focal or diffuse pain
	Focal or diffuse weakness
Neurologic	Visual disturbances (transient or progressive)
	Progressive hearing loss
	Unsteadiness and/or falls
	Transient focal symptoms
Psychological	Depression
	Anxiety and/or agitation
	Paranoia
	Forgetfulness and/or confusion

At the other end of the spectrum, geriatric patients with multiple complaints can frustrate the health care professional who is trying to sort them all out. The multiplicity of complaints can relate to the prevalence of coexisting chronic and acute conditions in many geriatric patients. These complaints may, however, be deceiving. Somatic symptoms may be manifestations of underlying emotional distress rather than symptoms of a physical illness, and symptoms of physical conditions may be exaggerated by emotional distress (see Chap. 5). Getting to know patients and their complaints and paying particular attention to new or changing symptoms are helpful in detecting potentially treatable conditions.

Table 3-3 lists aspects of the history that are especially important in geriatric patients. It is often not feasible to gather all information in one session; shorter interviews in a few separate sessions may prove more effective in gathering these data from some geriatric patients. Often shortchanged in medical evaluations, the social history is a critical component. Understanding the patient's socioeconomic environment and ability to function within it is crucial in determining the potential impact of an illness on an individual's overall health and need for health services. Especially important is the assessment of the family's feelings and expectations. Many family caregivers of frail geriatric patients have feelings of both anger (at having to care for a dependent family member) and guilt (over not being able or willing to do enough), and have unrealistic expectations. Such unrealistic expectations are often based on a lack of information and can interfere with care if not discussed. Unlike younger patients, older patients often have had multiple prior illnesses. The past medical history is, therefore, important in putting the patient's current problems in perspective; this can also be diagnostically important. For example, vomiting in an elderly patient who has had previous intraabdominal surgery should raise the suspicion of intestinal obstruction from adhesions; nonspecific constitutional symptoms (such as fatigue, anorexia, and weight loss) in a patient with a history of depression should prompt consideration of a relapse. Because older individuals are often treated with multiple medications, they are at increased risk of noncompliance and adverse effects (see Chap. 13). A detailed medication history (including both prescribed and over-the-counter drugs) is essential. The "brown bag" technique is very helpful in this regard; have the patient or caregiver empty the patient's medicine cabinet into a brown paper bag and bring it at each visit. More often than not, one or more of these medications can, at least in theory, contribute to geriatric patient's symptoms.

A complete systems review, focusing on potentially important and prevalent symptoms in the elderly, can help overcome many of the difficulties described above. Although not intended to be all-inclusive, Table 3-3 lists several of these symptoms.

General symptoms can be especially difficult to interpret. Fatigue can result from a number of common conditions such as depression, congestive heart failure, anemia, and hypothyroidism. Anorexia and weight loss can be symptoms of an underlying malignancy, depression, or poorly fitting dentures and diminished taste sensation. Age-related

changes in sleep patterns, anxiety, gastroesophageal reflux, congestive heart failure with orthopnea, or nocturia can underlie complaints of insomnia. Because many frail geriatric patients limit their activity, some important symptoms may be missed. For example, such patients may deny angina and dyspnea but restrict their activity to avoid the symptoms. Questions such as "How far do you walk in a typical day?" and "What is the most activity you carry out in a typical day?" can be helpful in patients suspected of limiting their activities to avoid certain symptoms.

THE PHYSICAL EXAMINATION

The common occurrence of multiple pathologic physical findings superimposed on age-related physical changes complicates interpretation of the physical examination. Table 3-4 lists common physical findings and their potential significance in the geriatric population. An awareness of age-related physical changes is important to the interpretation of many physical findings and therefore subsequent

(*Text continues on page 57*)

Table 3-4 Common physical findings and their potential significance in geriatrics

Physical findings	Potential significance
Vital signs	
Elevated blood pressure	Increased risk for cardiovascular morbidity; therapy should be considered if repeated measurements are high (see Chap. 10)
Postural changes in blood pressure	May be asymptomatic and occur in the absence of dehydration Aging changes, deconditioning, and drugs may play a role Can be exaggerated after meals Can be worsened and become symptomatic with antihypertensive, vasodilator, and tricyclic antidepressant therapy

(*continued*)

Table 3-4 Common physical findings and their potential significance in geriatrics *(Continued)*

Physical findings	Potential significance
Vital signs	
Irregular pulse	Arrhythmias are relatively common in otherwise asymptomatic elderly; seldom need specific evaluation or treatment (see Chap. 10)
Tachypnea	Baseline rate should be accurately recorded to help assess future complaints (such as dyspnea) or conditions (such as pneumonia or heart failure)
Weight changes	Weight gain should prompt search for edema or ascites Gradual loss of small amounts of weight common; losses in excess of 10% of usual body weight over 3 months or less should prompt search of underlying disease
General appearance and behavior	
Poor personal grooming and hygiene (e.g., poorly shaven, unkempt hair, soiled clothing)	Can be signs of poor overall function, caregiver neglect, and/or depression; often indicates a need for intervention
Slow thought processes and speech	Usually represents an aging change; Parkinson's disease and depression can also cause these signs
Ulcerations	Lower extremity vascular and neuropathic ulcers common Pressure ulcers common and easily overlooked in immobile patients
Diminished turgor	Often results from atrophy of subcutaneous tissues rather than volume depletion; when dehydration suspected, skin turgor over chest and abdomen most reliable

(continued)

Table 3-4 Common physical findings and their potential significance in geriatrics *(Continued)*

Physical findings	Potential significance
Ears (see Chap. 12)	
Diminished hearing	High-frequency hearing loss common; patients with difficulty hearing normal conversation or a whispered phrase next to the ear should be evaluated further Portable audioscopes can be helpful in screening for impairment
Eyes (see Chap. 12)	
Decreased visual acuity (often despite corrective lenses)	May have multiple causes, all patients should have thorough optometric or ophthalmologic examination Hemianopsia is easily overlooked and can usually be ruled out by simple confrontation testing
Cataracts and other abnormalities of the pupil and lens	Fundoscopic examination often difficult and limited; if retinal pathology suspected, thorough ophthalmologic examination necessary
Mouth	
Missing teeth	Dentures often present; they should be removed to check for evidence of poor fit and other pathology in oral cavity Area under the tongue is a common site for early malignancies
Skin	
Multiple lesions	Actinic keratoses and basal cell carcinomas common; most other lesions benign

(continued)

Table 3-4 Common physical findings and their potential significance in geriatrics *(Continued)*

Physical findings	Potential significance
Chest	
Abnormal lung sounds	Crackles can be heard in the absence of pulmonary disease and heart failure; often indicate atelectasis
Cardiovascular (see Chap. 10)	
Irregular rhythms	See vital signs, above
Systolic murmurs	Common and most often benign; clinical history and bedside maneuvers can help to differentiate those needing further evaluation Carotid bruits may need further evaluation
Vascular bruits	Femoral bruits often present in patients with symptomatic peripheral vascular disease
Diminished distal pulses	Presence or absence should be recorded, as this information may be diagnostically useful at a later time (e.g., if symptoms of claudication or an embolism develop)
Abdomen	
Prominent aortic pulsation	Suspected abdominal aneurysms should be evaluated by ultrasound
Genitourinary (see Chap. 7)	
Atrophy	Testicular atrophy normal; atrophic vaginal tissue may cause symptoms (such as dyspareunia and dysuria) and treatment may be beneficial
Pelvic prolapse (cystocele, rectocele)	Common and may be unrelated to symptoms; gynecologic evaluation helpful if patient has bothersome, potentially related symptoms

(continued)

Table 3-4 Common physical findings and their potential significance in geriatrics *(Continued)*

Physical findings	Potential significance
Extremities	
Periarticular pain	Can result from a variety of causes and is not always the result of degenerative joint disease; each area of pain should be carefully evaluated and treated (see Chap. 9)
Limited ranged of motion	Often caused by pain resulting from active inflammation, scarring from old injury, or neurologic disease; if limitations impair function, a rehabilitation therapist could be consulted
Edema	Can result from venous insufficiency and/or heart failure; mild edema often a cosmetic problem; treatment necessary if impairing ambulation, contributing to nocturia, predisposing to skin breakdown, or causing discomfort Unilateral edema should prompt search for a proximal obstructive process
Neurologic	
Abnormal mental status (i.e., confusion, depressed affect)	See Chaps. 4 and 5
Weakness	Arm drift may be the only sign of residual weakness from a stroke Proximal muscle weakness (e.g., inability to get out of chair) should be further evaluated; physical therapy may be appropriate

decision making. For example, age-related changes in the skin and postural reflexes can influence the evaluation of hydration; age-related changes in the lung and lower extremity edema secondary to venous insufficiency can complicate the evaluation of symptoms of heart failure.

Certain aspects of the physical examination are of particular importance in the geriatric population. Detection and further evaluation of impairments of vision and hearing can lead to improvements in quality of life. Evaluation of gait may uncover correctable causes of unsteadiness and thereby prevent potentially devastating falls (see Chap. 7). Careful palpation of the abdomen may reveal an aortic aneurysm, which, if large enough, might warrant consideration of surgical removal. The mental status examination is especially important; this aspect of the physical examination is discussed further below and in Chaps. 4 and 5.

LABORATORY ASSESSMENT

Abnormal laboratory findings are often attributed to "old age." While it is true that abnormal findings are common in geriatric patients, few are true aging changes. Misinterpretation of an abnormal laboratory value as an aging change may result in underdiagnosis and undertreatment of conditions such as anemia.

Table 3-5 lists those laboratory parameters unchanged in the elderly and those commonly abnormal. Abnormalities in the former

Table 3-5 Laboratory assessment of geriatric patients

Laboratory parameters unchanged*
Hemoglobin and hematocrit
White blood cell count
Platelet count
Electrolytes (sodium, potassium, chloride, bicarbonate)
Blood urea nitrogen
Liver function tests (transaminases, bilirubin, prothrombin time)
Free thyroxine index
Thyroid-stimulating hormone
Calcium
Phosphorus

(*continued*)

Table 3-5 Laboratory assessment of geriatric patients *(Continued)*

Common abnormal laboratory parameters[†]

Parameter	Clinical significance
Sedimentation rate	Mild elevations (10–20 mm) may be an age-related change.
Glucose	Glucose tolerance decreases (see Chap. 11); elevations during acute illness are common.
Creatinine	Because lean body mass and daily endogenous creatinine production decline, high-normal and minimally elevated values may indicate substantially reduced renal function.
Albumin	Average values decline (<0.5 g/mL) with age, especially in acutely ill, but generally indicate undernutrition.
Alkaline phosphatase	Mild asymptomatic elevations common; liver and Paget's disease should be considered if moderately elevated.
Serum iron, iron-binding capacity, ferritin	Decreased values are not an aging change and usually indicate undernutrition and/or gastrointestinal blood loss.
Prostate-specific antigen	May be elevated in patients with benign prostatic hyperplasia. Marked elevation or increasing values when followed over time should prompt consideration of further evaluation in patients for whom specific therapy for prostate cancer would be undertaken if cancer were diagnosed.
Urinalysis	Asymptomatic pyuria and bacteriuria are common and rarely warrant treatment; hematuria is abnormal and needs further evaluation (see Chap. 7).
Chest radiographs	Interstitial changes are a common age-related finding; diffusely diminished bone density generally indicates advanced osteoporosis (see Chap. 11).
Electrocardiogram	ST-segment and T-wave changes, atrial and ventricular arrhythmias, and various blocks are common in asymptomatic elderly and may not need specific evaluation or treatment (see Chap. 10).

* Aging changes do not occur in these parameters; abnormal values should prompt further evaluation.
† Includes normal aging and other age-related changes.

group should prompt further evaluation; abnormalities in the latter group should be interpreted carefully. Important considerations in interpreting commonly abnormal laboratory values are also noted in Table 3-5.

FUNCTIONAL ASSESSMENT

General Concepts

Ability to function should be a central focus of the evaluation of geriatric patients (Fig. 3-1). Medical history, physical examination, and laboratory findings are all of obvious importance in diagnosing and managing acute and chronic medical conditions in older people, as they are in all age groups. But once the dust settles, functional abilities are just as, if not more, important to the overall health, well-being, and potential need for services of the older individuals. For example, in a patient with hemiparesis, the nature, location, and extent of the lesion may be important in the management, but whether the patient is continent and can climb the steps to an apartment will make the difference between going home to live or going to a nursing home.

The concern about function as a core component of geriatrics deserves special comment. Functioning is the end result of the various efforts of the geriatric approach to care. Optimizing function necessitates integrating efforts on several fronts. It is helpful to think of functioning as an equation:

$$\text{Function} = \frac{\text{physical capabilities} \times \text{medical management} \times \text{motivation}}{\text{social, psychological, and physical environment}}$$

This admitted oversimplification is meant as a reminder that function can be influenced on at least three levels. The first is to remediate the remediable. Careful medical diagnosis and appropriate treatment are essential in good geriatric care. Adequate medical management, however, is necessary but not sufficient. Once those conditions amenable to treatment have been addressed, the next step is to develop the environment that will best support the patient's autonomous function. Environmental barriers can be both physical and psychological. It is easier to recognize the former: stairs for the person with dyspnea, inaccessible cabinets for the wheelchair-bound, and so on. Psychological barriers refer especially to the dangers of risk aversion. Those

most concerned about the patient may restrict activity in the name of protecting the patient or the institution. For example, hospitals are notoriously averse to risk; older patients will be restricted to a wheelchair rather than risk them falling when walking.

This risk averse behavior may be compounded by concerns about efficiency. Personal care is personnel-intensive. It takes much more time and patience to work with patients to encourage them to do things for themselves than to step in and do the task. But that pseudo-efficiency breeds dependence.

The third factor relates to the concept of motivation. If the care providers believe that the patient cannot improve, they will likely induce despair and discouragement in their charges. The tendency toward functional decline may become a self-fulfilling prophecy. Indeed, the opposite belief—that improvement is quite likely with appropriate intervention—may be the critical element in the success of geriatric evaluation units. Belief in the possibility of improvement can play another critical role in geriatric care. Psychologists have developed a useful paradigm referred to as "the innocent victim" (Lerner and Simmons, 1966). The basic concept is that caregivers respond in a hostile manner to those they feel impotent to help. If given a sense of empowerment, perhaps by using assessment tools and intervention strategies such as the ones provided in this book, for approaching the complex problems of older persons, care providers are likely to feel more positive toward those individuals and be more willing to work with them rather than avoiding them. The more an information system can provide feedback on accomplishments and progress toward improved function, the more the provider will feel positively about the older patient.

Several other important concepts about comprehensive functional assessment in the geriatric population, which were identified in a Consensus Development Conference at the National Institutes of Health (NIH, 1988), are summarized in Table 3-6. To a large extent the purpose, setting, and timing of the assessment dictate the nature of the assessment process. Table 3-7 lists the different purposes and objectives of functional status measures. Generally, functional assessment begins with a case-finding or screening approach in order to identify individuals for whom more in-depth and interdisciplinary assessment might be of benefit. Assessment is often carried out at points of transition, such as a threatened or actual decline in health status or impending change in living situation. Without this type of

Table 3-6 Important concepts for geriatric functional assessment

1. The nature of the assessment should be dictated by its purpose, setting, and timing (see Table 3-7).
2. Input from multiple disciplines is often helpful, but routine multidisciplinary assessment is not cost-effective.
3. Assessments should be targeted:
   a. Initial screening to identify disciplines needed.
   b. Times of threatened or actual decline in status, impending change in living situation, and other stressful situations.
4. Standard instruments are useful, but there are numerous potential pitfalls:
   a. Instruments should be reliable, sensitive, and valid for the purposes and setting of the assessment.
   b. How questions are asked can be critically important (e.g., performance vs. capability).
   c. Discrepancies can arise between different informants (e.g., self-report vs. caregiver's report).
   d. Self or caregiver report of performance, or direct observation of performance may not reflect what the individual does in everyday life.
   e. Many standard instruments have not been adequately tested for reliability and sensitivity to changes over time.
5. Open-ended questions are helpful in complementing information from standardized instruments.
6. The family's expectations, capabilities, and willingness to provide care must be explored.
7. The patient's preferences and expectations should be elicited and considered paramount in planning services.
8. A strong link must exist between the assessment process and follow-up in the provision of services.

targeting, the assessment of older people may be time-consuming and not cost-effective. Numerous standardized instruments are available to assist in the assessment process. Several examples of these instruments are discussed in this chapter and included in the Appendix. There are numerous potential pitfalls in the use of standardized assessment instruments (Kane and Kane, 1981; see Table 3-6). The critical concept in using standardized instruments is that they should fit the purposes and setting for which they are intended, and there must be a solid link between the assessment process and the follow-up provision of services. In addition, the assessment process should include a clear discussion of the patient's preferences and expectations, as well

Table 3-7 Purposes and objectives of functional status measures

Purpose	Objectives
Description	Develop normative data
	Depict geriatric population along selected parameters
	Assess needs
	Describe outcomes associated with various interventions
Screening	Identify from among population at risk those individuals who should receive further assessment and by whom
Assessment	Make diagnosis
	Assign treatment
Monitoring	Observe changes in untreated conditions
	Review progress of those receiving treatment
Prediction	Permit scientifically based clinical interventions
	Make prognostic statements of expected outcomes on the basis of given conditions

as the family's expectations and willingness to provide care. The importance of functional status assessment has recently been highlighted by data documenting the ability of functional status measures to predict mortality in older hospitalized patients (Inouye et al., 1998).

Assessment Tools for Functional Status

In this chapter, we focus on the assessment of physical and mental function. The latter is also discussed in Chap. 4. Examples of measures of physical functioning are shown in Table 3-8. Physical functioning is measured along a spectrum. For disabled persons, one may focus on the ability to perform basic self-care tasks, often referred to as *activities of daily living* (ADL). The patient is assessed on ability to conduct each of a series of basic activities. Data usually come from the patient or from a caregiver (e.g., a nurse or family member) who has had a sufficient opportunity to observe the patient. In some cases, it may be more useful to have the patient actually demonstrate the ability to perform key tasks. Grading of performance is usually divided into three levels of dependency: (1) ability to perform the task without human assistance (one may wish to distinguish those persons who need mechanical aids like a walker but are still independent),

Table 3-8 Examples of measures of physical functioning

Basic activities of daily living (ADL)
  Feeding
  Dressing
  Ambulation
  Toileting
  Bathing
  Transfer (from bed and toilet)
  Continence
  Grooming
  Communication

Instrumental activities of daily living (IADL)
  Writing
  Reading
  Cooking
  Cleaning
  Shopping
  Doing laundry
  Climbing stairs
  Using telephone
  Managing medication
  Managing money
  Ability to perform paid employment duties or outside work (e.g., gardening)
  Ability to travel (use public transportation, go out of town)

(2) ability to perform the task with some human assistance, and (3) inability to perform, even with assistance. Recent research suggests that distinguishing "independent without difficulty" from "independent *with* difficulty" may provide complementing prognostic information (Gill et al., 1998).

Commonly used tools for assessing physical function are included in the Appendix. These include the following:

1. The Katz Index of basic activities of daily living
2. The Lawton-Brody instrumental activities of daily living scale

With the exception of some items on the Barthel Index, these functional status measures are based on self and/or caregiver report. There may be discrepancies between such reports and what individuals actually do in their everyday life. Moreover, there may be differences

between reported physical functional status and actual measures of physical performance. Reuben's Physical Performance Test (PPT) is one example of a practical assessment that provides insights into actual performance and prognostic information (Reuben et al., 1992). (The PPT is included in the Appendix.) Other performance-based assessments of gait and balance are discussed in Chap. 8.

In addition to these general geriatric measures of functional status, other functional assessment tools are commonly used in different settings. Examples include the following:

1. The Short Form 36—a global measure of function and well-being which is increasingly being used in outpatient settings. This measure has a disadvantage in the frail geriatric population because of a ceiling effect—i.e., it does not distinguish well between sick and very sick older people.
2. The Minimum Data Set (MDS)—a comprehensive assessment mandated on admission with quarterly updates in Medicare/Medicaid certified nursing facilities. (See also Chaps. 4 and 15 and the Appendix.)
3. The Functional Independence Measure (FIM)—a detailed assessment tool commonly used to monitor functional status progress in rehabilitation settings.

A structured assessment of cognitive function should be part of every complete geriatric functional assessment. Because of the high prevalence of cognitive impairment, the potential impact of such impairment on overall function and safety and the ability of patients with early impairments to mask their deficits, clinicians must specifically attend to this aspect of functional assessment. At a minimum, assessment should include a test for orientation and memory. A standardized geriatric mental status test is included in the Appendix (the Folstein Mini-Mental Status Examination). Although these tests do not probe the variety of intellectual functions appropriate for a more detailed assessment, they are quick, easy, scorable, and reliable. More detailed assessment of cognitive function is discussed in Chap. 4.

ENVIRONMENTAL ASSESSMENT

We have emphasized earlier that patient function is the result of innate ability and environment. The clinician must therefore be particularly concerned with the older patient's environment. For many patients, an

assessment should include an evaluation of the available and potential resources to maintain functioning. Just as physicians comfortably prescribe drugs, they should also be prepared to prescribe environmental interventions when necessary.

Rehabilitation therapists (i.e., physical, occupational, speech) are especially skilled at functional assessment, developing and implementing rehabilitative plans of care targeted at potentially remediable functional impairments, and making specific recommendations about environmental modifications that can enhance safety and functional ability. An example of such an environmental assessment related to safety and falls is discussed in Chap. 9. (See also the Fall Hazard Checklist in the Appendix.) An environmental prescription may include alterations in the physical environment (e.g., ramps, grab bars, and elevated toilet seats), special services (e.g., "meals on wheels," homemaking, home nursing), increased social contact (e.g., friendly visiting, telephone reassurance, participation in recreational activities), or provision of critical elements (e.g., food or money).

The ability to identify the environmental interventions and function supports needed to maintain in the community may be the essential difference between enabling an older person to remain at home versus transferring that person to an institution. Although identifying the need is not tantamount to providing the resource, it is an important first step.

GERIATRIC CONSULTATION

Geriatric consultation may be requested to address specific clinical issues (e.g., confusion, incontinence, recurrent falling), to perform a comprehensive geriatric assessment (often in the context of determining the need for placement in a difficult living setting), or to perform a preoperative evaluation of a high-risk geriatric patient. In this chapter, we discuss the latter two types of consultation.

Comprehensive Geriatric Consultation

A comprehensive geriatric consultation includes the following:

1. A geriatric oriented history and physical examination attending to the issues reviewed earlier in this chapter.
2. Medication review

In addition, geriatric patients should be questioned about alcohol abuse. An example of a commonly used screening tool for alcohol abuse is included in the Appendix.

3. Functional assessment
4. Environmental and social assessment, focusing especially on care-giver support and other resources available to meet the patient's needs
5. Discussion of advance directives
6. A complete list of the patient's medical, functional, and psychosocial problems.
7. Specific recommendations in each domain

A systematic screening process to identify potentially remediable geriatric problems may be a useful tool for the comprehensive consultation. One such screening strategy is illustrated in Table 3-9 (Moore and

Table 3-9 Example of a screening tool to identify potentially remediable geriatric problems

Problem	Screening measure	Positive result
Poor vision	Ask, "Do you have difficulty driving, watching television, reading, or doing any of your daily activities because of your eyesight?" If yes, then test acuity with Snellen chart, with corrective lenses	Inability to read better than 20/40 on Snellen chart
Poor hearing	With audioscope set at 40 dB, test hearing at 1000 and 2000 Hz	Inability to hear 1000 or 2000 Hz in both ears or either frequency in one ear
Poor leg mobility	Time the patient after asking, "Rise from the chair. Walk 20 feet briskly, turn, walk back to the chair, and sit down."	Unable to complete task in 15 s

(*continued*)

Table 3-9 Example of a screening tool to identify potentially remediable geriatric problems *(Continued)*

Problem	Screening measure	Positive result
Urinary incontinence	Ask, "In the past year, have you ever lost your urine and gotten wet?" If yes, then ask, "Have you lost urine on at least 6 separate days?"	Yes to both questions
Malnutrition and weight loss	Ask, "Have you lost 10 pounds over the past 6 months without trying to do so?" and then weigh the patient	Yes to the question or weight <100 Lb
Memory loss	Three-item recall	Unable to remember all three items after 1 min
Depression	Ask, "Do you often feel sad or depressed?"	Yes to the question
Physical disability	Ask six questions: "Are you able to "Do strenuous activities such as fast walking or bicycling? "Do heavy work around the house like washing windows, walls, or floors? "Go shopping for groceries or clothes? "Get to places that are out of walking distance? "Bathe: either a sponge bath, tub bath, or shower? "Dress, including putting on a shirt, buttoning and zipping, and putting on shoes?"	No to any question

Source: From Moore and Siu, 1996, with permission.

Siu, 1996). Examples of tools for functional, environmental, and social assessment are included in the Appendix. It may also be useful, especially in capitated systems, to use a tool that identifies risk for crises and expensive health care utilization. The Pra instrument is one such tool (Table 3-10; Pacala et al., 1997). Among frail, dependent geriatric patients, screening for risk factors and elder abuse is important. Elder abuse is more common among older people who are in poor health and who are physically and cognitively impaired. Additional risk factors include shared living arrangements with a relative or friend suspected of alcohol or substance abuse, mental illness, or a history of violence. Frequent emergency room visits for injury or exacerbations of chronic illness should also raise suspicion for abuse. Table 3-11 illustrates an example of an effective format for documenting the results of the consultation, listing the problems and recommendations first.

Table 3-10 Questions on the Pra instrument for identifying geriatric patients at risk for health service utilization

1. In general, would you say your health is:
   (excellent; very good; good; fair; poor)

2. In the previous 12 months, have you stayed overnight as a patient in a hospital?
   (not at all; one time; two or three times; more than three times)

3. In the previous 12 months, how many times did you visit a physician or clinic?
   (not at all; one time; two or three times; four to six times; more than six times)

4. In the prvious 12 months, did you have diabetes?
   (yes; no)

5. Have you ever had: Coronary heart disease? (yes; no)
   Angina pectoris? (yes; no)
   A myocardial infarction? (yes; no)
   Any other heart attack? (yes; no)

6. Your sex?
   (male; female)

7. Is there a friend, relative, or neighbor who would take care of you for a few days if necessary?
   (yes; no)

8. Your date of birth?
   (month   ; day   ; year   )

Source: From Pacala et al., 1997, with permission.

Table 3-11 Suggested format for summarizing the results of a comprehensive geriatric consultation

1. Identifying data, including referring physician
2. Reason(s) for consultation
3. Problems
   a. Medical Problem List
   b. Functional Problem List
   c. Psychosocial Problem List
4. Recommendations
5. Standard documentation
   a. History, including medications, significant past medical and surgical history, system review
   b. Social and environmental information
   c. Functional assessment
   d. Advance directive status
   e. Physical exam

PREOPERATIVE EVALUATION

Geriatricians are often called upon by surgeons and anesthesiologists to assess elderly patients before surgical procedures. Table 3-12 lists several of the key factors involved in the preoperative evaluation of geriatric patients. Although numerous studies have examined the relative risk of various surgical procedures in elderly compared with younger populations, none have shown convincingly that age alone increases risk of surgical morbidity and mortality (Hosking et al., 1989). Morbidity and mortality, however, are influenced by the presence and severity of systemic illnesses and whether the procedure is elective versus emergent. Thus, evaluating a geriatric patient's preoperative status and risk for surgery necessitates a thorough assessment of cardiopulmonary and renal function as well as nutritional and hydration status (Freeman et al., 1989). Patients with a recent history of myocardial infarction, active angina, pulmonary edema, and severe aortic stenosis are at especially high risk (Goldman, 1983; Kroenke, 1987; Gerson et al., 1990; Mangano and Goldman, 1995). Because physiologic reserve declines with age, especially in the cardiovascular, pulmonary, and renal systems, routine preoperative measurement of physiologic capacity is helpful in certain situations. A baseline arterial blood gas, assessment of pulmonary function, measurement of

Table 3-12 Key factors in the preoperative evaluation of the geriatric patient

1. Age >70 is associated with an increased risk of complications and death
   a. Risk varies with the type of procedure and local complication rates
   b. Emergency procedures are associated with much higher risk
   c. Comorbid conditions, especially cardiovascular, are more important risk factors than age per se
2. The appropriateness and risk-benefit ratio of the proposed surgery must be carefully considered
3. Underlying conditions must be evaluated and optimally managed before nonemergency surgery, e.g.:
   a. Cardiovascular disease, especially heart failure
   b. Pulmonary status
   c. Renal function
   d. Diabetes mellitus
   e. Thyroid disease (which is often occult)
   f. Anemia
   g. Nutrition
   h. Hydration, especially in patients on diuretics
4. Medication regimens should be carefully planned; some drugs should be continued, others should be withheld, and some necessitate dosage adjustments
5. Several cardiovascular conditions substantially increase risk, including:
   a. Myocardial infarction within 6 months
   b. Pulmonary edema
   c. Angina (especially if unstable)
   d. Severe aortic stenosis
6. Specific laboratory evaluations may be helpful in some situations, e.g.:
   a. Pulmonary function tests and arterial blood gas with respiratory symptoms, obesity, chest deformity (e.g., kyphoscoliosis), abnormal chest radiographs, planned thoracic or upper abdominal procedure
   b. Exercise test or dipyridamole-thallium scanning with uncertain or borderline cardiovascular status
   c. Creatinine clearance with unstable or borderline renal function, or the use of nephrotoxic or renally excreted drugs
7. The documented effectiveness, risks, and benefits of perioperative prophylactic measures should be considered.
   a. Antithrombotic prophylaxis*
   b. Antimicrobial prophylaxis†

---

* See Weinman and Salzman, 1994.
† See Medical Letter, 1995.

creatinine clearance, and in some patients modified exercise testing and/or dipyridamole thallium scanning may be indicated if specific indications exist.

Underlying conditions that are prevalent in the geriatric population, such as hypertension, congestive heart failure, chronic obstructive lung disease, diabetes mellitus, anemia, and undernutrition, need particularly careful management in the preoperative period (Thomas and Ritchie, 1995; Schiff and Emanuele, 1995). Medication regimens should be scrutinized in order to determine whether specific drugs should be continued or withheld (Cygan and Waitzkin, 1987; Kroenke, 1987). Careful consideration should also be given to perioperative prophylactic measures for the prevention of thromboembolism and infection, many of which have documented efficacy in specific situations (Medical Letter, 1995; Weinman and Salzman, 1994).

Many surgeons and anesthesiologists tend to favor regional over general anesthesia for geriatric patients. Regional anesthesia (e.g., epidural), however, may have several potential disadvantages. Patients may require added intravenous sedation and/or analgesia, thus increasing the risks of perioperative cardiovascular and mental status changes. Significant cardiovascular changes can, in fact, occur during regional anesthesia; thus invasive monitoring may be required in some patients. Neither the incidence of deep vein thrombosis nor the amount of blood loss seems to be substantially decreased compared to general anesthesia. Thus, decisions about the type of anesthesia should be carefully individualized on the basis of patient factors, the nature of the procedure, and the preferences of the surgical team.

REFERENCES

American College of Physicians: Guidelines for assessing and managing the perioperative risk from coronary artery disease associated with major noncardiac surgery. *Ann Intern Med* 127:309–312, 1997.

Brody EM, Kleban MH, Moles E: What older people do about their day-to-day mental and physical health symptoms. *J Amer Geriatr Soc* 31:489–498, 1983.

Cygan R, Waitzkin H: Stopping and restarting medications in the perioperative period. *J Gen Intern Med* 2:270–283, 1987.

Folstein MF, Folstein S, McHuth PR: Mini-Mental State: A practical method for grading the cognitive state of patients for the clinician. *J Psychiatr Res* 12:189–198, 1975.

Freeman W, Gibbons R, Shub C: Preoperative assessment of cardiac patients undergoing noncardiac surgical procedures. *Mayo Clin Proc* 64:1105–1117, 1989.

Gerson MC, Hurst JM, Hertzberg VS, et al: Prediction of cardiac and pulmonary complications related to elective abdominal and noncardiac thoracic surgery in geriatric patients. *Am J Med* 88:101–107, 1990.

Gill TM, Robison JT, Tinetti ME: Difficulty and dependence: Two components of the disability continuum among community-living older persons. *Ann Intern Med* 128:96–101, 1998.

Goldman L: Cardiac risks and complications of noncardiac surgery. *Ann Intern Med* 98:504–513, 1983.

Inouye SK, Peduzzi PN, Robison JT, et al: Importance of functional measures in predicting mortality among older hospitalized patients. *JAMA* 279:1187–1993, 1998.

Hosking MP, Wamer MA, Lobdell CM, et al: Outcomes of surgery in patients 90 years and older. *JAMA* 261:1909–1915, 1989.

Kane RL, Kane RA: *Assessing the Elderly: A Practical Guide to Measurement.* Lexington, MA, Heath, 1981.

Katz S, Ford A, Moskowitz R, et al: The index of ADL: A standardized measure of biological and psychosocial function. *JAMA* 185:914–919, 1963.

Kroenke MK: Preoperative evaluation: The assessment and management of surgical risk. *J Gen Intern Med* 2:257–269, 1987.

Landefeld CS, Palmer RM, Kresevic DM, et al: A randomized trial of care in hospital medical unit especially designed to improve the functional outcomes of acutely ill older patients. *N Engl J Med* 332:1338–1344, 1995.

Lerner MJ, Simmons CH: Observer's reaction to the "innocent victim": Compassion or rejection? *J Pers Soc Psychol* 4:203–210, 1966.

Mangano DT, Goldman L: Preoperative assessment of patients with known or suspected coronary disease. *N Engl J Med* 333:1750–1756, 1995.

Medical Letter on Drugs and Therapeutics: Antimicrobial prophylaxis in surgery. *Med Lett* 37(957):79–82, 1995.

Moore AA, Siu AL: Screening for common problems in ambulatory elderly: Clinical confirmation of a screening instrument. *Am J Med* 100:438–443, 1996.

NIH Consensus Development Conference Statement: Geriatric assessment methods for clinical decision-making. *J Am Geriatr Soc* 36:342–347, 1988.

Pacala JT, Boult C, Reed RL, Aliberti E: Predictive validity of the P_{ra} instrument among older recipients of managed care. *J Am Geriatr Soc* 45:614–617, 1997.

Reuben DB, Siu A, Kimpau S: The predictive validity of self-report and performance-based measures of function and health. *J Gerontol Med Sci* 47:106–110, 1992.

Reuben DB, Borok GM, Wolde-Tsadik G, et al: A randomized trial of comprehensive geriatric assessment in the care of hospitalized patients. *N Engl J Med* 332:1345–1350, 1995.

Rubenstein LZ, Stuck AE, Sill AL, Wieland D: Impacts of geriatric evaluation and management programs on defined outcomes: Overview of the evidence. *J Am Geriatr Soc* 39(suppl):85–165, 1991.

Schiff RL, Emanuele MA: The surgical patient with diabetes mellitus: Guidelines for management. *J Gen Intern Med* 10:154–161, 1995.

Stuck AE, Aronow HU, Steiner A, et al: A trial of annual in-home comprehensive geriatric assessments for elderly people living in the community. *N Engl J Med* 333:1184–1189, 1995.

Thomas DR, Ritchie CS: Preoperative assessment of older adults. *J Am Geriatr Soc* 43:811–821, 1995.
Weinmann EE, Salzman EW: Deep-vein thrombosis. *N Engl J Med* 331:1630–1641, 1994.

SUGGESTED READINGS

Applegate WB, Blass JP, Williams TF: Instruments for functional assessment of older patients. *N Engl J Med* 322:1207–1214, 1990.
Beck A, Scott J, Williams P, et al: A randomized trial of group outpatient visits for chronically ill older HMO members: The cooperative health care clinic. *J Am Geriatr Soc* 45:543–549, 1997.
Crum RM, Anthony SC, Bassett SS, Folstein MF: Population-based norms for the Mini-Mental State Examination by age and educational level. *JAMA* 269:2386–2391, 1993.
Feinstein AR, Josephy BR, Wells CK: Scientific and clinical problems in indexes of functional disability. *Ann Intern Med* 105:413–420, 1986.
Finch M, Kane RL, Philp I: Developing a New Metric for ADLs. *J Am Geriatr Soc* 43:877–884, 1995.
Fleming KC, Evans JM, Weber DC, Chutka DS: Practical functional assessment of elderly persons: A primary-care approach. *Mayo Clin Proc* 70:890–910, 1995.
Gill TM, Feinstein AR: A critical appraisal of the quality of quality-of-life measurements. *JAMA* 272:619–626, 1994.
Katz S, Branch LG, Branson MH, et al: Active life expectancy. *N Engl J Med* 309:1218–1224, 1983.
Palda VA, Detsky AS: Perioperative assessment and management of risk from coronary artery disease. *Ann Intern Med* 127:313–328, 1997.
Reuben DB, Siu AL: An objective measure of physical function of elderly persons: The physical performance test. *J Am Geriatr Soc* 38:1105–1112, 1990.
Scheitel SM, Fleming KC, Chutka DS, Evans JM: Geriatric health maintenance. *Mayo Clin Proc* 71:289–302, 1996.
Siu A: Screening for dementia and its causes. *Ann Intern Med* 115:122–132, 1991.
Williams ME, Hadler N, Earp JA: Manual ability as a mark of dependency in geriatric women. *J Chronic Dis* 40:481–489, 1987.

FOUR

DEVELOPING CLINICAL EXPECTATIONS

Attitudes about older patients tend to carry over into their care. Elderly patients are in danger of being dismissed as hopeless or not worth the effort. The physician faced with the question of how much time and resources to spend in searching for a diagnosis will want to consider the probability of benefit for the investment. In some cases, older patients are better investments than younger ones. This apparent paradox occurs in the case of some preventive strategies when high risk of susceptibility and the discounted benefits of future health favor older persons. But it also arises in situations where small increments of change can yield dramatic differences.

Perhaps the most striking example of the latter is found in the case of nursing home patients. Very modest changes in their routine—such as introducing a pet, giving them a plant to tend, or increasing their sense of control over their environment—can produce dramatic improvements in mood and morale (Kane and Kane, 1987).

At the same time, the ratio of risk to benefit is different with older patients. Treatments that might be easily tolerated in younger patients may pose a much greater risk of producing harmful effects in older patients. In effect, the dosage that will produce a positive effect more closely approaches one that can lead to a toxic effect. As

noted earlier, one of the hallmarks of aging is a loss of responsiveness to stress. In this context, treatment may be viewed as a stress.

Those who treat older patients must also consider the theory of competitive risks. Because older persons often suffer from multiple problems, treating one problem may provide an opportunity for more adverse effects from another. In essence, eliminating one cause of death increases the likelihood of death from another.

Creating a more proactive attitude among those who care for older persons may be enhanced by the use of flowcharts. The data selected should represent those parameters that are both significant and most likely to be affected. Because the changes are likely to be subtle, it is often helpful to establish treatment goals with time frames for achieving them. Both the health care team and the patient can then agree on expectations and follow progress toward the goal. It is important that the goals be achievable. Small successes are very important and reinforcing. Thus the units of measurement should be capable of detecting small but meaningful changes. In many instances, small gains can, in fact, make an enormous difference. The stroke patient, for example, who regains the use of hand muscles has a greatly improved ability to function. Being able to change position in bed may mean the difference between getting pressure sores and not. Regaining a method of communication, whether by speech or some other means, can restore social contact.

By introducing gradual, small steps, a functional task may appear more achievable. We have all had some experience in getting a bedridden patient to resume a more active role. For an older person who has been at bed rest for a long period, this task requires overcoming both physiological and psychological problems. Small steps will often ease the transition and provide an opportunity to monitor the effects at each stage to minimize risk.

CLINICAL GLIDEPATHS

We noted earlier in this book that care for chronic disease is conceptually different than that for acute disease. To provide effective chronic care, one needs a longitudinally oriented information system that is sensitive to change. Each clinical encounter with a chronically ill patient is essentially a part of a continuing episode of care; it has a history and a future. Caring for a chronically ill patient, especially

one with multiple problems, demands an enormous feat of memory as the patient's list of problems is unearthed and the history, treatments, and expectations associated with each are reviewed. Clinicians caring for such patients (often under enormous time pressures) may find themselves either overwhelmed with large volumes of data from which they must quickly extract the most salient facts or, alternatively, relying on inadequate data from which to reconstruct the patient's clinical course. What is needed in chronic care is a simple information system that can focus the clinician's attention on salient parameters.

One approach to help to focus clinicians' attention on the salient parameters of a chronic condition is the clinical glidepath. This technique is modeled on the way one lands an airplane. The goal is to establish a flight path that will lead to a safe landing. Information about the plane's position is provided regularly to allow the pilot to make small corrections in order to avoid making drastic adjustments at the last minute or crashing. In a similar vein, one can manage chronic illnesses by establishing the salient parameters, the indications that the patient's clinical course is being achieved. For each chronic problem, the clinician should identify the one or two parameters (physiologic or functional) that will best indicate when things are going well. Information on these is then systematically collected (by the clinician or by other staff) and charted graphically. As long as the patient's course is as good as or better than predicted, no adjustments need be made; but indications that the course is beginning to slip below that expected should trigger an early reassessment, in the same way that a pilot is warned when the plane begins to move out of the glidepath box. Figure 4-1 shows an example of a glidepath.

The choice of the parameters to be tracked for each problem can either be left up to each practitioner or the practitioner can choose from a window of pertinent options. In most cases, the latter makes the most sense. It provides some structure but permits an individualized approach.

The clinical glidepath approach combines making a prognosis about a patient's expected course with the collection of systematic information on salient parameters. The prognosis can be generated intuitively or derived from statistical data. Unfortunately we do not yet have systematic data collection from which to generate such statistics. Implementing a glidepath system will have to rely on clinical judgment about prognosis. This judgment can be made by each clinician, or one can rely on the systematic judgment of experts. Initially the value of

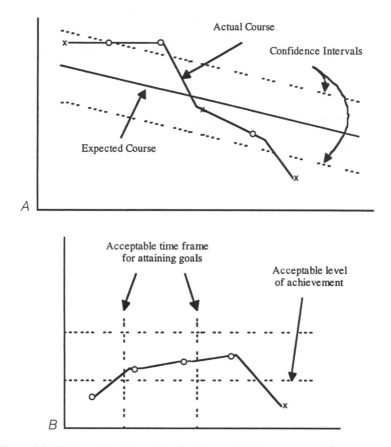

Figure 4-1 Clinical glidepath models. In this model (A), the expected course (solid line) calls for gradual decline. The confidence intervals are shown as dotted lines. Actual measures that are within or better than the glidepath are shown as O. When the patient's course is worse than expected, the O changes to an x. The design shown uses confidence intervals with upper and lower bounds, but actually only the lower bound is pertinent. Any performance above the upper confidence interval boundary is very acceptable. The design of the glidepath can also take another form (B). It may be preferable to think in terms of reaching a threshold level within a given time window (e.g., in recuperating from an illness) and then maintaining that level.

the glidepath system will come less from assessing the rate of achieving the expected path than from the systematic attention to patients' courses. Rendering a great deal of complex information more coherently and setting expectations should have a positive effect on chronic care.

It is important to distinguish the clinical glidepath approach from clinical pathways. The latter specify an expected course with specific milestones and dictates what care should be provided at specific junctures. This approach works well in very predictable situations such as postoperative recovery and even some instances of rehabilitation, but most of chronic care management is not as predictable. The glidepath method specifies what data should be collected, not what actions should be taken. Its underlying premise holds that when clinicians can be aided in focusing their attention on a patient's salient parameters, they will be able to manage the chronic problems better.

DISEASE MANAGEMENT

Focusing attention on the management of specific problems has become a consistent theme in efforts to improve the management of chronic illness. Disease management can exist in several forms. Most of the disease management approaches make heavy use of extant computerized data, which tends to come from drug records and lab tests. This information can be combined with diagnostic data (usually obtained from billing records) to create a system that can look for errors of both omission and commission. In some cases, potential complications can be flagged and checks built in to try to avoid untoward events such as drug interactions.

Some disease management has taken a more active approach than relying simply on information systems to detect potential problems. Case managers may be assigned to patients who are determined to need special attention either because they have a diagnosis that suggests high risk of subsequent utilization or their history indicates problems in controlling their disease(s). These case managers work with the patients to be sure that they understand their regimens. They encourage the patients to raise any questions early. They may make home visits to ascertain how the patients are doing and to ensure that they can function effectively in their natural habitats. The positive

reports from trials of this approach have encouraged many replications (Rich et al., 1995).

Another variation on disease management is being practiced in a few managed care organizations. Here patients with a given disease are brought together for periodic sessions that include health education and group support. It has proven more efficient to use groups in this way. The same sessions can draw upon specialists to see problematic cases more efficiently (Beck et al., 1997).

Particularly in the context of managed care, there is a strong incentive to try to identify high-risk patients in order to attend to them before they develop into high-cost cases. Various predictive models have been developed to identify such cases. One of the ones that has been widely used is the Pra (probability of repeat admissions). This tool uses an eight-item questionnaire to flag older patients who are most likely to have two or more hospital admissions in the next several years (Boult et al., 1993). A modification of this method has been developed to utilize administrative data bases as well (Coleman et al., 1998). A similar approach is being developed to identify those at high risk for needing long-term care. Once these patients have been targeted, an intervention is needed to change the predicted course. The Pra does not specify what actions should be taken, but it was initially developed as a method for identifying those in need of a comprehensive geriatric examination. The benefit of such an intervention is still being assessed, but preliminary data are encouraging (Boult et al., 1998), and at least one metanalysis of geriatric assessment declared it a substantial boon to care (Stuck et al., 1993). Function has proven to be an important predictive risk factor for both subsequent utilization of expensive services and or outcomes in general. Poor functional status in hospital patients predicts later mortality over and above the effects of burden-of-illness measures (Inouye et al., 1998).

BENCHMARKS

The clinical glidepath system is closely related to another approach that combines a set of prognoses and the criteria for predicted progress. The latter are termed *benchmarks*. Ideally each physician would evaluate each patient as a unique combination of problems and potential. However, the costs involved may prove prohibitive in view of

time pressures. An alternative is to use a previously conceived set of basic benchmarks geared to the common problems of geriatrics. The generation of a problem list then leads to the implementation of the appropriate benchmarks. These can be modified to fit the more specific characteristics of a given patient. A great advantage of this approach lies in its capacity to enhance delegation. The benchmarks provide a structure to guide ongoing information gathering. They target the pertinent information and can even offer general guidelines about what steps to take when the observed results deviate from those expected. (These actions are usually couched in terms of varying stages of urgency for seeking help.) The benchmark system does not preclude gathering additional data or recognizing the development of a new problem.

One setting ideally suited to such an approach is the nursing home. Because the system guides the collection of information and relates each item to one or more specific problems, it has an educational role as well as a clinical one. Nursing home staff who may feel isolated from the infrequently seen physician now have a more effective means of communication. They know what information is being sought and why. They have a format for recording those data, which offers desired information.

The benchmark system was, in fact, developed for use in the nursing home and has been used effectively in that setting (Woolley et al., 1974). Because the general level of literacy among the nursing home aides was quite low, the system was specifically designed to require minimal narrative by using symbols in a flowchart format.

Table 4-1 presents a sample set of benchmark criteria for hip fracture. The two scales referred to—independence and behavior—were specially developed for the project but could be replaced by measures of activities of daily living and a standardized mood scale such as that for depression. Other clinicians may choose to add, delete, or modify items to fit their pattern of practice. Figure 4-2 offers a hypothetical chart for recording data pertinent to this problem. Specific narrative notes are made only when an event warrants them. The flowchart format readily shows when a change in pattern occurs and intervention is indicated.*

This basic approach has been taken a step farther. "Extended care pathways" have been developed, largely in the arena of nursing,

---

*A complete copy of the system is available from the authors.

Table 4-1 Example of benchmark instructions: hip fracture

Observation	Frequency	Benchmark	Action
1. Independence scale score	Every 2 weeks	Decreased score or no change within 6 weeks after therapy is begun	Inform physician
2. Behavioral scale score	Every 2 weeks	Decreased score or no change within 6 weeks after therapy is begun	Inform physician
3. Soreness in either calf (use: R5 right soreness, L5 left soreness)	Daily; check by pushing foot up with knee extended	Present Notify physician	Place patient on bed rest
4. Temperature (°F) pain, malaise	Increased hip pain, calf pain in afternoon	Above 100.8° orally for 8–16 h	Notify physician Take temperature every 4–8 h if elevated
5. Contracture or stiff joint, especially foot drop, hip flexion, knee flexion, hip abducted or turned out (+ or −)	Daily	Present	Continue to position properly and give range of motion to tolerance; inform physician; chart location of contracture
6. Distance walked at one time (in yards)	Daily	Decrease over 3 days or no improvement within 1 week after therapy is begun	Inform physician
7. Pain in hip (+ for pain)	Afternoon	No relief by medication after 24 h of administration	Notify physician

Source: From Pepper et al., 1972, with permission.

DATE	8/12	9/13	9/14	9/15	8/16	8/17	8/18	3/19	8/20	8/21	F/22	8/23	8/24	6/25	6/26	8/27
Hip Fracture																
1. Independence Scale Score	20															
2. Behavior Scale Score								40								
3. Soreness in either calf (-, R or L)	-	-	-	-	-	-	-	*R	R							
4. Contracture (+ or -)	-	-	+c	+	+*	+	+	+	-	-	-	-	-	-	-	-
5. Distance Walked (yds.)	10	10	11	12	13	14	15	C	N							
6. Temperature (°F) prn								101°/F	F							

Figure 4-2 Hypothetical example of benchmark chart. The data charted correspond to those outlined in Table 4-1. C = See nurse's notes in chart, as some information about this observation was charted here on this date. F = See form appropriate for charting this observation elsewhere (e.g., I & O; diabetic record; TPR graphic; etc.). * = Physician informed concerning this observation on this day. N = Not determined. *(From Pepper et al, 1972, with permission.)*

whereby specific outcomes are defined and timelines laid out by which they should be met. Charting is done for exceptions. Treatments and next steps are usually indicated.

Neither the benchmark system nor the extended care pathways fit easily into the current system of regulations for physician attendance to nursing home patients. The present rules are designed to achieve at least a minimal frequency of contact with these patients (usually once a month). Unfortunately, the result is too often superficial attention to the patient's chart. The doctor's signature is the ticket to continued coverage under Medicaid. Particularly when the same system discourages frequent visits, the care of nursing home patients is neglected.

Nursing home care has never attracted a great deal of physician enthusiasm, but this need not continue to be the case. If we can implement a new form of record keeping that provides better information to staff and demands better performance from them, we should see an improvement in morale and hence a more attractive atmosphere in which to practice. It is also worth noting here that the benchmark system was originally developed for use with a nurse practitioner as the person giving primary care under supervision of physicians. Nurse practitioners have proved themselves very effective in such roles for nursing home patients, and the care they provide is now covered by Medicare Part B.

MINIMUM DATA SET FOR NURSING HOMES

The Omnibus Budget Reconciliation Act of 1987 (OBRA '87) produced many changes in the way nursing homes were regulated. Perhaps none was as influential as the requirement that all nursing home residents covered by federal funds be assessed regularly using a standardized form, the Minimum Data Set for Nursing Home Resident Assessment and Care Screening (MDS) (see Chap. 15 for a more complete discussion of the MDS). This information is designed to be completed by a nurse, but it draws on data from a number of disciplines. The MDS summarizes a number of facets about each resident, including functional levels, cognitive and behavioral problems, special care needs, skin condition, nutritional status, and psychosocial wellbeing. In addition to serving as a basic data set, problems identified

trigger more detailed required documentation, called *Resident Assessment Protocols* (RAPs), in 18 areas:

- Delirium
- Visual function
- ADL functional/rehabilitation potential
- Psychosocial well-being
- Behavior problem
- Falls
- Feeding tubes
- Dental care
- Psychotropic drug use
- Cognitive loss/dementia
- Communication
- Urinary incontinence
- Mood state
- Activities
- Nutritional status
- Dehydration/fluid maintenance
- Pressure ulcers
- Physical restraints

The MDS is intended to provide a basis for developing better plans of care and for assessing the changes in functional levels over time. A copy of the MDS is shown in the Appendix.

The MDS can also prove a useful tool for physicians. It is a compact source of information about various aspects of each nursing home resident. If the pertinent parameters for goals determined to be achieved in the care plan were systematically charted in a flow sheet, it would be possible to see progress at a glance or to recognize the need for a change in the plan of care. Physicians can play a key role in helping nursing home staff to see how such information can be used to improve care, not just to meet external mandates for better documentation.

However, several important shortcomings of the MDS must be acknowledged. The MDS was designed to be a means of recording judgments. These judgments inevitably pass through several hands. The persons with the most direct opportunity to observe behavior are the nurses aides, who then communicate their observations to the nurses completing the forms. The overall reliance on observations

means that, in effect, all nursing home residents are being assessed as though they were cognitively impaired. This limitation is especially severe, because the MDS purports to measure critical elements of quality of life. Assuming that one can truly infer another person's emotional state, the degree to which they are engaged in meaningful activities or whether they have real social relationships seems like an act of hubris. Even using observations to determine a person's cognitive capacity seems to require heroic assumptions (Morris et al., 1994). It may be possible to detect extremes of behavior, but no one would want to argue that such an approach is the best way to assess many of these critical domains. Nonetheless, the MDS does not use specific questions put to those patients who can respond. Moreover, the proponents of the MDS have made broad claims that they are, indeed, able to tap many of the domains that constitute a central portion of what we commonly term *quality of life* (Hawes, 1996).

The MDS has also been used as the basis for assessing the quality of nursing home care (Zimmerman et al., 1995). The outcomes and processes of care reflected in various measures have been matched to various clinical subgroups derived from the same data to permit more valid comparisons across more homogenous groupings (Arling et al., 1997).

ROLE OF OUTCOMES IN ASSURING QUALITY OF LONG-TERM CARE

Quality of care remains a critical, if elusive, goal for long-term care. As we consider steps for resource allocation, we might first address the question of whether we are spending our current funds most wisely. There is at once a growing demand for more creativity and more accountability in long-term care. It may be possible to reduce the regulatory burden, increase the meaningful accountability, and make the incentives within the system more rational.

Before we can talk about how to package it or how to buy it cheaper, we need a better understanding of what we are really buying. One hears more and more about the value of shifting attention from the process of care to the actual outcomes achieved in acute care (Ellwood, 1988; Institute of Medicine, 1990). These arguments apply at least as strongly to long-term care. There are several reasons for looking toward outcomes as the way to assess and assure quality.

- Outcomes encourage creativity by avoiding domination by current professional orthodoxies or powerful constituencies
- Outcomes permit flexibility in the modality of care
- Outcomes permit comparisons of efficacy across modalities of care.
- Outcomes permit more flexible responses to different levels of performance, and thus avoid the "all-or-none" difficulties of many sanctions

At the same time, outcomes have some limitations.

- Outcomes necessitate a single point of accountability; all the actors—facility operators, agencies, staff, physicians, patients, and family—contribute to them. Under this approach the role of the provider includes motivating others.
- Outcomes are largely influenced by the patient's status at the beginning of treatment. The easiest and most direct way to address this issue is to think of the relationship between achieved and expected outcomes as the measure of success. Henceforth in this section the term *outcomes* is used to mean that relationship between achieved and expected.
- Outcomes must also take cognizance of case mix. Predicting outcomes necessitates information about disease characteristics (e.g., diagnosis, severity, comorbidity) and patient characteristics (e.g., demographic factors, prior history, and social support).

Clinicians frequently balk at being judged on the basis of outcomes. This discomfort can be traced to several issues.

1. Virtually all of clinical training addresses the process of care. Clinicians are schooled in what to do for whom. They reasonably believe, therefore, that if they do the right thing well, they have provided a quality service. They do not like to discuss clusters of patients, preferring to review their care one patient at a time.
2. Many factors can affect the outcomes of care that are out of the clinicians' control. They have difficulty with the concept of probability and prefer to either be responsible or not.
3. Outcomes are by their nature post hoc. Often a long period can elapse between the time of an action and the report of its success. It is thus too late to intervene in that case.

4. Outcomes indicate a problem but offer no solution. Outcomes do not often point to specific actions that must be taken to correct the problems.

Hence, introducing outcomes, however rational, has not been easy. Making clinicians comfortable with an outcomes philosophy will require substantial training and new incentives. Physicians need to be trained to think in terms of both condition-specific and generic outcomes. They need access to data systems that can display the outcomes of their care for clinically relevant groups of patients under their care and compare them with what are reasonable outcomes for comparable patients receiving good care. Table 4-2 summarizes the key issues in outcomes measurement and its applications.

Outcomes should be used as the basis for quality assurance in long-term care. The outcome approach can be used in several ways.

1. As reflected in the 1987 OBRA regulations [which, in turn, were stimulated by the Institute of Medicine's 1986 report (Institute of Medicine, 1986)], there is already growing national interest in increasing the emphasis on outcomes in regulatory activities. Outcome measures can be substituted for most of the current structure and process measures. It is appropriate to continue regulation in areas such as life safety. Concomitant with an outcomes emphasis would be the reduction of regulatory burden. It is important to recognize, however, that it is *not* appropriate to dictate structure, process, and outcome at the same time. Such a policy removes all degrees of freedom and stifles creativity at the point when we want to encourage it. Under an outcome-regulated approach, providers whose patients do better than expected are rewarded and are less worried about their style of caregiving, whereas those whose patients do relatively poorly are investigated more closely.
2. Outcomes can be incorporated into the payment structure to link payment with effects of care. Payments, either in the form of bonuses and penalties or as a more fundamental part of the payment structure, can be used to reward and penalize good and bad outcomes, respectively. (For example, an outcome approach might use a factor reflecting the overall achieved/expected ratio for a patient as a multiplier against the costs of care to develop a total price paid for that period of time; or one might use a similar ratio to weigh the amount of money going to a given provider from a

Table 4-2 Outcomes measurement issues

Issue	Comments
Need outcome measures that are both clinically meaningful and psychometrically sound.	Use combination of condition-specific and generic measures. Usually better to adapt extant measures than to develop measures de novo.
Outcomes are always post hoc.	Expand outcomes information systems to include data on risk factors. These data should be useful in guiding clinicians to collect information that will identify potential problems. Use these data to create risk warnings to flag high-risk cases.
Every physician has all the tough cases.	Need to include a wide variety of case-mix adjusters for severity and comorbidity. Ask clinicians in advance to identify potential risk adjusters. Collect almost any item that a clinician might want to see. Test the ability of the potential risk factor to predict outcomes and discard if it has little predictive power.
Because no two clinicians see the same cases, comparisons are unfair.	Use risk adjustment. Create clinically homogeneous subgroups; use risk propensities (groups of patients with same a priori likelihood of developing the outcome).
Cannot control for selection bias; patients may receive different treatments because of subtle differences.	Adjust for all clinically identifiable differences. Use statistical methods (e.g., instrumental variables) to adjust for unmeasured differences.

fixed pool of dollars committed to such care.) Such an approach must be viewed carefully within the context of our present case-mix reimbursement scheme for nursing homes, because the latter indirectly rewards deterioration in function. An outcome approach to payment is compatible with a case-mix approach that is used on admission only.

3. An outcomes approach can be incorporated into the basic caring process. Where the information base used in assessing patients and developing care plans is structured, the emphasis on outcomes can become a proactive force to guide care. Optimally, the information used to assess outcomes will come from the clinical records and will be the same information used to guide care. Using available computer technology, it is now feasible to collect such data, translate them into care plans, and aggregate these data for quality assurance at minimal additional cost. The great advantage of such a scheme is its potential both to provide a better information base with which to plan care and to reinforce the creative use of such information to achieve improvements in function. Much of the current efforts going into more traditional regulatory activities might be redirected to this effort, with assessors used to validate the assessment and to focus more intense efforts on the miscreants.

We have generally good consensus on the components of outcomes and less about how to sum them. The gerontologic literature is consistent in citing the following as outcomes: physiologic function (e.g., blood pressure control, lack of decubiti), functional status (usually a measure of ADL), pain and discomfort, cognition (intellectual activity), affect (emotional activity), social participation (based on preferences), social relations (at least one person who can act as a confidant), and satisfaction (with care and living environment). To these must be added more global outcomes, such as death and admission to hospital.

There is already work available with nursing home residents to show that these factors can be predicted with sufficient accuracy to be used in a regulatory model. There is similar work to show that there is reasonable consensus across a variety of constituencies about the relative weights to be placed on them for different kinds of patients (e.g., different levels of physical and cognitive function at baseline).

The outcomes approach offers significant assistance with a recurrent problem in regulation—the development of standards. This ap-

proach may avoid many of these difficulties by relying on empiric standards. Rather than arguing about what is a reasonable expectation, the standard can be empirically determined. Expectations can be derived from the actual outcomes associated with real care given by those felt to represent a reasonable level of practice. This could include the entire field or a designated subset. Under this arrangement, providers would be comparing their achievements to each other's past records, with the possibility that everyone can do better.

TECHNOLOGY FOR QUALITY IMPROVEMENT

Ideally, one would like to see a measurement approach that

- Can cover the spectrum of performance
- Is easy and rapid to administer
- Is sensitive to meaningful change in performance
- Is stable within the same patient over time
- Performs consistently in different hands
- Cannot be manipulated to meet the needs of either the provider or the patient

The solution to this challenge is to create an assessment approach that incorporates the features designed to maximize these elements. To cover the broad spectrum sought and still be relatively quickly administered, an instrument should have multiple branch points. These permit the user to focus on the area along the continuum where the patient is most likely to function and to expand that part of the scale to measure meaningful levels of performance. Branching can also ensure that the assessment is comprehensive but not burdensome. By using key questions to screen an area, interviewers can ascertain whether to obtain more detailed information in each relevant domain. Where the initial response is negative, they can go on to the next branch point.

Reliability is more likely to be achieved when the items are expressed in a standardized fashion tied closely to explicit behaviors. Whenever possible, performance is preferred over reports of behavior. One cannot expect to totally avoid the gaming of an assessment. If the patient knows that poor performance is needed to ensure eligibility, he or she may be motivated to achieve the requisite low level. One can

use some test of ripeness bias, such as measures of social desirability, but they will not prevent gaming the system or detect all cheating.

Redundancy can be dramatically reduced by using computer technology. Properly mobilized, computers can provide the structure needed to assure a comprehensive assessment with no duplication of effort. Because they are interactive, they can carry out much of the desired branching and can even use simple algorithms to clarify areas of ambiguity and retest areas where some unreliability is suspected. Similar algorithms can look for inconsistency to screen for cheating.

Data stored on computers can be aggregated to look at performance across patients by provider (e.g., physician, nursing home, or agency). Data on a patient can be traced across time to look at changes in function and, in turn, can be aggregated.

The next important step in the progression is to move the focus from a single point of care to the linking of related elements of care. In an ideal system, patient information would be linked to permit tracing changes in status for that individual as he or she moves from one treatment modality to another. Thus, hospital admission and discharge information, long-term-care information, and primary care information would be merged into a common, computer-linked record, which allows one to trace the patient's movements and status. Finally, it would be desirable to have data on the process of care as well as the outcomes. This combination would permit analyses of what elements of care made a difference for which patients.

Such an approach to assuring quality is within our grasp if we are prepared to invest in data systems and to commit ourselves to collecting standardized information. It necessitates a shift in some of our fundamental paradigms from thinking about whether we did the right thing to deciding if it made any difference after all.

Two basic changes in thinking are necessary for an outcome-based philosophy, both of which are difficult for clinicians:

1. Thinking in the aggregate, using averages instead of examining each case; outcomes do not work well for individual cases because there is always a chance that something will go wrong, and life does not provide a control group.
2. Attributing responsibility to the whole enterprise rather than placing blame on an individual; a pattern of poor outcomes will mandate closer inspection of the process of care, but outcomes per se are a collective responsibility.

Computerized records greatly facilitate the task of monitoring the outcomes of care. Ideally, such a record system should be proactive, directing the collection of clinical information to encourage adequate coverage of relevant material. Long-term care is actually ahead of acute care in this regard, with the federal requirement for computerized versions of the MDS. Unfortunately, most of the systems in use are simply inputting mechanisms. They do not begin to tap the real potential of a computerized information system. Because long-term care depends heavily on poorly educated personnel for so much of its core services, the availability of an information support system, which can provide feedback and direction, is especially appropriate.

The computer can provide both the flexibility and the brevity sought by using branching logic to expand a category when there is reason to explore it more thoroughly. It can avoid duplication by displaying data already collected by others while still permitting the second observer to correct and challenge earlier entries. More important, it can display information to show change over time, thus permitting both the regulators and the caregivers to look at the effects of care.

Once the data are in electronic form, they are easily transmitted and manipulated. It is not hard to envision a large set of data derived from these systematic observations that would permit calculations of expected courses for different types of long-term-care patients. These could then be compared to individual patient's courses to assess the potential impact of care on outcomes.

The computer's ability to compare observed and expected outcomes extends beyond its role as a regulatory device. It could be a major source of assistance to caregivers. One of the great frustrations in long-term care, especially in the trenches, is the difficulty in sensing whether the caregiver is making a difference. Because so many patients enter care when they are already declining, the benefits of care are often best expressed as a slowing of that decline curve. Without some measure of expected course in the absence of good care, those who render care daily may not appreciate how much they are accomplishing and thereby may forgo one of the important rewards of their labors.

To display information about the change in patient condition over time, a simple task for a computer, will assist the long-term caregiver to think more in terms of the overall picture rather than a series of separate snapshots in time. Given the computer's ability to translate data into graphics, it is a simple procedure to develop pictorial repre-

sentations of the changes occurring for a given patient or group of patients and to contrast those with what might be reasonably expected.

Again the effort is directed toward changing perceptions about older persons, especially those in long-term care. For too long, long-term care has worked in a negative spiral—a self-fulfilling prophecy that expected patients to deteriorate served to discourage both care providers and patients. Such an attitude is hardly likely to attract the best and the brightest in any of the health professions. As noted earlier in this chapter, nursing home patients are among the most responsive to almost any form of intervention. Any information system that can reinforce a prospective view of long-term care, especially one that can display patient progress, represents an important adjunct to such care.

PREVENTION

General Principles

The physician's concern about a patient's future and the value of that future is reflected in the patient's actions with regard to preventive activities. Enthusiasm for prevention is based on beliefs about the following:

1. The efficacy of the intervention in preventing disease or dysfunction in the future. This includes an estimate of the likelihood of the patient's following the preventive regimen.
2. The value of the health gained. In the case of older patients, this includes concerns about the likelihood of other problems reducing the benefit.
3. The cost of the preventive activity. This includes both the direct cost and the indirect costs, such as anxiety, restricted lifestyle, and false-positive results.

Perhaps the most preventable problem connected with caring for older persons is iatrogenic disease. Here some of the major issues and strategies surrounding more conventional preventive activities are discussed. The major thesis here, as with much covered elsewhere in this volume, is that age alone should not be a predominant factor in choosing an approach to a patient. A number of preventive strategies

deserve serious consideration in light of their immediate and future benefits for many elderly patients.

Preventive activities can be divided into three types: primary prevention, where some specific action is taken to render the patient more resistant or the environment less harmful; secondary prevention, or screening and early detection for asymptomatic disease or early disease; and tertiary prevention, or efforts to improve care to avoid later complications. Table 4-3 offers examples of activities in each category. Not all the items indicated in Table 4-3 are supported by clear research findings. In some cases—such as seat belts, exercise, and social support—they are based on prudent judgment.

In addressing prevention for older persons, it is important to bear in mind the goals pursued. The World Health Organization has provided a useful continuum, which progresses from disease to impairment to disability to handicap (WHO, 1980). Preventive efforts for older people can be productively targeted at several points along this spectrum. Efforts can seek to prevent disease, but they can also be designed to minimize its consequences, by reducing the progression to disability. This is, in essence, the heart of geriatrics.

Grimley Evans has identified several ways in which preventive efforts on behalf of elderly patients are special, beyond the emphasis on function (Evans, 1984). The narrowing of the therapeutic window, discussed in Chap. 13, means that older persons may be susceptible

Table 4-3 Preventive strategies for older persons

Primary	Secondary	Tertiary
Immunization	Pap smear	Assessment
Influenza	Breast exam	Foot care
Pneumococcal	Breast self-exam	Dental care
Tetanus	Mammography	Toileting efforts
Blood pressure	Fecal blood	
Smoking	Hypothyroidism	
Exercise	Depression	
Obesity	Vision	
Cholesterol	Hearing	
Sodium	Oral cavity	
Social support	Tuberculosis	
Environment		
Seat belts		

to the side effects of prevention as well as treatment. Some risk factors that strongly predict the onset of disease may not be appropriate for modification in older persons. Perhaps the condition has already become well established and is resistant to change, or the factor may have already exerted its influence at an earlier stage of life.

Clearly, primary prevention is the most desirable. If a brief encounter can confer some form of long-lasting protection at minimal risk, such a strategy will be actively pursued. Unfortunately, the number of activities that are both safe and effective is small. More often, we must rely on the other two strategies, each of which comes at a cost. Screening for one or another condition is useful where the disease process can be detected in advance of the condition's clinical appearance, but this may be excessively costly if the number of treatable cases detected is low. Screening is usually judged on the criteria of sensitivity and specificity. The former refers to the proportion of actual cases correctly identified and the latter to the accuracy of labeling of noncases (normal individuals). Alas, the two factors are usually linked, so that an improvement in one comes at the cost of a decrement in the other. The decision about where to set them relative to each other depends on the expected prevalence of the problem and the consequences of a false-positive and a false-negative finding with respect to a given clinical condition.

While older persons have been traditionally excluded from preventive trials, that situation is changing. As it does, findings suggest that primary prevention is appropriate for older persons as well, but the problems associated with translating the results of clinical trials into practice are at least as great as with younger persons. Active treatment of hypertension (both systolic and diastolic) is associated with reduced cardiovascular complications (Staessen et al., 1997). Control of systolic blood pressure was associated with preventing heart failure (Kostis et al., 1997).

Even more broadly, the value of geriatric assessment suggests that important problems in primary care of older persons are being ignored or undertreated. Reports that a yearly visit by a nurse practitioner to unselected persons aged 75 and older can lead to substantial functional improvement and reduced nursing home admissions raise serious questions about how well the current primary care system is working (Stuck et al., 1993). The concept of geriatric assessment has given way to a model of geriatric evaluation and management (GEM), which allows for the geriatric team to assume responsibility for the

patient's care for a period sufficient to permit stabilization of the patient's condition and, in some instance, therapeutic trials. The problem still remains that when the patient is returned to the care of his or her primary care physician, the benefits of this rehabilitation may be lost unless provision is made to sustain the therapeutic changes. In the absence of this continuity, the investment represented by geriatric assessment may be threatened.

Effectiveness of Prevention in Older People

In evaluating the efficacy of preventive activities for older persons, we must confront a dilemma. Because older people were systematically excluded from many trials of prevention strategies, there are few hard data on which to base judgments. At the same time, there are strong feelings from both sides about the value of prevention. Active advocates for wellness among elderly people urge strenuous efforts to promote major life changes. They are allied with those who view many of the accoutrements of aging as acquired and hence capable of modification. They cite data showing that muscle strength and endurance can be regained with active training even at advanced ages. Another group argues that older people have already reached a stage in life where they have demonstrated a capacity to cope. They would accept many of the consequences of aging and note that the demonstrated gains are less strongly associated with major improvements in morbidity and function than with values derived from testing.

The U.S. Preventive Services Task Force attempted to assess available scientific information on the efficacy of preventive efforts for persons at all ages (U.S. Preventive Services Task Force, 1996). Table 4-4 summarizes the major recommendations from the Task Force and other sources for screening activities for those aged 65 and over. Many of these recommendations are based on expert judgment in lieu of hard data. Another area of concern pertains to foot care. Although there are no formal studies to confirm the effects, clinical experience strongly suggests the benefits of podiatry in improving the ambulation of many elderly patients. Not only diabetics should receive attention to their feet; each elderly person should be carefully asked about foot pain and discomfort and checked for bunions and corns. Appropriate treatment can do a great deal to keep such patients ambulatory and stable. The U.S. Task Force avoided the debate about false-positive results with regard to screening for glaucoma by

Table 4-4 Summary of preventive recommendations for older adults

Maneuver	Recommendation (source)
Screening[a]	
Blood pressure	Every exam, at least every 1–2 years (USPSTF, AHA)
Physician breast exam	Annually >40 (ACS, USPSTF)
Mammogram	Annually >40 (ACS) or every 1–2 years, age 50–69 (USPSTF, ACP); Continue every 1–3 years, age 70–85, in willing/appropriate patients (AGS, USPSTF)
Pelvic exam/Pap smear	Every 2–3 years after three negaive annual exams; can then ↓ or discontinue after age 65–69 (ACS, USPSTF, CTF, AGS)
Cholesterol	Adults every 5 years (NCEP, ACP, USPSTF)
Rectal exam/fecal occult blood test	Annually >5 (ACS, AHCPR, Win)
Sigmoidoscopy	Every 5 years >50 years of age or colonoscopy/BE every 10 years (ACS)
Visual acuity test	Periodically in older adults (various)
Test/inquire for hearing impairment	Periodically in older adults (various)
Mouth, nodes, testes, skin, heart, lung exams	Annually (ACS, AHA)
Glucose	Periodic in high-risk groups (USPSTF); every 3 years (ADA)
Thyroid function	Clinically prudent for elderly, especially women (USPSTF)
Electrocardiogram	Periodically > age 40–50 (AHA)
Glaucoma screening	Periodically by eye specialist > age 65 (USPSTF)
Mental/functional status	As needed; be alert for decline (USPSTF)
Osteoporosis (bone densitometry)	If needed for treatment decision (USPSTF)
Prostate exam/prostate-specific antigen	Annually > age 50 (ACS); NR[b] especially > age 70 (USPSTF, ACP)
Chest x-ray	NR/as needed (USPSTF)
Prophylaxis/counseling	
Exercise	Encourage aerobic and resistance exercise as tolerated (AHA)

(continued)

Table 4-4 Summary of preventive recommendations for older adults *(Continued)*

Maneuver	Recommendation (source)
Prophylaxis/counseling (*Continued*)	
Tetanus-diphtheria vaccine	1° series then booster every 10 years (ACP, USPSTF)
Influenza vaccine	Annually > age 65 or chronically ill (ACP, USPSTF)
Pneumovax	23-Valent at least once > age 65 (ACP, USPSTF)
Calcium	800–1500 mg/day (various)
Estrogen	Postmenopausal women (various)
Aspirin	Men > age 50, 80–325 mg per day or on alternate days (various)
Vitamin E, red wine	?

[a] Screening recommendations apply only to asymptomatic individuals; specific clinical circumstances may necessitate different testing and treatment schedules. Where no upper age limits are listed, screening should continue until approximately age 85 or when the patient is not a treatment candidate because of limited active life expectancy/quality.

[b] NR = Not recommended for routine screening in asymptomatic individuals, though may be useful when clinically indicated.

Source: From Goldberg and Chavin, 1997. Reproduced with permission of the author and updated by the author on the Internet (URL: http/members.aol.com/TGoldberg/prevrecs.htm). Based on recommendations from American College of Physicians (ACP), American Cancer Society (ACS), American Geriatrics Society (AGS), American Heart Association (AHA), Canadian Task Force on the Periodic Health Examination (CTF), National Cholesterol Education Program (NCEP), U.S. Preventive Services Task Force (USPSTF), American Diabetes Association (ADA), Winawer et al., 1997 (Win); and the authors' interpretations of the literature.

recommending that the decision be made by an ophthalmologist, but the importance of vision in the overall functioning of the elderly patient argues strongly for attention to this area. In a similar vein, the potential for improving function by replacing cataracts with implanted lenses mandates greater attention to visual problems as well as concern about the excess use of surgery (Applegate et al., 1987). However, the functional benefit is not realized by cognitively impaired persons (Elam et al., 1988). Pneumococcal vaccines are now in widespread use, and many consider them to be useful in the care of elderly persons at risk, especially those in institutions, but there remains an active controversy

about their cost-effectiveness (Simberkoff et al., 1986; Forrester et al., 1987; Sims et al., 1988). Tuberculosis remains a problem among older people, especially those in institutions. Special care must be taken in interpreting a lack of reaction to tuberculin skin tests in elderly persons because of the risk of anergy (Stead et al., 1987a; 1987b).

In addition to specific recommendations for preventive actions, a number of areas can be usefully examined as part of routine care. Table 4-5 offers examples of such geriatric health maintenance activities. It is important to recognize that these recommendations as well as those from the Task Force are intended to be carried out as part of regular primary care. No special visits for prevention are implied. Particularly in our current system, where Medicare Part B does not pay for many preventive services, it is important to appreciate that much can be done in prevention without special visits for that purpose. Most, if not all, of the procedures can be performed by an appropriately trained nonphysician.

Table 4-5 Geriatric health maintenance items worth including in a routine screening program

Historical information
  Tobacco

Physical examination
  Height and weight
  Blood pressure
  Hearing and vision
  Gait and fall assessment

Diagnostic tests
  Mammography
  Papanicolaou smear in underscreened women
  Flexible sigmoidoscopy

Interventions
  Aspirin therapy to prevent coronary artery disease (CAD)
  Estrogen replacement therapy
  For prevention of osteoporosis in women at risk
  For reduction of CAD in women at risk or who have undergone hysterectomy

Immunizations
  Influenza
  Tetanus

Source: From Scheitel et al., 1996, with permission.

In some cases, care must be taken to avoid penalizing older persons on the basis of stereotypes. For example, the U.S. Preventive Services Task Force was skeptical about the usefulness of breast self-examination in elderly women (O'Malley et al., 1987). Moreover, physicians tend to be less enthusiastic about treating older patients with breast cancer (Greenfield et al., 1987).

At the same time, some areas are well served by increased clinical attention. Greater physician sensitivity to identifying depression in older persons can detect an often remediable condition. Detection of mental problems is greatly enhanced by structured screening data (German et al., 1987). Awareness of the likelihood of alcoholism can lead to recognition of a problem that can be corrected. There is more controversy about the desirability of increasing the recognition of cognitive deficiency. Although standardized testing can detect cases that might otherwise be masked in older persons who have skillfully compensated for their loss, it is not immediately clear that there is great benefit in such early uncovering.

Routine screening for geriatric populations tends to uncover problems that are already known. Among a group of elderly persons coming for a health screening, 95 percent had at least one positive finding. About 55 percent were referred to a physician for further evaluation and 15 percent were treated for the finding (Rubenstein et al., 1986). Routine annual laboratory testing of nursing home residents has received mixed reviews. A modest panel—including a complete blood count, electrolytes, renal and thyroid function tests, and a urinalysis—may be useful (Levinstein et al., 1987).

Behavior change represents at once the most promising and the most frustrating component of prevention. While some may argue that "you can't teach an old dog new tricks" or that engrained habit patterns are hard to break, there is no evidence to support such pessimism. Quite to the contrary, anecdotal data about elderly people taking up exercise programs and changing their dietary habits provide reason for more optimism. The critical issue here is the degree to which such changes will sufficiently modify risk factors to justify the disturbance.

In general, moderation seems safest. For example, data from the Alameda County study suggest that not smoking, modest physical activity, moderate weight, and regular meals are associated with lower mortality risks among older populations (Kaplan et al., 1987). As shown in Fig. 4-3, older persons' health habits are generally as good

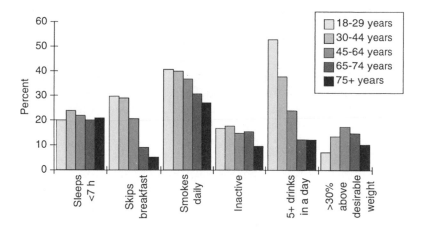

Figure 4-3 Personal health habits of people aged 65 and over, 1995. An older person's health habits are generally as good as or better than those of younger people. *(From U.S. Senate, 1991.)*

as or better than those of younger people. Although our data are scant, the degree of enthusiasm for active modification will likely vary with the topic addressed.

In general, the best preventive strategies for older persons are those associated with the least risk. The findings from the TONE study, suggesting that weight loss and sodium restriction could effectively lower blood pressure in older persons, is a good example of such an approach (Whelton et al., 1998). Reducing dietary salt intake was shown to lower blood pressure in another study as well (Cappuccio et al., 1997). Along the same lines, antioxidant vitamins have been suggested by epidemiologic evidence as a means of reducing cardiovascular disease (Gey, 1995). Similar suggestions have been made for using vitamin E to prevent Alzheimer's disease (Sano et al., 1997). Hormone replacement therapy in women has been widely hailed as having multiple benefits including delaying osteoporosis, lowered cholesterol, and prevention of Alzheimer's disease (Paganini-Hill et al., 1996). Although the quality of the evidence for all these effects varies, the growing evidence for the benefits of hormone replacement therapy needs to be seriously weighed against the increased risk of breast and uterine cancer.

An effort to develop a more comprehensive approach to health promotion in a group of older people met with less success. The first lesson to come out of the project was that older persons have their own agenda about what is important to them and what they believe will benefit them. Even after they reached a compromise agenda that included elements both subjects and health professionals felt were valuable, the changes in functioning were not greater than those for the control group (Omenn et al., 1997).

One area that has received considerable attention, and perhaps created confusion in the minds of both older persons and their clinicians, is exercise. Overall, there is widespread belief that exercise will benefit the individual. However, exercise is not a unidimensional activity. There are various types, and each is directed at a specific target. Table 4-6 summarizes the major types of exercise and the intended benefits of each type. Different approaches to exercise should be pursued to achieve specific goals. Although its role in osteoporosis prevention remains controversial (Block et al., 1987), exercise is generally recommended as a safe approach, with more possible benefits than risks (Rodysill, 1987). Less than a third of older persons report regular exercise, to say nothing of vigorous activity (LaCroix, 1987). Although evidence suggests that active aerobic exercise is necessary to reduce risk of cardiovascular accidents, even modest amounts of exercise will improve strength, keep joints more limber, promote a sense of well-being, and improve sleep. Recent work has indicated that even severely compromised nursing home residents can benefit from carefully supervised and graded strength-training exercise. Both the direct benefits (e.g., improved muscle strength and activity tolerance) and indirect effects (e.g., being treated with more esteem) allowed residents to function more autonomously (Fiatarone

Table 4-6 Types of exercise

Type	Purpose/expected benefit
Aerobic/anaerobic	Cardiovascular conditioning
Resistance/weights	Strength, tone, muscle mass
Antigravity	Prevent osteoporosis
Balance	Prevent falls
Stretching	Flexibility

et al., 1994). Exercise appears to improve both overall well-being and older persons' sense of self-worth. Likewise, occupational therapy has been shown to produce beneficial results for a group of independently living older adults (Clark et al., 1997). In a manner similar to that represented in the positive results of screening home visits by a geriatric nurse practitioner (Stuck et al., 1995; Alessi et al., 1997), modest efforts can yield substantial rewards in terms of improved function and reduced use of long-term care. Surprisingly, change in activities of daily living (ADL) status is not a better predictor of ADL dependency than a one-time measure (Gill et al., 1997).

Epidemiologic data suggest that even among quite elderly persons, cessation of smoking will reduce mortality to levels of nonsmokers in a sufficiently short time to justify actively encouraging quitting (Jaijich et al., 1984). From 1979 to 1985, the prevalence of elderly current smokers increased among older males but decreased among younger males and the youngest females (Havlik et al., 1987). These changes likely reflect differences in cohorts as well as changes in behavior. In each age group, the rate of former smokers was higher in 1985 than in 1979. Smoking cessation will have rapid benefits for risks of both vascular and lung disease. Wearing seat belts is of immediate benefit in reducing automobile fatalities. Despite the recent controversy over large-scale clinical trials, there is growing enthusiasm for controlling even modest levels of hypertension. Increased calcium has been recommended to prevent osteoporosis, but no clearly efficacious regimen has yet been established. Low-dosage estrogens have been shown capable of halting bone loss. The increased risk of uterine cancer has thwarted their adoption as a preventive strategy, but this risk is substantially reduced if progesterone is added.

There is growing enthusiasm for treating both diastolic and systolic hypertension among the elderly. The European Working Party on High Blood Pressure in the Elderly showed that treatment was associated with a significant reduction in cardiac mortality, a nonsignificant reduction in cerebrovascular mortality, but no reduction in overall mortality (Amery et al., 1985). The results from the Systolic Hypertension in the Elderly Program (SHEP) suggest that lowering isolated systolic hypertension can lead to reduced rates of fatal and nonfatal endpoints for stroke, coronary heart disease, and cardiovascular disease (SHEP Cooperative Research Group, 1991; Petrovitch et al., 1992). It is important to distinguish carefully between the value of uncovering elevated blood pressure and the need to control it over

a sustained period. Most older persons with hypertension are aware of it; the challenge is to maintain them in a safe range without producing significant side effects. Hypertension is very common among the elderly. Black females have the highest rates, and among white males the rate approaches 40 percent.

The effects of dietary changes are less certain. Weight loss for obese persons makes sense in terms of reducing cardiovascular load and in the management of adult-onset diabetes and hypertension, but hard data suggest that the benefit may be oversold, certainly for the former. The efficacy of changing diet, especially to reduce the amount of fat consumed, has not yet been clearly established.

Cholesterol has been shown to be a risk factor for heart disease for general populations but has not been specifically tested in the elderly. Females are at particular risk for this problem. Over 30 percent of white females have high-risk cholesterol levels (greater than 268 mg/dL) (Havlik et al., 1987). Cholesterol-lowering therapy has been shown to work in older persons as well as the middle aged generally included in such trials (Miettinen et al., 1997). Recommendations for using lipid-lowering drugs in older patients with a history of cardiac or vascular disease (Johannesson et al., 1997; Santanello et al., 1997) are countered by other claims that cholesterol is not a significant risk factor in older persons (Krumholz et al., 1994). At the same time, only about 50 percent of older persons put on lipid-lowering medications remain on the regimen after 5 years (Avorn et al., 1998).

In areas such as weight, cholesterol, and even blood pressure, the clinician must weigh the benefits of intervention against the costs (risks). There is a compelling argument that overzealous activity in the name of prevention may cost more in quality of life than it gains in quality years. Some have suggested that the survivor effect should be taken more seriously. Persons who survive to old age may have demonstrated a biological ability that deserves more respect. At the very least, any determination to change lifestyle at this stage of life should be made by the patient after suitable counseling. Nonetheless, older persons should not be denied the opportunity to actively consider the benefits of primary prevention. The growing body of evidence about at least the art of the possible imposes on clinicians a responsibility to provide them with such information.

One area of behavior with great theoretical promise but little immediate practical application is social support. There is some evi-

dence to suggest that those older persons with strong social support systems, or at least perceived support, are at less risk for adverse events (Zuckerman et al., 1984), but it is not yet clear how to build such a support system for those without one naturally. Social support likely plays at least two distinct roles: (1) Having (or perhaps just believing one has) a strong support system may reduce the risk of adverse events (through a yet to be elucidated mechanism that likely involves stress). (2) For persons who are disabled and require assistance, having a real support system may prove the difference between staying in the community and needing to enter an institution. It is difficult to assess the availability of that support system in advance. The perception, even the promise, of such support does not guarantee that the necessary support will be consistently and conveniently available when it is needed. Even well-intentioned family members may find the task too daunting to be able to maintain it.

Preventing Disability

Although discussions of prevention tend to focus on the prevention of disease, the context of geriatrics—with its emphasis on functioning—urges a broader approach. When caring for older patients, equal attention must be paid to seeking means to keep them as active as possible. While there may be little that can be done to prevent the occurrence of a disease in an elderly person, much can be done to minimize the impact of that disease. Impairments cannot be allowed to become disabilities.

A major component of the efforts to avoid this transition are contained in geriatric assessment programs. The general approaches of such programs are reviewed in Chap. 3. It is important to note that these programs have been very varied in their composition. Table 3-1 in Chap. 3 summarizes the major randomized controlled trials using different approaches to assessment.

A promising line of work has been begun by Williams (1987). In addition to relying more on demonstrated performance than simply on patient report, he has used the time required to complete the task as part of the measure. This additional component provides a way to achieve more variability and may lead to better prediction. It offers a means to detect more subtle change.

The overarching goal of geriatric practice is the improvement, or at least the preservation, of patients' function. In general, function can be thought of as being determined by three principal forces:

1. The patient's overall physical health
2. The environment
3. The patient's motivation

Much of the discussion in this book deals with ways to maximize the patient's health status by proper diagnosis and treatment. Such steps are necessary but not sufficient for good geriatric care. It is essential to appreciate that a person's environment can play a critical role in affecting his or her functioning. Just imagine for a minute what it would be like to be in a country where you did not speak the language or even understand its symbols. Although your capabilities are intact, you cannot function effectively. By a similar token, even after therapy has achieved its maximal effect, a patient's environment can be crucial.

Environment in this case refers to both the physical and psychological setting. It is fairly easy to imagine the physical barriers to functioning. Narrow doorways, poor lighting, and stairs can all serve as barriers. Occupational therapists can be especially helpful in assessing the patient's environment to suggest modifications and adaptive equipment (see Chap. 8, especially Table 8-18). The Appendix contains a simple environmental assessment form useful in uncovering hazards.

The psychological barriers are more subtle but perhaps more important. They refer to the way patients are treated and, especially, the extent to which they are encouraged to do as much for themselves as they can. We have noted earlier that a risk-averse environment can engender excessive dependency—so, too, can the pressure to be productive. As long as time is at a premium, care providers will be motivated to do things for patients rather than encouraging them to perform those tasks themselves, especially if the latter course takes considerably longer. In the name of efficiency, we may be creating dependency. The efforts to encourage self-sufficiency are precisely what is usually called rehabilitation, even when it occurs in a plain wrapper.

The third element of functional effects is the patient's motivation. Today's older patients place especially high trust in their physicians, whom they view as figures of authority. Thus, one of the most subtle but nonetheless important aspects of this approach to prevention—the prevention of inactivity and despair—is the physician's attitude. For the patient, a gain in function or an ability to deal with a chronic problem is essential. It is surely no mean feat. Such behavior should

be encouraged and rewarded. Indifference may be enough to discourage the patient from trying.

Other programs can be mobilized in the patient's behalf. Self-help groups are available in many communities to offer support with chronic illness, including stress management and drugless pain-control techniques. Social activity can play an essential role in maintaining function. Pets have proved to be very effective in improving morale and maintaining function.

Special efforts may be necessary to deal with members of the patient's family. Their concern over potentially dangerous accidents may lead them to become overprotective and thus exaggerate the condition of dependency.

IATROGENESIS

Probably the most important preventable problems faced by older persons today are those associated with treatment. Many iatrogenic problems result from the care that has been provided. In some cases these problems can be traced to oversights and omissions. In other cases overzealous care can be blamed. Some of the problem is attributable to lack of expertise in managing older persons, but a substantial portion is caused by the inevitable problems of trying to titrate therapy in an environment that is considerably less resilient to error. The more aggressive the treatment, the greater the chance that it will produce adverse effects. Figure 4-4 portrays in a conceptual manner this narrowing of the therapeutic window (i.e., the space between a therapeutic dose and a toxic dose) with age. As the response to therapy decreases, the susceptibility to toxic side effects increases. These changes are attributable to many factors, including the ability to metabolize drugs, changes in receptor behavior, and an altered chemical environment produced by other simultaneous drugs.

This narrowing of the therapeutic window is perhaps most easily recognized in the pharmacologic treatment of older patients. In the face of reduced capacity for metabolizing and excreting many drugs, the older patient can develop high blood levels on "normal" dosages. Changes in receptors may alter sensitivity to chemicals in either direction. Use of numerous drugs transforms the elderly patient into a living chemistry set. Because of their prevalence and importance, drugs are discussed separately in Chap. 13. Here we focus attention

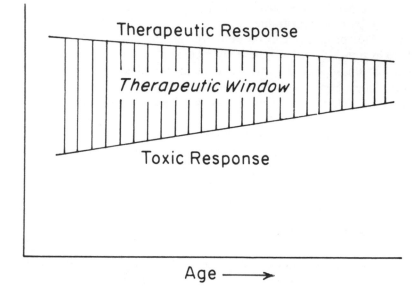

Figure 4-4 Narrowing of the therapeutic window. This diagram portrays in a conceptual manner the space between a therapeutic dose and a toxic dose as it narrows with age.

on some of the more subtle ways in which other types of treatment can adversely affect older people. In general, many drugs can be discontinued safely (Graves et al., 1997). One caveat, however: in the fear of overmedicating older patients, doctors may be tempted to discontinue drugs that were begun at an earlier time. While such a reevaluation is prudent, the decision to discontinue should be made carefully. One study showed that stopping long-term diuretic medications in elderly patients resulted in an exacerbation of heart failure symptoms and a rise in their blood pressure (Walma et al., 1997).

On a more philosophical plane, one can think about aging as a continuously changing relationship between an organism and its environment. As noted in Chap. 1, aging is typified by a decreased capacity to respond to stress. A person's environment can do much to reduce or create stress. Whereas a mature adult is likely to adapt to or alter the environment, the aged individual is greatly affected by changes of setting. In infancy, a person is readily influenced by his or her environment. One of the signs of maturation is the person's ability

to function independently of that environment and ultimately to influence that environment. Indeed, one of the attributes that distinguishes humans from other animals is precisely this capacity to shape the environment. With increased age, the delicate balance shifts again to the point where advanced age often means that the individual is heavily affected by the environment. It is hardly surprising, then, that the elderly patient is vulnerable to the variety of stresses imposed by modern medical care. Table 4-7 lists some of the iatrogenic problems elderly patients may suffer.

Special Risks of Hospitals

Hospitals are dangerous places for any patient. Most of us are resilient enough to enter an acute care hospital and suffer the vicissitudes of care with the expectation that we will emerge better (certainly in the long run). The calculation of benefits received for risks undertaken needs to be more carefully thought through with older patients. Just a little thought reveals the litany of familiar hazards of hospitalization—from the risk of nosocomial infection to getting the wrong drug to the stress of major surgery or the danger of certain diagnostic procedures. The high rate of adverse drug reactions in hospitalized patients in general is estimated at almost 7% in one metanalysis (Lazarou et al., 1998). All these are imposed on the

Table 4-7 Common iatrogenic problems of older persons

Overzealous labeling
   Dementia
   Incontinence

Underdiagnosis

Bed rest

Polypharmacy

Enforced dependency

Environmental hazards

Transfer trauma

general hazards of bed rest discussed in Chap. 9. Table 4-8 offers some examples of potential hazards in the hospital. They include problems of both overtreatment and undertreatment (Gorbien et al., 1992).

Elderly patients are more likely to experience an untoward event during a hospital stay. In part, this is because they present with more physical problems, but they are also more vulnerable. Among 815 consecutive admissions to a hospital's general medical service, an overall rate of 497 iatrogenic events developed, involving 36 percent

Table 4-8 The hazards of hospitalization

Diagnostic procedures
  Cardiac catheterization
  Arteriography

Therapeutic procedures
  Intravenous therapy
  Urinary catheters
  Nasogastric tube
  Dialysis
  Transfusion

Drugs
  Medication error
  Drug-drug interaction
  Drug reaction
  Drug side effect

Surgery
  Anesthesia
  Infection
  Metabolic imbalance
  Malnutrition
  Hypovolemia

Bed rest
  Hypovolemia and hypertension
  Calcium metabolism
  Fecal impaction
  Urine incontinence
  Thromboembolism

Nosocomial infection

Falls

Table 4-9 Risk factors for iatrogenic hospital events

Admission from nursing home or other hospital
Physician's assessment of overall condition on admission
Age
Number of drugs
Length of stay

of patients; 9 percent of the patients had complications classified as major, and in 2 percent the complications contributed to death. Patient characteristics associated with increased risk of iatrogenic complications are listed in Table 4-9. Of these, only the first two, source of admission and condition on admission, remained significant when other factors were controlled (Steel et al., 1981). Because elderly patients are more likely to come from nursing homes and to be in poor condition on admission, they should be considered at high risk for iatrogenic complications.

In a study of patients hospitalized on a general medical service, the incidence of functional symptoms unrelated to diagnosis was over four times higher among patients aged 70 and over than among younger patients. Younger patients were more likely to be treated for symptoms of confusion, but older patients were more likely to be treated for problems of not eating and incontinence (Gillick et al., 1982). A simple rapid screening test for identifying older patients at risk of functional decline in the hospital is shown in Table 4-10. Delirium can be a serious problem in elderly hospitalized patients (see Chap. 5 for a discussion of this condition).

The elderly patient's vulnerability extends to a more subtle level. Admission to a hospital means entering an unfamiliar world. Moreover, the patient enters the hospital at a time of great stress. The anxiety of unknown consequences exists in addition to the physical stress of the illness.

The hospital presents physical and organizational barriers to which the patient must adapt. Not only the geography but the routines are different. The things we rely on to preserve our sense of identity are among the first things taken away: our clothing, our personal effects. It is hardly surprising, then, that many elderly persons who are able to function in their familiar surroundings become disoriented

Table 4-10 Risk factors for functional decline in elderly hospitalized patients

Age 75+
Missing >15 of the first 21 MMSE items
Dependence in 2+ IADLs prior to admission
Pressure sore
Baseline functional dependency
History of low social activity

Key: MMSE, Mini-Mental State Examination; IADLs, independent activities of daily living.
Sources: Adapted from Sager et al., 1996, and Inouye et al., 1996.

and often agitated in the hospital. Just as a blind person can move flawlessly in familiar surroundings, an older person may have developed a host of adaptive mechanisms to function in his or her home situation, overcoming problems of memory loss and impaired vision. Transferred into the sterile, rigid hospital room, such an individual may decompensate. The syndrome of "sundowning," whereby older patients in the hospital become agitated and disoriented as dusk falls, is likely a function of visual or hearing impairments, diminished sensory stimuli, and resultant disorientation.

The older person accustomed to coping with nocturia may wander at night in the dark to where the bathroom at home ought to be and wet the floor. In the crisis of urinary urgency, the patient may be unable to scale the side rails and make it to the bathroom in time. To label an individual who suffers such environmentally exacerbated accidents as incontinent is to inflict double jeopardy.

We fail to appreciate the dangers of bed rest for the elderly people. Bed is actually a very dangerous place for an older person. Besides the risk of falling out of bed, enforced immobility can produce many harms. Complications of bed rest are summarized in Table 4-11 and detailed in Chap. 9.

The hospital breeds dependency. Even with younger patients, hospital personnel are accustomed to performing basic functions for the patient. Use of the bathroom is by prescription only. Bathing is

**Table 4-11 Potential
complications of bed rest
in older persons**

Pressure sores
Bone resorption
Hypercalcemia
Postural hypotension
Atelectasis and pneumonia
Thrombophlebitis and thromboembolism
Urinary incontinence
Constipation and fecal impaction
Decreased muscle strength
Decreased physical work capacity
Contractures
Depression and anxiety

often a supervised event. Patients are transported from one location to another. Although most of us as patients may have enjoyed being indulged for a while, we soon begin to rail against the imposed dependency. In older patients who need to be urged, encouraged, and cajoled into doing as much for themselves as possible, such an atmosphere can be especially debilitating.

Encouraging patients to act independently necessitates patience and time; unfortunately, both are scarce in the acute care hospital. It is much faster and easier to do a task for a person who performs slowly and uncertainly than to take the time to encourage that person to do that task independently. Moreover, the result of a professionally performed task is usually neater and more in keeping with hospital standards. Thus, well-meaning staff bowing to the pressures for efficiency may be inclined to do things for elderly patients rather than urging the patients to do as much as possible for themselves. This well-intentioned behavior fosters dependency at a time when independent function is crucial.

The hospital is notoriously averse to risk taking. Hospital policies are designed to err on the side of caution. Such behavior can further compromise the independent functioning of older patients. Patients who are not allowed to bathe themselves or who are wheeled rather than walked are likely to become less motivated to use their full capacities. Any fears about their ability are likely to increase.

In light of the multiple adverse consequences that may be associated with hospitalizing older people, we might pause to ask why we have not done more to make hospitals more hospitable for them. Ironically, we have invested great care in minimizing the trauma of hospitalization for children. Creativity in architecture and programs has gone into making pediatric wards as nonthreatening and homelike as possible. Although children are rarely hospitalized and geriatric patients are frequently hospitalized, no similar investment of creativity has been devoted to making the hospital less stressful for frail elderly patients. We know enough about perceptual and functional problems of aging to recognize that even simple architectural modifications can make a hospital stay easier. Use of primary colors, windows at lower heights, better-designed furniture, use of textures and patterns, and better design of rooms can all help the older patient retain maximum functioning capacity.

Special units for managing geriatric patients are beginning to emerge (Landefeld et al., 1995). Staffed by an interdisciplinary team composed of nurses, social worker, physician, and physical or occupational therapist, these units apply techniques of multidimensional functional evaluation to assess the capacity of the geriatric patient. Likewise, the reports of geriatric assessment units that took patients who had completed a course of acute care hospitalization and were otherwise destined for a nursing home and dramatically altered both their clinical state and their long-term care course, even reducing mortality rates, suggest that much more can be done for older persons while they are in a hospital (Stuck et al., 1993). Such geriatric units can uncover treatable conditions, provide rehabilitation to improve functional capacity, and develop a plan of care that will allow elderly patients to remain in the community (Rubenstein et al., 1982).

An iatrogenic danger to the elderly patient thus lies in underdiagnosis, especially of mundane but critical conditions involving hearing, vision, and dentition. In addition, even more clinically important problems such as thyroid disease or aortic aneurysms may be overlooked unless a careful examination is performed.

Labeling

Perhaps even more dangerous than the cases of underdiagnosis are those of overdiagnosis. The physician who too readily labels a disoriented patient as senile or demented or who classifies a urinary accident

as incontinence may be sealing the fate of that patient unnecessarily. These two diagnoses are strongly associated with an increased likelihood of nursing home admission and thus should not be made lightly.

Physicians admitting patients to nursing homes are responsible for assuring both themselves and their patients on several scores:

1. The patient truly needs care in such a setting and cannot reasonably get such care elsewhere
2. The institution is capable of providing the needed care
3. The patient is prepared for a transfer to the nursing home

Too frequently, hospital discharge to the nursing home compounds the trauma. Discharge planning is often begun too late. There is not sufficient time to find the best facility for the patient's needs or to allow the patient and the patient's family a sufficient role in making the decision for nursing home placement.

Good discharge planning includes at least five critical steps:

1. Adequate identification of those at risk of needing special arrangements on discharge
2. Assessment to identify problems and strengths
3. Determination of the risks and benefits associated with alternative modalities of care
4. Determination of the most suitable vendor among the modality of care selected
5. Transmission of adequate information to assure a successful transition

Patients and their families should play an active role in steps 3 and 4. Ideally, they should make the choice after the information has been provided by professionals. In practice, this is rarely the case. Adequate information about the risks and benefits of alternative modalities is not presented (it may not be known). No encouragement or assistance is provided to help patients and families determine precisely what outcomes they seek to maximize. Little time is allowed to weigh the complexities of the choice. When it comes to choosing among vendors of a given service, real choices may not exist because of the constraints of payment arrangements, including managed care.

As discussed in Chap. 14, the nature of nursing home care is changing. The pressure for earlier discharges from hospitals has

created a new demand for what has been termed *subacute care*—in essence, care that was formerly provided in hospitals.

TERMINAL CARE

The physician's concern with the patient's functioning continues throughout the course of the chronic disease. Elderly patients will die. In many cases, death is not a reflection of medical failure. The approach to the dying patient will often raise difficult dilemmas. No simple answers suffice. Perhaps the best advice is not to take on the whole burden. Too often the dying patient is treated as an object. Ignored and isolated, the patient may be discussed in the third person. Physicians must come to terms with death if they are to treat elderly patients. Often the patients are more comfortable with the subject than are their physicians. Fleeing from the dying patient is inexcusable. Enough has been written on this subject by Kubler-Ross (1969) and others (Duff et al., 1968) to make that point clear. Dying patients need their doctors. At a very basic level, everything should be done to keep the patient as comfortable as possible. One simple step is to identify the pattern of discomforting symptoms and arrange the dosage schedule of palliatives to prevent rather than respond to the symptoms (Foley, 1985).

Patients need an opportunity to talk about their death. Not everyone will take advantage of that chance, but a surprising number will respond to a genuine offer made without time pressure. Such discussions are not conducted on the run. Often several invitations accompanied by appropriate behavior (i.e., sitting down at the bedside) are necessary.

Some physicians are unable to confront this aspect of practice. For them, the challenge is to recognize their own behavior and get appropriate help. Such help is available at various levels: help for the physician and for the patient. Groups and therapy are readily available to assist doctors to deal with their feelings. Patients of doctors who fear death need the help of other caregivers. Often other professionals—nurses, social workers—who are working with these patients already can play the lead role in helping them work through their feelings. But the active intervention of another caregiver is not justification to ignore the patient.

The rise of the hospice movement has created a growing cadre of persons and settings to help with the dying patient. The lessons coming from this experience suggest that much can be done to facilitate this stage of life (Saunders, 1978; Fennell, 1980; Zimmerman, 1984), although the formal studies done to evaluate hospice care do not show dramatic benefits (Greer et al., 1986; Kane et al., 1984). Patients should be encouraged to be as active as possible and as interactive as they wish. Even more than in other aspects of care, the unique condition of the dying patient necessitates that the physician be prepared to listen carefully to the patient and to share in decision making about how and when to do things.

SUMMARY

Physicians caring for older patients need to think in prospective terms. They will enjoy their practices more if they can learn to set reasonable goals for patients, to record progress toward these goals, and to use the failure to achieve progress as an important clinical sign of the need for reevaluation. Prospective medicine should also carry over into prevention. Many useful steps can be taken to improve and protect the health of elderly patients.

The elderly patient represents a different risk-benefit ratio than the younger patient. Actions well tolerated in others may produce serious consequences in the old. Bed is a dangerous place for the older patient; confinement to bed rest should be avoided whenever possible.

The physician must guard against several potential iatrogenic problems with elderly patients. Diagnostic labels implying incurable problems (like dementia and incontinence) should not be used until a careful search for correctable causes has been undertaken. Special attention should be given to the tendency to create dependency through well-intentioned care. By keeping in mind the need to maintain the patient's functioning, the physician can remain sensitive to the effects of the environment to enhance or impede such activity.

REFERENCES

Alessi CA, Stuck AE, Aronow HU, et al: The process of care in preventive in-home comprehensive geriatric assessment. *J Am Geriatr Soc* 45:1044–1050, 1997.

Amery A, Birkenhager W, Brixko P, et al: Mortality and morbidity results from the European Working Party on high blood pressure in the elderly trial. *Lancet* 1:1349–1354, 1985.

Applegate WB, Miller ST, Elam ET, et al: Impact of cataract surgery with lens implantation on vision and physican function in elderly patients. *JAMA* 257:1064–1066, 1987.

Arling G, Karon SL, Sainfort F, et al: Risk adjustment of nursing home quality indicators. *Gerontologist* 37:757–766, 1997.

Avorn J, Monette J, Lacour A, et al: Persistence of use of lipid-lowering medications: A cross-national study. *JAMA* 279:1458–1462, 1998.

Beck A, Scott J, Williams P, et al: A randomized trial of group outpatient visits for chronically ill older HMO members: The cooperative health care clinic. *J Am Geriatr Soc* 45:543–549, 1997.

Block JE, Smith R, Black D, et al: Does exercise prevent osteoporosis? *JAMA* 257:3115–3117, 1987.

Boult C, Dowd B, McCaffrey D, et al: Screening elders for risk of hospital admission. *J Am Geriatr Soc* 41:811–817, 1993.

Boult C, Boult L, Morishita L, et al: Outpatient geriatric evaluation and management. *J Am Geriatr Soc* 46:296–302, 1998.

Cappuccio FP, Markandu ND, Carney C, et al: Double-blind randomised trial of modest salt restriction in older people. *Lancet* 350:850–854, 1997.

Clark F, Azen SP, Zemke R, et al: Occupational therapy for independent-living older adults: A randomized controlled trial. *JAMA* 278:1321–1326, 1997.

Coleman EA, Wagner EH, Grothaus LC, et al: Predicting hospitalization and functional decline in older health plan enrollees: Are administrative data as accurate as self-report? *J Am Geriatr Soc* 46:419–425, 1998.

Duff RS, Hollingshead AB: *Sickness and Society.* New York, Harper & Row, 1968.

Elam JT, Graney MJ, Applegate WB, et al: Functional outcome one year following cataract surgery in elderly persons. *J Gerontol* 43:122–126, 1988.

Ellwood PM. (1988). Outcomes management: A technology of patient experience. *N Engl J Med* 318:1549–1556, 1988.

Evans JG: Prevention of age-associated loss of autonomy: Epidemiological approaches. *J Chronic Dis* 37:353–363, 1984.

Fennell FB: The need for hospice. *N Engl J Med* 303:158–161, 1980.

Fiatarone MA, O'Neil EF, Ryan ND, et al: Exercise training and nutritional supplementation for physical frailty in very elderly people. *N Engl J Med* 330:1769–1775, 1994.

Foley KM: The treatment of cancer pain. *N Engl J Med* 313:84–95, 1985.

Forrester HL, Jahnigen DW, LaForce FM: Inefficacy of pneumococcal vaccine in a high-risk population. *Am J Med* 83:425–430, 1987.

German PS, Shapiro S, Skinner EA, et al: Detection and management of mental health problems of older people by primary care providers. *JAMA* 257:489–493, 1987.

Gey KF: Cardiovascular disease and vitamins: Concurrent correction of "suboptima" plasma antioxidant levels may, as important part of "optimal" nutrition, help to prevent early stages *Human Nutrition.* Basel, Karger, 1995, pp. 75–91.

Gill TM, Williams CS, Mendes de Leon CF, et al: The role of change in physical performance in determining risk for dependence in activities of daily living among nondisabled community-living elderly persons. *J Clin Epidemiol* 50:765–777, 1997.

Gillick MR, Serrell NA, Gillick LS: Adverse consequences of hospitalization in the elderly. *Soc Sci Med* 16:1033–1038, 1982.

Goldberg TH, Chavin SI: Preventive medicine and screening in older adults. *J Am Geriatr Soc* 43:344–354, 1997.

Gorbien M, Bishop J, Beers M, et al: Iatrogenic illness in hospitalized elderly people. *J Am Geriatr Soc* 40:1031–1042, 1992.

Graves T, Hanlon JT, Schmader KE, et al: Adverse events after discontinuing medications in elderly outpatients. *Arch Intern Med* 157:2205–2210, 1997.

Greenfield S, Blanco DM, Elashoff RM, et al: Patterns of care related to age of breast cancer patients. *JAMA* 257:2766–2770, 1987.

Greer DS, Mor V, Morris JN, et al: An alternative in terminal care: Results of the national hospice study. *J Chronic Dis* 39:9–26, 1986.

Havlik RJ, Liu BM, Kovan MG, et al: Health statistics on older persons, United States, 1986, in J. VanNostrand (ed): *Vital and Health Statistics, Series 3,* Washington, DC: U.S. Government Printing Office, 1987.

Hawes C: Quality of life in nursing homes: What are potential indicators on the nursing home Resident Assessment Instrument (RAI)? Paper presented at the Health Standards and Quality Bureau of the Health Care Financing Administration, Baltimore, MD, July 11–12, 1996.

Inouye SK, Charpentier PA: Precipitating factors for delerium in hospitalized elderly persons. *JAMA* 275:852–857, 1996.

Inouye SK, Peduzzi PN, Robinson JT, et al: Importance of functional measures in predicting mortality among older hospitalized patients. *JAMA* 279:1187–1193, 1998.

Institute of Medicine: *Improving the Quality of Care in Nursing Homes.* Washington, DC, National Press, 1986.

Institute of Medicine: *Medicare: A Strategy for Quality Assurance.* Vo. 1. Washington, DC: National Academy Press, 1990.

Jaijich CL, Ostfeld AM, Freeman DH: Smoking and coronary heart disease mortality in the elderly. *JAMA* 252:2831–2834, 1984.

Johannesson M, Jonsson B, Kjekshus J, et al: Cost effectiveness of simvastatin treatment to lower cholesterol levels in patients with coronary heart disease. *N Engl J Med* 336:332–336, 1997.

Kane RA, Kane RL: *Long-Term Care: Principles, Programs, and Policies.* New York. Springer-Verlag, 1987.

Kane RL, Wales J, Bernstein L, et al: A randomized controlled trial of hospice care. *Lancet* 1:890–894, 1984.

Kaplan G, Seeman T, Cohen R, et al: Mortality among the elderly in the Alameda County Study: Behavioral and demographic risk factors. *Am Public Health* 77:307–312, 1987.

Kostis JB, Davis BR, Cutley J, et al: Prevention of heart failure by antihypertensive drug treatment in older persons with isolated systolic hypertension. *JAMA* 278:212–216, 1997.

Krumholz HM, Seeman TE, Merrill SS, et al: Lack of association between cholesterol and coronary heart disease mortality and morbidity and all-cause mortality in persons older than 70 years. *JAMA* 272:1335–1340, 1994.

Kubler-Ross E: *On Death and Dying,* New York: Macmillan, 1969.

LaCroix AZ: Determinants of health—Exercise and activities of daily living, in Havlik RJ, Liu M, Kovar G, et al (eds): *Health Statistics on Older Persons, United States,*

1986 (Public Health Service ed., Vol. Series 3). Washington, DC: U.S. Government Printing Office, 1987.

Landefeld CS, Palmer RM, Kresevic DM, et al: A randomized trial of care in a hospital medical unit especially designed to improve the functional outcomes of acutely ill older patients. *N Engl J Med* 332:1338–1344, 1995.

Lazarou J, Pomeranz BH, Corey PN: Incidence of adverse drug reactions in hospitalized patients: A metal-analysis of prospective studies. *JAMA* 279:1200–1205, 1998.

Levinstein MR, Ouslander JG, Rubenstein LZ, et al: Yield of routine annual laboratory tests in a skilled nursing home population. *JAMA* 258:1909–1915, 1987.

Miettinen TA, Pyorala K, Olsson AG, et al: Cholesterol-lowering therapy in women and elderly patients with myocardial infarction or angina pectoris: Findings from the Scandinavian Simvastatin Survival Study (4S). *Circulation* 96:4211–4218, 1997.

Morris JN, Fries BE, Mehr DR, et al: MDS cognitive performance scale. *J Gerontol Med Sci* 49:M174–M182, 1994.

O'Malley MS, Fletcher SW: Screening for breast cancer with breast self-examination: A critical review. *JAMA* 257:2197–2203, 1987.

Omenn GS, Beresford SM, Buchner DM, et al: Evidence of modifiable risk factors in older adults as a basis for health promotion/disease prevention programs, in Hickey T, Speers MA, Prohaska TR, (eds): *Public Health and Aging.* Baltimore, MD, Johns Hopkins University Press, 1997, pp. 107–127.

Paganini-Hill A, Dworsky R, Krauss RM: Hormone replacement therapy, hormone levels, and lipoprotein cholesterol concentrations in elderly women. *Am J Obstet Gynecol* 174:897–902, 1996.

Pepper GA, Jorgensen LB, Kane RL, et al: *Problem-Oriented Process: Nurse's Manual.* Salt Lake City, University of Utah, 1972.

Petrovitch H, Vogt T, Berge K: Isolated systolic hypertension: Lowering the risk of stroke in older patients. *Geriatrics* 47:30–38, 1992.

Rich MW, Beckham V, Wittenberg C, et al: A multidisciplinary intervention to prevent the readmission of elderly patients with congestive heart failure. *N Engl J Med* 333:1190–1195, 1995.

Rodysill KJ: Postmenopausal osteoporosis—Intervention and prophylaxis: A review. *J Chronic Dis* 40:743–760, 1987.

Rubenstein LZ, Josephson KR, Nichol-Seamons M, et al: Comprehensive health screening of well elderly adults: An analysis of a community program. *J Gerontol* 41:342–352, 1986.

Rubenstein LZ, Rhee L, Kane RL: The role of geriatric assessment units in caring for the elderly: An analytic review. *J Gerontol* 37:513–521, 1982.

Sager MA, Rudberg MA, Jalaluddin M, et al: Hospital admission risk profile (HARP): Identifying older patients at risk for functional decline following acute medical illness and hospitalization. *J Am Geriatr Soc* 44:251–257, 1996.

Sano M, Ernesto C, Thomas RG, et al: A controlled trial of selegiline, alpha-tocopherol, or both as treatment for Alzheimer's disease: The Alzheimer's Disease Cooperative Study. *N Engl J Med* 336:1245–1247, 1997.

Santanello NC, Barber BL, Applegate WB, et al: Effect of pharmacologic lipid lowering on health-related quality of life in older persons: Results from the Cholesterol Reduction in Seniors Program (CRISP) pilot study. *J Am Geriatr Soc* 45:8–14, 1997.

Saunders C: Hospice care. *Am J Med* 65:726–728, 1978.

Scheitel SM, Fleming KC, Chutka DS, et al: Geriatric health maintenance. *Mayo Clin Proc* 71:289–302, 1996.

SHEP Cooperative Research Group: Prevention of stroke by antihypertensive drug treatment in older persons with isolated systolic hypertension: Final results of the Systolic Hypertension in the Elderly Program. *JAMA* 265:3255–3264, 1991.

Simberkoff MS, Cross AP, Al-Ibrahim M, et al: Efficacy of pneumococcal vaccine in high-risk patients: Results of a Veterans Administration Cooperative Study. *N Engl J Med* 315:1318–1327, 1986.

Sims RV, Steinmann WC, McConville JH, et al: The clinical effectiveness of pneumococcal vaccine in the elderly. *Ann Intern Med* 108:653–657, 1988.

Staessen JA, Fagard R, Thijs L, et al: Randomised double-blind comparison of placebo and active treatment for older patients with isolated systolic hypertension. *Lancet* 350:757–764, 1997.

Stead WW, To T: The significance of the tuberculin skin test in elderly persons. *Ann Intern Med* 107:837–842, 1987a.

Stead WW, To T, Harrison RW, et al: Benefit-risk considerations in preventive treatment for tuberculosis in elderly persons. *Ann Intern Med* 107:843–845, 1987b.

Steel K, Gertman PM, Crescenzi C, et al: Iatrogenic illness on a general medical service at a university hospital. *N Engl J Med* 304:638–642, 1981.

Stuck AE, Aronow HU, Steiner A, et al: A trial of annual in-home comprehensive geriatic assessments for elderly people living in the community. *N Engl J Med* 333:1184–1189, 1995.

Stuck AE, Siu AL, Wieland GD, et al: Comprehensive geriatric assessment: A meta-analysis of controlled trials. *Lancet* 342:1032–1036, 1993.

U.S. Preventive Services Task Force: *Guide to Clinical Preventive Services: Report of the U.S. Preventive Services Task Force, 2nd ed.* Baltimore, MD: Williams & Wilkins, 1996.

Walma EP, Hoes AW, van Dooren C, et al: Withdrawal of long term diuretic medication in elderly patients: A double blind randomised trial. *BMJ* 315:464–468, 1997.

Whelton PK, Appel LJ, Espeland MA, et al: Sodium reduction and weight loss in the treatment of hypertension in older persons: A randomized controlled trial on nonpharmacologic interventions in the elderly (TONE). *JAMA* 279:839–846, 1998.

WHO: *International Classification of Impairments, Disabilities, and Handicaps: A Manual of Classification Relating to the Consequences of Disease.* Geneva, World Health Organization, 1980.

Williams ME: Identifying the older person likely to require long-term care services. *J Am Geriatr Soc* 33:761–766, 1987.

Winawer SJ, Fletcher RH, Miller L: Colorectal screening clinical guidelines and rationale. *Gastroenterology* 112:59–62, 1997.

Woolley FR, Warnick R, Kane RL, et al: *Problem-Oriented Nursing.* New York, Springer-Verlag, 1974.

Zimmerman DR, Karon SL, Arling G, et al: Development and testing of nursing home quality indicators. *Health Care Fin Rev* 16(4):107–127, 1995.

Zimmerman JM: *Hospice.* Baltimore, Urban & Schwartzenberg, 1984.

Zuckerman DM, Kasl SV, Ostfeld AM: Psychosocial predictors of mortality among the elderly poor: The role of religion, well-being, and social contacts. *Am J Epidemiol* 119:410–423, 1984.

SUGGESTED READINGS

Institute of Medicine: *Disability in America: Toward a National Agenda for Prevention.* Washington, DC: National Academy Press, 1991.

Kane RL, Kane RA: *Values and Long-Term Care.* Lexington, MA, Heath, 1982.

World Health Organization: *Preventing Disability in the Elderly.* Copenhagen, Regional Office for Europe, 1982.

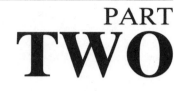

PART
TWO

DIFFERENTIAL DIAGNOSIS AND MANAGEMENT

CHAPTER FIVE

CONFUSION

The appropriate diagnosis and management of geriatric patients exhibiting symptoms and signs of confusion can make a critical difference to their overall health and ability to function independently. Among community-dwelling older people, about 5 to 10 percent of those above age 65 and close to 20 percent of those over 75 have some degree of clinically detectable impairment of cognitive function. As more people live into the tenth decade of life, the chance that they will develop some form of dementia increases substantially. Community-based studies report a prevalence of dementia as high as 47 percent among those 85 years of age and older (Evans et al., 1989; Bachman et al., 1992). Prevalence rates are, however, highly dependent on the criteria used to define dementia (Erkinjuntti et al., 1997). In nursing homes, 50 to 80 percent of those above age 65 have some degree of cognitive impairment (Rovner et al., 1990). Between one-third and one-half of older patients admitted to acute care medical and surgical services will also exhibit varying degrees of confusion (Francis et al., 1990).

Misdiagnosis and inappropriate management of confusion in geriatric patients can cause substantial morbidity among the patients, hardship to their families, and millions of dollars in health care expen-

diture. This chapter provides a practical framework for diagnosing and managing geriatric patients who appear confused. We focus on the most common causes of confusion in the geriatric population—delirium and dementia—though a variety of other disorders can cause confusion. Details of the anatomy, biochemistry, and pathophysiology of various forms of dementia can be found in the Suggested Readings at the end of this chapter.

DEFINING CONFUSION

Imprecise definition of the abnormalities of cognitive function in older patients labeled as "confused" has led to problems in the diagnosis and management of these patients. *Confusion* has been defined as a "mental state in which reactions to environmental stimuli are inappropriate; a state in which the person is bewildered or perplexed or unable to orientate himself" (*Stedman's Medical Dictionary,* 1976). This type of definition, although descriptive, is too broad and imprecise to be clinically useful. Documentation such as "confused" or "confused at times" is also imprecise. Descriptions such as "impairment of mental function" or "cognitive impairment" coupled with careful documentation of the timing and nature of specific abnormalities provides more precise and clinically useful information. Such documentation is best accomplished by means of a thorough mental status examination.

A thorough mental status examination has several components (Table 5-1). In evaluating older patients who appear confused, atten-

Table 5-1 Key aspects of mental status examinations

State of consciousness
General appearance and behavior
Orientation
Memory (short- and long-term)
Language
Visuospatial functions
Other cognitive functions (e.g., calculations, proverb interpretation)
Insight and judgment
Thought content
Mood and affect

tion should focus on each of these components in a systematic manner. Recording observations in each area is critical to recognizing and evaluating changes over time. Standardized and validated measures of cognitive function such as the Mini-Mental State Examination (see Appendix) can be helpful screening tools in these assessments as well as in subsequent monitoring. Several factors may influence performance and interpretation of standard mental status tests, such as prior low educational level, primary language other than English, severely impaired hearing, or poor baseline intellectual function. Thus, scores on one or more of these tests should not be used to replace a more comprehensive examination that includes all the components listed in Table 5-1.

Important information can be gleaned unobtrusively from simply observing and interacting with the patient during the history. Is the patient alert and attentive? Does the patient respond appropriately to questions? How is the patient dressed and groomed? Does the patient repeat himself or herself or give an imprecise medical history, suggesting memory impairment? Orientation to person, place, time, and situation can sometimes be assessed during the history as well.

Questions relating to specific areas of cognitive functioning should be introduced in a nonthreatening manner, because many patients with early deficits respond defensively. Each of the three basic components of memory should be tested: immediate recall (e.g., repeating digits), recent memory (e.g., recalling three objects after a few minutes), and remote memory (e.g., ability to give details of early life). Language and other cognitive functions should be carefully evaluated. Is the patient's speech clear? Can the patient read (and understand) and write? Does there seem to be a good general fund of knowledge (e.g., current events)? Other cognitive functions that can be tested easily include the ability to perform simple calculations (one that relates to making change while shopping, for example) and to copy diagrams. The ability to interpret proverbs abstractly and to list the names of animals (12 names in 1 min is normal) are sensitive indicators of cognitive function and are easy to test.

Judgment and insight can usually be assessed during the examination without asking specific questions, though input from family members or other caregivers can be helpful and sometimes necessary. Any abnormal thought content should also be noted during the examination; bizarre ideas, mood-incongruent thoughts, and delusions (especially paranoid delusions) may be prominent in older patients with

cognitive impairment and are important both diagnostically and therapeutically.

Throughout the examination, the patient's mood and affect should be assessed. Depression and emotional lability are common in older patients with cognitive impairment, and failure to recognize these abnormalities can lead to improper diagnosis and management. In some—such as very intelligent or poorly educated patients, or individuals with low intelligence, and those in whom depression is suspected—more detailed neuropsychological testing by an experienced psychologist is helpful in more precisely defining abnormalities in cognitive function and in differentiating between the many and often interacting underlying causes.

DIFFERENTIAL DIAGNOSIS OF CONFUSION IN GERIATRIC PATIENTS

The causes of confusion in the geriatric population are myriad. The differential diagnosis in an older patient who presents with confusion includes disorders of the brain (e.g., stroke, dementia), a systemic illness presenting atypically (e.g., infection, metabolic disturbance, myocardial infarction, congestive heart failure), sensory impairment, (e.g., hearing loss), and adverse effects of a variety of drugs or alcohol.

Similar to many other disorders in geriatric patients, confusion often results from multiple interacting processes rather than a single causative factor. Accurate diagnosis depends on specifically defining abnormalities in mental status and cognitive function and on consistent definitions for clinical syndromes. Disorders causing confusion in the geriatric population can be broadly categorized into three groups:

1. Acute disorders, usually associated with acute illness, drugs, and environmental factors (i.e., delirium)
2. More slowly progressive impairment of cognitive function, as seen in most dementia and amnestic syndromes
3. Impaired cognitive function associated with affective disorders and psychoses

Old age alone does not cause impairment of cognitive function of sufficient severity to render an individual dysfunctional. Mild, recent memory loss and slowed thinking and reaction time are common. Older patients are often labeled "senile" because they are unable to

answer a question or because they are not given adequate time to respond. Other age-associated disorders such as impaired hearing can also lead to mislabeling an older patient as "confused" or "senile."

Three questions are helpful in making an accurate diagnosis of the underlying cause(s) of confusion:

- Has the onset of abnormalities been acute (i.e., over a few hours or a few days)?
- Are there physical factors (i.e., medical illness, sensory deprivation, drugs) that may contribute to the abnormalities?
- Are psychological factors (i.e., depression and/or psychosis) contributing to or complicating the impairments in cognitive function?

These questions focus on identifying treatable conditions, which, when diagnosed and treated, might result in substantially improved cognitive function. The Suggested Readings at the end of this chapter provide more detailed discussions of these disorders as well as other conditions causing confusion in the geriatric population.

DELIRIUM

Delirium is an acute or subacute alteration in mental status especially common in the geriatric population. The prevalence of delirium in hospitalized geriatric patients is about 15 percent on admission (Francis, 1992), and the incidence in this setting may be close to one-third (Schor et al., 1992). In the past, a variety of labels have been used to describe delirious patients (including acute confusional state, acute brain syndrome, metabolic encephalopathy, and toxic psychosis). The *Diagnostic and Statistical Manual of Mental Disorders* (DSM-IV) (American Psychiatric Association, 1994) defines diagnostic criteria for delirium (Table 5-2). The key features of this disorder include the following:

- Disturbance of consciousness
- Change in cognition not better accounted for by dementia
- Symptoms and signs developing over a short period of time (hours to days)
- Fluctuation of the symptoms and signs
- Evidence that the disturbances are caused by the physiologic consequences of a medical condition

Table 5-2 Diagnostic criteria for delirium

1. Disturbance of consciousness (that is, reduced clarity of awareness of the environment) in conjunction with reduced ability to focus, sustain, or shift attention
2. A change in cognition (such as memory deficit, disorientation, or language disturbance) or the development of a perceptual disturbance that is not better accounted for by a preexisting, established, or evolving dementia
3. Development of the disturbance during a brief period (usually hours to days) and a tendency for fluctuation during the course of the day
4. Evidence from the history, physical examination, or laboratory findings that the disturbance is caused by:
   a. A general medical condition
   b. A substance intoxication, side effect, or withdrawal

Source: From the American Psychiatric Association, 1994, with permission.

The disturbances of consciousness and attention, with the suddenness of onset and the fluctuating cognitive status, are the major features that distinguish delirium from other causes of impaired cognitive function. Delirium is characterized by difficulty in sustaining attention to external and internal stimuli, sensory misperceptions (e.g., illusions), and a fragmented or disordered stream of thought. Disturbances of psychomotor activity (such as restlessness, picking at bedclothes, attempting to get out of bed, sluggishness, drowsiness, and generally decreased psychomotor activity) and emotional disturbances (anxiety, fear, irritability, anger, apathy) are very common in delirious patients. Neurologic signs (except asterixis) are uncommon in delirium. Many hospitalized patients have delirium on only a single day, but the severity and time course delirium varies considerably (Rudberg et al., 1997). Many factors predispose geriatric patients to the development of delirium, including impaired sensory functioning and sensory deprivation, sleep deprivation, immobilization, transfer to an unfamiliar environment, and psychosocial stresses such as bereavement. Among hospitalized geriatric patients, several factors are associated with the development of delirium (Schor et al., 1992; Inouye and Charpentier 1996; Elie et al., 1998). Delirium as a complication of hospitalization is discussed in Chap. 4.

The following factors may predispose a patient to develop delirium:

- Age over 80
- Male sex
- Preexisting dementia
- Fracture
- Symptomatic infection
- Malnutrition
- Addition of three or more medications
- Use of neuroleptics and narcotics
- Use of restraints
- Bladder catheters
- Iatrogenic events

Rapid recognition of delirium is critical because it is often related to other reversible conditions and its development may be a poor prognostic sign. Inouye and colleagues have described a strategy to identify delirium, termed the Confusion Assessment Method (CAM) (Inouye et al., 1990). The diagnosis of delirium by the CAM requires the presence of items 1 and 2, and either 3 or 4 listed below:

1. Acute onset and fluctuating course
2. Inattention
3. Disorganized thinking
4. Altered level of conciousness

It is also important to differentiate delirium from dementia, because the latter is not immediately life-threatening, and inappropriately labeling a delirious patient as demented may delay the diagnosis of serious and treatable conditions. It is not possible to make the diagnosis of dementia when delirium is present in a patient with previously normal or unknown cognitive function. The diagnosis of dementia must await the treatment of all of the potentially reversible causes of delirium, as discussed below. Table 5-3 shows some of the key clinical features that are helpful in differentiating delirium from dementia. *Sundowning* is a term that describes an increase in confusion which commonly occurs in geriatric patients, especially those with preexisting dementia, at night. This condition is probably related to sensory deprivation in unfamiliar surroundings (such as the acute

Table 5-3   Key features differentiating delirium from dementia

Feature	Delirium	Dementia
Onset	Acute, often at night	Insidious
Course	Fluctuating, with lucid intervals, during day; worse at night	Generally stable over course of day
Duration	Hours to weeks	Months to years
Awareness	Reduced	Clear
Alertness	Abnormally low or high	Usually normal
Attention	Hypoalert or hyperalert, distractible; fluctuates over course of day	Usually normal
Orientation	Usually impaired for time, tendency to mistake unfamiliar for familiar place and persons	Often impaired
Memory	Immediate and recent impaired	Recent and remote impaired
Thinking	Disorganized	Impoverished
Perception	Illusions and hallucinations (usually visual) relatively common	Usually normal
Speech	Incoherent, hesitant, slow or rapid	Difficulty in finding words
Sleep-wake cycle	Always disrupted	Often fragmented sleep
Physical illness or drug toxicity	Either or both present	Often absent, especially in Alzheimer's disease

Source: From Lipkowski, 1987, with permission.

care hospital) and patients who "sundown" may actually meet the criteria for delirium.

A complete list of conditions that can cause delirium in the geriatric population would be too long to be useful in a clinical setting. Table 5-4 lists some of the common causes of this disorder. Several of them deserve further attention.

Table 5-4   Common causes of delirium in geriatric patients

Metabolic disorders
  Electrolyte abnormalities
  Acid-base disturbances
  Hypoxia
  Hypercarbia
  Hypo- or hyperglycemia
  Azotemia

Infections

Decreased cardiac output
  Dehydration
  Acute blood loss
  Acute myocardial infarction
  Congestive heart failure

Stroke (small cortical)

Drugs (see Table 4-5)

Intoxication (alcohol, other)

Hypo- or hyperthermia

Acute psychoses

Transfer to unfamiliar surroundings (especially when sensory input is diminished)

Other
  Fecal impaction
  Urinary retention

Each geriatric patient who becomes acutely "confused" should be evaluated to rule out treatable conditions such as metabolic disorders, infections, and causes for decreased cardiac output (i.e., dehydration, acute blood loss, heart failure). Sometimes this workup is unrevealing. Small cortical strokes, which do not produce focal symptoms or signs, can cause delirium. These events may be difficult or impossible to diagnose with certainty, but there should be a high index of suspicion for this diagnosis in certain subgroups of patients—especially those with a history of hypertension, previous strokes, transient ischemic attacks, or cardiac arrhythmias. If delirium recurs, a source of emboli should be sought and associated conditions (such as hypertension) should be treated optimally. Fecal impaction and urinary retention, common in geriatric patients (especially those in acute care hospitals), can have dramatic effects on cognitive function and may be causes

Table 5-5 Drugs that can cause or contribute to delirium and dementia*

Analgesics	Cardiovascular
Narcotic	Antiarrhythmics
Nonnarcotic	Digoxin
Nonsteroidal anti-inflammatory agents	H_2 receptor antagonists
Anticholinergics/antihistamines	Psychotropic drugs
Anticonvulsants	Antianxiety drugs
Antihypertensives	Antidepressant drugs
	Antipsychotics
Antimicrobials	Sedative/hypnotics
Antiparkinsonism drugs	Skeletal muscle relaxants
	Steroids

* See AHCPR guidelines (Costa et al., 1996) for a more complete list.

of acute confusion. The response to relief from these conditions can be just as impressive.

Drugs are a major cause of acute as well as chronic impairment of cognitive function in older patients (Larson et al., 1987). Table 5-5 lists commonly prescribed drugs that can cause or contribute to delirium (as well as dementia). Every attempt should be made to avoid or discontinue any medication that may be worsening cognitive function in a delirious geriatric patient. Environmental factors, especially rapid changes in location (such as being hospitalized, going on vacation, or entering a nursing home) and sensory deprivation, can precipitate delirium. This is especially true of those with early forms of dementia (see below). The "sundowner syndrome" (confusion and agitation with the onset of evening) is a familiar example of this problem (Evans, 1987). Measures such as preparing older patients for changes in location, placing familiar objects in the surroundings, and maximizing sensory input with lighting, clocks, and calendars may help prevent or manage delirium in some patients.

DEMENTIA

Dementia is a clinical syndrome involving a sustained loss of intellectual functions and memory of sufficient severity to cause dysfunction in daily living. Its key features include:

- A gradually progressing course (usually over months to years)
- No disturbance of consciousness

Dementia in the geriatric population can be grouped into two broad categories:

1. Reversible or partially reversible dementias
2. Nonreversible dementias

Reversible Dementias

While it is especially important to rule out treatable and potentially reversible causes of dementia in individual patients, these dementias account for less than 20 percent of all causes of dementia in most series (Costa et al., 1996; Clarfield, 1988). Moreover, finding a reversible cause does not guarantee that the dementia will improve after the putative cause has been treated.

Causes of reversible dementia are outlined in Table 5-6. These disorders can be detected by careful history, physical examination, and selected laboratory studies. Drugs known to cause abnormalities in cognitive function (Table 5-5) should be discontinued whenever feasible. There should be a high index of suspicion regarding excessive alcohol intake in older patients. The incidence of alcohol consumption varies considerably in different populations but is easily missed and can cause dementia as well as delirium, depression, falls, and other medical complications.

Table 5-6 Causes of potentially reversible dementias

Neoplasms	Autoimmune disorders
Metabolic disorders	Central nervous system vasculitis, temporal arteritis
	Disseminated lupus erythematosus
Trauma	Multiple sclerosis
Toxins	Drugs (see Table 5-5)
Alcoholism	
Heavy metals	Nutritional disorders
Organic poisons	Psychiatric disorders
Infections	Depression
	Other disorders (e.g., normal-pressure hydrocephalus)

Sources: From Costa et al., 1996, and Katzman et al., 1988, with permission.

One particular disorder, *depressive pseudodementia,* deserves special emphasis. This term has been used to refer to patients who have reversible or partially reversible impairments of cognitive function caused by depression. Depression may coexist with dementia in over one-third of outpatients with dementia and an even greater proportion in nursing homes (Rovner et al., 1990; Lazarus et al., 1987; Merriam et al., 1988). The interrelationship between depression and dementia is complex. Many patients with early forms of dementia become depressed. Sorting out how much of the cognitive impairment is caused by depression and how much by an organic factor(s) can be difficult. Table 5-7 compares some clinical characteristics that can be helpful in diagnosing depressive pseudodementia. In addition to these characteristics, detailed neuropsychological testing, performed by a psychologist or other health care professional skilled in the use of these tools, can be helpful in many patients. At times, even after a complete assessment, uncertainty still exists regarding the role of depression in producing intellectual deficits. Under these circumstances, a careful trial of antidepressants (in rare instances, electroconvulsive therapy) is justified to facilitate the diagnosis and may help improve overall (but not cognitive) functioning (Reifler et al., 1986). Older patients who develop reversible cognitive impairment while depressed appear at relatively high risk for developing dementia over the following few years, and their cognitive function should be followed closely over time.

Nonreversible Dementias

Several different classifications have been recommended for the nonreversible dementias. The AHCPR guideline on Alzheimer's and related dementias (Costa et al., 1996) lists four basic categories, based on the work of Katzman et al., 1988 (Table 5-8):

- Degenerative diseases of the central nervous system
- Vascular disorders
- Trauma
- Infections

Alzheimer's disease, other degenerative disorders, and vascular dementias account for a vast majority of dementias in the geriatric population, and are the focus of discussion in this chapter.

Table 5-7 Dementia versus depressive pseudodementia: Comparison of clinical characteristics

Characteristics	Dementia	Depressive pseudodementia
A. History		
1. Onset can be dated with some precision	Unusual	Usual
2. Duration of symptoms before physician consulted	Long	Short
3. Rapid progression of symptoms	Unusual	Usual
4. Patient's complaints of cognitive loss	Variable (minimized in later stages)	Usual
5. Patient's description of cognitive loss	Vague	Detailed
6. Family aware of dysfunction and severity	Variable (usual in later stages)	
7. Loss of social skills	Late	Early
8. History of psychopathology	Uncommon	Common
B. Examination		
1. Memory loss for recent versus remote events	Greater	About equal
2. Specific memory loss ("patchy" deficits)	Uncommon	Common
3. Attention and concentration	Often poor	Often good
4. "Don't know" answers	Uncommon	Common
5. "Near miss" answers	Variable (common in later stages)	Uncommon
6. Performance on tasks of similar difficulty	Consistent	Variable
7. Patient's emotional reaction to symptoms	Variable (unconcerned in later stages)	Great distress
8. Patient's affect	Labile, blunted, or depressed	Depressed
9. Patient's effort in attempting to perform tasks	Great	Small
10. Patient's efforts to cope with dysfunction	Maximal	Minimal

Source: From Small et al., 1981, with permission.

Table 5-8 Causes of nonreversible dementias

Degenerative diseases
 Alzheimer's disease
 Dementia associated with Lewy bodies
 Pick's disease
 Huntington's disease
 Progressive supranuclear palsy
 Parkinson's disease
 Others

Vascular dementias
 Occlusive cerebrovascular disease (multi-infarct dementia)
 Binswanger's disease
 Cerebral embolism(s)
 Arteritis
 Anoxia secondary to cardiac arrest, cardiac failure of carbon monoxide
  intoxication

Traumatic dementia
 Craniocerebral injury
 Dementia pugilistica

Infections
 Acquired immunodeficiency syndrome
 Opportunistic infections
 Creutzfeldt-Jakob disease
 Progressive multifocal leukoencephalopathy
 Postencephalitic dementia

Sources: From Costa et al., 1996, and Katzman et al., 1988, with permission.

Alzheimer's and Other Degenerative Diseases

Alzheimer's disease accounts for close to two-thirds of dementias in the geriatric population. Recently, dementia associated with Lewy bodies (DLB) has received increased attention. Autopsy studies suggest that DLB may account for 25 percent of dementias and may overlap with Alzheimer's and Parkinson's dementia (Small et al., 1997; McKeith et al., 1996). In addition to the characteristic pathologic findings, DLB is characterized by

- Detailed visual hallucinations
- Parkinsonian signs
- Alterations of alertness and attention

DLB should especially be suspected in patients who present with early signs of parkinsonian and more prominent dementia and in dementia patients who are very sensitive to the extrapyramidal effects of antipsychotic agents.

Diagnostic criteria for Alzheimer's disease (AD) are outlined in Table 5-9. Family history and increasing age are the primary risk factors for AD. About 6 to 8 percent of persons above age 65 have AD. The prevalence doubles every 5 years, so that nearly 30 percent of the population above age 85 has AD. By the age of 90, almost 50 percent of persons with a first-degree relative suffering from AD may develop the disease themselves. Rare genetic mutations on chromosomes 1, 14, and 21 cause early-onset familial forms of AD, and some

Table 5-9 Diagnostic criteria for Alzheimer's dementia

A. The development of multiple cognitive deficits manifested by both:
  1. Memory impairment (impaired ability to learn new information or to recall previously learned information)
  2. One (or more) of the following cognitive disturbances:
    a. Aphasia (language disturbance)
    b. Apraxia (impaired ability to perform motor activities despite intact motor function)
    c. Agnosia (failure to recognize or identify objects despite intact sensory function)
    d. Disturbance in executive functioning (that is, planning, organizing, sequencing, abstracting)
B. The cognitive deficits in criteria A1 and A2 each cause severe impairment in social or occupational functioning and represent a major decline from a previous level of functioning
C. The course is characterized by gradual onset and continuing cognitive decline
D. The cognitive deficits in criteria A1 and A2 are not due to any of the following:
  1. Other central nervous system conditions that cause progressive deficits in memory and cognition (e.g., cerebrovascular disease, Parkinson's disease, Huntington's disease, subdural hematoma, normal-pressure hydrocephalus, brain tumor
  2. Systemic conditions known to cause dementia (for example, hypothyroidism, vitamin deficiencies, hypercalcemia, neurosyphilis, HIV infection)
E. The deficits do not occur exclusively during the course of a delirium
F. The disturbance is not better accounted for by another axis I disorder (for example, major depressive disorder, schizophrenia)

Source: From the American Psychiatric Association, 1994, with permission.

forms of late-onset AD have been linked to chromosome 12 (Small et al., 1997).

The strongest genetic linkage with late-onset AD identified thus far is the apolipoprotein E-4 (APOE-E4) allele on chromosome 19. The relative risk of AD associated with one or more copies of this allele in whites is about 2.5. However, APOE-E4 does not appear to confer increased risk for AD among African Americans or Hispanics. One study suggests, however, that the cumulative risks of AD to age 90, adjusted for education and sex, are four times higher for African Americans and two times higher for Hispanics than for whites (Tang et al., 1998). Because the presence of one or more APOE-E4 alleles is neither sensitive nor specific, there is disagreement on recommending it as a screening test for AD (Small et al., 1997; Mayeux et al., 1998). Until more sensitive and specific tests become available, routine screening, even among high-risk populations, is generally not recommended.

Other possible risk factors for AD include previous head injury, female sex, lower education level, and other yet to be identified susceptibility genes. Possible protective factors include the use of estrogen and nonsteriodal anti-inflammatory drugs. The clinical significance of these protective effects, however, remains to be proven.

Vascular Dementias

Vascular dementias, predominately due to multiple infarcts *(multi-infarct dementia),* account for about 15 percent of dementia in the geriatric population. Multi-infarct dementia can occur alone or in combination with other disorders that cause dementia. Autopsy studies suggest that cerebrovascular disease may play an important role in the presence and severity of symptoms of AD (Snowdon et al., 1997). Multi-infarct dementia results when a patient has sustained recurrent cortical or subcortial strokes. Many of these strokes are too small to cause permanent or residual focal neurologic deficits or evidence of strokes on computed tomography (CT). Magnetic resonance imaging (MRI) may be more sensitive in detecting small infarcts, but there has been a tendency to overinterpret some of these findings as more MRI scans are being done. Table 5-10 identifies characteristics of patients likely to have multi-infarct dementia and compares the clinical characteristics of primary degenerative and multi-infarct dementias. A key feature of multi-infarct dementia is

Table 5-10 Alzheimer's disease versus multi-infarct dementia: Comparison of clinical characteristics

Characteristics	Alzheimer's disease	Multi-infarct dementia
A. Demographic		
1. Sex	Women more commonly affected	Men more commonly affected
2. Age	Generally over age 75	Generally over age 60
B. History		
1. Time course of deficits	Gradually progressive	Stuttering or episodic, with stepwise deterioration
2. History of hypertension	Less common	Common
3. History of stroke(s) transient ischemic attack(s), or other focal neurologic symptoms	Less common	Common
C. Examination		
1. Hypertension	Less common	Common
2. Focal neurologic signs	Uncommon	Common
3. Signs of atherosclerotic cardiovascular disease	Less common	Common
4. Emotional lability	Less common	More common

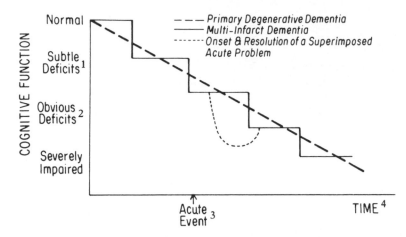

Figure 5-1 Primary degenerative dementia versus multi-infarct dementia: comparison of time courses. 1, Recognized by patient, but only detectable on detailed testing. 2, Deficits recognized by family and friends. 3, See text for explanation. 4, Exact time courses are variable; see text.

the stepwise deterioration in cognitive functioning, as illustrated in Fig. 5-1. Another form of vascular form of dementia has been described, termed *senile dementia of the Binswanger type,* which may be impossible to differentiate clinically from multi-infarct dementia (Roman, 1987). It has become increasingly important to differentiate vascular from other dementias because patients with the former may benefit from more aggressive treatment of hypertension and other cardiovascular risk factors, whereas new pharmacologic treatments for AD may not help patients with vascular forms of dementias.

EVALUATION

The AHCPR practice guideline (Costa et al., 1996) and a consensus statement of the American Association of Geriatric Psychiatry, the Alzheimer's Association, and the American Geriatrics Society (Small et al., 1997) have updated recommendations for the evaluation of patients suspected of having a dementia syndrome. The first step is

to recognize clues that dementia may be present. Table 5-11 lists symptoms that should suggest further evaluation. Patients suspected of having dementia should undergo the following:

- Focused history and physical examination, including:
  Assessment for delirium and depression
  Identification of comorbid conditions (e.g., sensory impairment, physical disability)
- A functional status assessment (See Chap. 3)
- A mental status examination (see above and Table 5-1)
- Selected laboratory studies to rule out reversible dementia and delirium

Key aspects of the history are outlined in Table 5-12. Because many physical illnesses and drugs can cause cognitive dysfunction, active medical problems and use of prescription and nonprescription

Table 5-11 Symptoms that may indicate dementia

- Learning and retaining new information
  Is repetitious; has trouble remembering recent conversations, events, appointments; frequently misplaces objects.
- Handling complex tasks
  Has trouble following a complex train of thought or performing tasks that require many steps, such as balancing a checkbook or cooking a meal.
- Reasoning ability
  Is unable to respond with a reasonable plan to problems at work or home, such as knowing what to do if the bathroom is flooded; shows uncharacteristic disregard for rules of social conduct.
- Spatial ability and orientation
  Has trouble driving, organizing objects around the house, finding his or her way around familiar places.
- Language
  Has increasing difficulty with finding the words to express what he or she wants to say and with following conversations.
- Behavior
  Appears more passive and less responsive, is more irritable than usual, is more suspicious than usual, misinterprets visual or auditory stimuli.

Source: From Costa et al., 1996, with permission.

Table 5-12 Evaluating dementia: The history

Summarize active medical problems and current physical complaints
List drugs (including over-the-counter preparations and alcohol)
Cardiovascular and neurologic history
Characterize the symptoms
  Nature of deficits (memory versus other cognitive functions)
  Onset and rate of progression
  Associated psychological symptoms
    Depression
    Anxiety or agitation
    Paranoid ideation
    Psychotic thought processes (delusions and/or hallucinations)

Ask about special problems
  Wandering (and getting lost)
  Dangerous driving and car crashes
  Disruptive or self-endangering behaviors
  Verbal agitation
  Physical aggression
  Insomnia
  Poor hygiene
  Malnutrition
  Incontinence

Assess the social situation
  Living arrangements
  Social supports
  Availability of relatives and other caregivers
  Employment and health of caregivers

drugs (including alcohol) should be reviewed. The nature and severity of the symptoms should be characterized. What are the deficits? Does the patient admit to them or is the family member describing them? How is the patient reacting to the problems? The responses to these questions can be helpful in differentiating between dementia and depressive pseudodementia (see Table 5-7). The onset of symptoms and the rate of progression are particularly important. The sudden onset of cognitive impairment (over a few days) should prompt a search for one of the underlying causes of delirium listed in Table 5-4. Irregular, stepwise decrements in cognitive function (as opposed to a more even and gradual loss) favor a diagnosis of multi-infarct dementia (Table 5-10 and Fig. 5-1). Patients with dementia

are often brought for evaluation at a time of sudden worsening of cognitive function (as illustrated by the broken line in Fig. 5-1) and may even meet the criteria for delirium. These sudden changes may be triggered by a number of acute events (a small stroke without focal signs, acute physical illness, drugs, changes in environment, or personal loss such as the death or departure of a relative). Only a careful history (or familiarity with the patient) will help determine when an acute event has been superimposed on a preexisting dementia. Appropriate management of the acute event will, in many instances, result in improvement in cognitive function (Fig. 5-1, broken line).

The history should also include specific questions about common problems requiring special attention in patients with dementia. These problems may include wandering, dangerous driving and car crashes, disruptive behavior (e.g., verbal agitation, physical aggression, and nighttime agitation), delusions or hallucinations, insomnia, poor hygiene, malnutrition, and incontinence. They require careful management and most often substantial involvement of family or other caregivers.

A social history is especially important in patients with dementia. Living arrangements and social supports should be assessed. Along with functional status, these factors play a major role in the management of patients with dementia and are of critical importance in determining the necessity for institutionalization. A patient with dementia and weak social supports may require institutionalization at a higher level of function than will a patient with strong social supports. In addition to the lack of availability of a spouse, child, or other relative who can serve as a caregiver, the caregiver's employment and/or poor health can play an important role in determining the need for institutional care.

A general physical examination should focus particularly on cardiovascular and neurologic assessment. Hypertension and other cardiovascular findings and focal neurologic signs (such as unilateral weakness or sensory deficit, hemianopia, Babinski reflex) favor a diagnosis of multi-infarct dementia. Pathologic reflexes (such as the glabellar sign and grasp, snout, and palmomental reflexes) are nonspecific and occur in many forms of dementia as well as in a small proportion of normal aged persons. These frontal lobe release signs—as well as impaired stereognosis or graphesthesia, gait disorder, and abnormalities on cerebellar testing—are significantly more com-

mon in patients with Alzheimer's disease than in age-matched controls (Huff et al., 1987). Parkinsonian signs (tremor, bradykinesia, muscle rigidity) should be sought because they may indicate either dementia associated with Lewy bodies or frank Parkinson's disease.

A careful mental status examination (Table 5-1) and a standardized mental status test should be performed. Although the AHCPR guidelines indicate that no single test is clearly superior, the Mini-Mental State Examination is most widely used by geriatricians and is the most comprehensive test (see Appendix). Neuropsychological testing can be helpful when there is a normal mental status score but also functional and/or behavioral changes (this can occur in patients with high baseline intelligence) or when there is a low score without functional deficits (this can occur in patients with lower educational levels). Neuropsychological testing can also be helpful in differentiating depression and dementia and in pinpointing specific cognitive strengths and weaknesses for patients, families, and health providers.

Selected diagnostic studies are useful in ruling out reversible forms of dementia (Table 5-13). Most of these studies were recommended by a National Institutes of Health Consensus Conference (1987). Although CT and MRI scans of the head are expensive, many clinicians and experts order them for patients with dementia of recent

Table 5-13 Evaluating dementia: Diagnostic studies

Blood studies
  Complete blood count
  Glucose
  Urea nitrogen
  Electrolytes
  Calcium and phosphorous
  Liver function tests
  Thyroid stimulating hormone
  Vitamin B_{12} and folate
  Serologic test for syphilis
  Human immunodeficiency virus antibodies (if suspected)

Radiographic studies
  Computed tomography (or magnetic resonance imaging) of the head

Other studies
  Neuropsychological testing (selected patients; see text)

onset in whom no other clinical findings explain the dementia and in those with focal neurologic signs or symptoms. Cerebral atrophy on one of these scans does not establish the diagnosis of Alzheimer's disease; it can occur with normal aging as well as with several specific disease processes. The scan is thus recommended to rule out treatable causes (e.g., subdural hematoma, tumors, normal-pressure hydrocephalus). Both CT and MRI have advantages and disadvantages. They are roughly equivalent in the detection of most remediable structural lesions. MRI will demonstrate more lesions than CT in patients with multi-infarct dementia but will also demonstrate white matter changes of uncertain clinical significance (NIH Consensus Conference, 1988; Small et al., 1997). Position emission tomography (PET) scanning is increasingly available but remains largely a research tool. PET scanning quantitates glucose metabolism and reveals decreases in specific areas (e.g., frontotemporal) that are highly associated with Alzheimer's disease. Some studies now suggest that PET scan abnormalities can precede the development of clinical deficits by several years in patients at risk for Alzheimer's disease.

MANAGEMENT OF DEMENTIA

General Principles

Although complete cure is not available for most forms of dementia, optimal management can provide improvements in the ability of these patients to function as well as in their overall well-being and that of their families and other caregivers. Key principles for the management of dementia are outlined in Table 5-14.

If causes of reversible or partially reversible forms of dementia are identified (Table 5-6), they should be specifically treated. Small strokes (lacunar infarcts), which can cause further deterioration of cognitive function in patients with AD as well as those with vascular dementia, may be prevented by controlling hypertension; thus hypertension should be aggressively treated in patients with dementia as long as side effects can be avoided. Other specific diseases such as Parkinson's disease should be optimally managed. The treatment of these and other medical conditions is especially challenging because it (usually drugs) may have adverse effects on cognitive function.

Table 5-14 Key principles in the management of dementia

Optimize the patient's function
  Treatment underlying medical conditions (e.g., hypertension, Parkinson's disease)
  Avoid use of drugs with CNS side effects (unless required for management of
    psychological or behavioral disturbances—see Chap. 13)
  Assess the environment and suggest alterations if necessary
  Encourage physical and mental activity
  Avoid situations stressing intellectual capabilities; use memory aids whenever
    possible
  Prepare the patient for changes in location
  Emphasize good nutrition

Identify and manage complications
  Wandering
  Dangerous driving
  Behavioral disorders
  Depression (see Chap. 6)
  Agitation or aggressiveness
  Psychosis (delusions, hallucinations)
  Malnutrition
  Incontinence (see Chap. 7)

Provide ongoing care
  Reassessment of cognitive and physical function
  Treatment of medical conditions

Provide medical information to patient and family
  Nature of the disease
  Extent of impairment
  Prognosis

Provide social service information to patient and family
  Local Alzheimer's association
  Community health care resources (day centers, homemakers, home health aides)
  Legal and financial counseling

Provide family counseling for
  Identification and resolution of family conflicts
  Handling anger and guilt
  Decisions on respite or institutional care
  Legal concerns
  Ethical concerns (see Chap. 16)

Pharmacologic Treatment of Dementia

There are three basic approaches to the pharmacologic treatment of dementia:

1. Agents that enhance cognition and function
2. Drug treatment of coexisting depression
3. Pharmacologic treatment of complications such as paranoia, delusions, psychoses, and agitation (verbal and physical)

Drug treatment of depression is discussed in detail in Chap. 6. Pharmacologic treatments including antipsychotics and sedatives are discussed in Chap. 13.

The primary pharmacologic approach to the treatment of AD has been the use of cholinesterase inhibitors. At the time of this revision, there are two approved drugs of this class on the market. Tacrine is a centrally active but nonspecific cholinesterase inhibitor. When given 10 to 40 mg of tacrine four times daily, 20 to 30 percent of patients have shown clinical improvement, representing an average 6 months of deterioration, as compared with placebo-treated patients. However, about 30 percent of patients have adverse effects (especially gastrointestinal) and about 20 percent have reversible elevations (three times above normal) of serum transaminases. Although 90 percent of patients can tolerate the drug after withdrawal and a rechallenge, monitoring transaminases levels adds substantially to the cost and inconvenience of drug therapy. Donepezil is a second-generation cholinesterase inhibitor with greater brain specificity. In placebo-controlled trials, this drug appears to enhance memory, orientation, language, and reasoning without hepatotoxicty. It is also more convenient than tacrine because it can be given once a day. The recommended starting dose is 5 mg per day, which can be increased to 10 mg after a month. The higher dose is associated with more gastrointestinal side effects (Small, et al., 1997). Other cholinesterase inhibitors are also being developed and studied.

Other drugs are also being used widely, such as the botanical agent EGb, an extract of ginkgo biloba (LeBars et al., 1997). This agent appears to have modest effects and is available over the counter. Vitamin E (alpha-tocopherol) and selegiline (an inhibitor of monoamine oxidase type B, used for Parkinson's disease) have been reported to delay progression of AD (Sano et al., 1997). The use of

nonsteroidal anti-inflammatory drugs and estrogen is also being explored because they appear to be protective against AD in epidemiologic studies. Newer neuroprotective agents and nerve growth factors are being developed but are not available at this time.

Nonpharmacologic Management

A variety of supportive measures and other nonpharmacologic management techniques have been found to be useful in improving the overall function and well-being of patients with dementia and their families (Table 5-14). These interventions range from specific recommendations such as alterations in the physical environment, the use of memory aids, the avoidance of stressful tasks, and preparation for the patient's move to another living setting with a higher level of care, to more general techniques such as providing information and counseling to the patient's family. Many nursing homes have developed "special care units" for dementia patients. With few exceptions, however (Rovner, 1996), there is little evidence that such units improve these patients' outcomes (Phillips et al., 1997). Assisted living facilities are now establishing specialized dementia units, with optimally designed environments, trained staff, and intensive activities programming and without the more hospital-like environment typical of many nursing homes.

The provision of ongoing care is especially important in the management of dementia patients. They are often abandoned by health professionals who find their problems uninteresting and difficult to manage. Reassessment of the patient's cognitive abilities can be helpful in identifying potentially reversible causes for deteriorating function and in making specific recommendations to family and other caregivers. The family is the primary target of strategies to help manage dementia patients in noninstitutional settings. Caring for relatives with dementia is physically, emotionally, and financially stressful. Information on the disease itself and the extent of impairment and on community resources helpful in managing these patients can be of critical importance to family and caregivers. The local chapter of the Alzheimer's Association and the Area Agency on Aging are examples of community resources that can provide education and linkages with appropriate services. Anticipating and teaching family members strategies to cope with common behavioral problems associated with dementia—such as wandering, incontinence, day-night reversal, and

nighttime agitation—can be of critical importance. Hazardous driving that can result in car crashes is an especially troublesome problem. Several states now require reporting patients with dementia who maintain a drivers' licenses. There remain, however, no validated methods of assessing driving capabilities and safety among individuals with early dementia. Wandering may be especially hazardous for the dementia patient's safety and is associated with falls. Incontience is common and often very difficult for families to manage (see Chap. 7). Books providing information and suggestions for family management techniques are very useful (see Suggested Readings). Support groups for families of patients with Alzheimer's disease through the Alzheimer's Association are available in most large cities. Family counseling can be helpful in dealing with a variety of issues such as anger, guilt, decisions on institutionalization, handling the patient's assets, and terminal care. Dementia patients and their families should also be encouraged to discuss and document their wishes, using a durable power of attorney for health care or an equivalent mechanism early in the course of the illness (see Chap. 16). Family members should be encouraged to seek respite care periodically that they can have time for themselves. Some communities have formal respite care programs available. In the absence of such programs, informal arrangements can often be made to relieve the primary family caregivers for short periods of time at regular intervals. Such relief will help the caregiver to cope with what is generally a very stressful situation. Often a multidisciplinary group of health professionals—made up of a physician, a nurse, a social worker, and, when needed, rehabilitation therapists, a lawyer, and a clergy member—must coordinate efforts to manage these patients and provide support to family and caregivers.

REFERENCES

American Psychiatric Association: *Diagnostic and Statistical Manual of Mental Disorders,* 4th ed. Washington, DC, APA, 1994.

Bachman DL, Wolf PA, Linn R, et al: Prevalence of dementia and probable senile dementia of the Alzheimer type in the Framingham Study. *Neurology* 42:115–119, 1992.

Clarfield AM: The reversible dementias: Do they reverse? *Ann Intern Med* 109:476–186, 1988.

Costa PT Jr, Williams TF, Somerfield M, et al: *Recognition and Initial Assessment of Alzheimer's Disease and Related Dementias.* Clinical Practice Guideline No. 19. Rockville, MD: U.S. Department of Health and Human Services, Public Health

Service, Agency for Health Care Policy and Research. AHCPR Publication No. 97-0702. November 1996.

Cutler NR, Duara R, Creasey H, et al: Brain imaging: Aging and dementia. *Ann Intern Med* 101:355–369, 1984.

Elie M, Cole MG, Primeau FJ, et al: Delirium risk factors in elderly hospitalized patients. *J Gen Intern Med* 13:204–212, 1998.

Erkinjuntti T, Ostbye T, Steenhuis R, et al: The effect of different diagnostic criteria on the prevalence of dementia. *N Engl J Med* 337:1667–1674, 1997.

Evans LK: Sundown syndrome in institutionalized elderly. *J Am Geriatr Soc* 35:101–108, 1987.

Evans DA, Funkenstein HH, Albert MS, et al: Prevalence of Alzheimer's disease in a community population of older persons: Higher than previously reported. *JAMA* 262:2551–2556, 1989.

Francis J: Delirium in older patients. *J Am Geriatr Soc* 40:829–838, 1992.

Francis J, Martin D, Kapoor WN: A prospective study of delirium in hospitalized elderly. *JAMA* 263:1097–1101, 1990.

Huff JF, Boller F, Lucchelli F, et al: The neurologic examination in patients with probable Alzheimer's disease. *Arch Neurol* 44:929–932, 1987.

Inouye SK, Charpentier PA: Precipitating factors of delirium in hospitalized elderly persons: Predictive model and interrerlationship with baseline vulnerability. *JAMA* 275:852–857, 1996.

Inouye SK, van Dyck CH, Alessi CA, et al: Clarifying confusion: The confusion assessment method: A new method for detection of delirium. *Ann Intern Med* 113:941–948, 1990.

Katzman R, Lasker B, Bernstein N: Advances in the diagnosis of dementia: Accuracy of diagnosis and consequences of misdiagnosis of disorders causing dementia, in Terry RD (ed): *Aging and the Brain.* New York, Raven Press, 1988.

Larson EB, Kukull WA, Buchner D, et al: Adverse drug reactions associated with global cognitive impairment in elderly persons. *Ann Intern Med* 107:169–173, 1987.

Lazarus LW, Newton N, Cohler B, et al: Frequency and presentation of depressive symptoms in patients with primary degenerative dementia. *Am J Psychiatry* 144:41–45, 1987.

LeBars PL, Katz MM, Berman N, et al: A placebo-controlled, double-blind, randomized trial of an extract of ginkgo biloba for dementia. *JAMA* 278:1327–1332, 1997.

Lipowski ZJ: Delirium (acute confusional states). *JAMA* 258:1789–1792, 1987.

Mayeux R, Saunders AM, Shea S, et al: Utility of the apolipoprotein E genotype in the diagnosis of Alzheimer's disease. *N Engl J Med* 338:506–511, 1998.

McKeith LG, Galasko D, Kosaka K, et al: Consensus guidelines for the clinical and pathologic diagnosis of dementia with lewy bodies (DLB): Report on the Consortium of DLB International Workshop. *Neurology* 47:1113–1124, 1996.

Merriam AR, Aronson MK, Gaston P, et al: The psychiatric symptoms of Alzheimer's disease. *J Am Geriatr Soc* 36:7–12, 1988.

NIH Consensus Conference: Differential diagnosis of dementing diseases. *JAMA* 258:3411–3416, 1987.

Phillips C, Sloane P, Hawes C, et al: Effects of residence in Alzheimer disease special care units on functional outcomes. *JAMA* 278:1340–1344, 1997.

Reifler BV, Larson E, Teri L, et al: Dementia of the Alzheimer's type and depression. *J Am Geriatr Soc* 34:855–859, 1986.

Roman GC: Senile dementia of the Binswanger type: A vascular form of dementia in the elderly. *JAMA* 258:1780–1788, 1987.

Rovner BW, German PS, Broadhead J, et al: The prevalence and management of dementia and other psychiatric disorders in nursing homes. *Int Psychogeriatr* 2:13–24, 1990.

Rovner BW, Steele CD, Shmuely Y, Folstein MF: A randomized trial of dementia care in nursing homes. *J Am Geriatric Soc* 44:7–13, 1996.

Rudberg MA, Pompei P, Foreman MD, et al: The natural history of delirium in older hospitalized patients: A syndrome of heterogeneity. *Age Ageing* 26:169–174, 1997.

Sano M, Ernesto C, Thomas RG, et al: A controlled trial of selegiline, alpha-tocopherol, or both as treatment for Alzheimer's disease. *N Engl J Med* 336:1216–1222, 1997.

Schor JD, Levkoff SE, Lipsitz LA, et al: Risk factors for delirium in hospitalized elderly. *JAMA* 267:827–831, 1992.

Small GW, Liston EH, Jarvik LF: Diagnosis and treatment of dementia in the aged. *West J Med* 135:469–481, 1981.

Small GW, Rabins PV, Barry PP, et al: Diagnosis and treatment of Alzheimer disease and related disorders. *JAMA* 278:1363–1371, 1997.

Snowdon DA, Greiner LH, Mortimer JA, et al: Brain infarction and the clinical expression of Alzheimer's disease: The nun study. *JAMA* 277:813–817, 1997.

Stedman's Medical Dictionary, 23d ed. Baltimore, MD: Williams & Wilkins, 1976.

Tang MX, Stern Y, Marder K, et al: The ApoE-E4 allele and the risk of Alzheimer disease among African Americans, whites, and hispanics. *JAMA* 279:751–755, 1998.

SUGGESTED READINGS

Carlson DL, Fleming KC, Smith GE, Evans JM: Management of dementia-related behavioral disturbances: A nonpharmacologic approach. *Mayo Clin Proc* 70:1108–1115, 1995.

Crum RM, Anthony JC, Bassett SS, Folstein MF: Population-based norms for the Mini-Mental State Examination by age and education level. *JAMA* 269:2386–2391, 1993.

Cummings JL, Benson FD: *Dementia: A Clinical Approach,* 2nd ed. Boston: Butterworths-Heineman, 1992.

Geldmacher DS, Whitehouse PJ: Evaluation of dementia. *N Engl J Med* 335:330–336, 1996.

Green RC: Alzheimer's disease and other dementing disorders in adults, in Joynt RJ (ed): *Clinical Neurology.* New York, Lippincott-Raven, 1995.

Jarvik LF, Small GW: *Parentcare.* New York, Crown, 1988.

Mace NL, Rabins PV: *The 36-Hour Day: A Family Guide to Caring for Persons with Alzheimer's Disease, Related Dementing Illnesses, and Memory Loss in Later Life.* Baltimore, MD, Johns Hopkins University Press, 1981.

Siu AL: Screening for dementia and investigating its causes. *Ann Intern Med* 115:122–132, 1991.

Teri L, Larson EB, Reifler BV: Behavioral disturbance in dementia of the Alzheimer's type. *J Am Geriatr Soc* 36:1–6, 1988.

Williams ME: *The American Geriatric Society's Complete Guide to Aging and Health.* New York: Harmony Books, 1995.

CHAPTER SIX

DIAGNOSIS AND MANAGEMENT OF DEPRESSION

Depression is probably the most common example of the nonspecific and atypical presentation of illness in the geriatric population. The signs and symptoms can be the result of a variety of treatable physical illnesses or the presenting manifestations of depression or a related condition that requires specific diagnosis and management. Frequently depression and physical illness(es) coexist in older patients. Thus, it is not surprising that treatable depressions are often overlooked in geriatric patients with physical illnesses and that treatable physical illnesses are often not managed optimally in geriatric patients diagnosed as having depression.

Sorting out the complex interrelationships between symptoms and signs of depression caused by physical illnesses and those caused primarily by an affective disorder or related psychiatric diagnosis challenges individuals caring for the geriatric population. Recognition and appropriate management of the onset or recurrence of geriatric depression are critical for improving quality of life and function as well as for potentially preventing medical morbidity, optimizing health care utilization, and forestalling premature death. This chapter ad-

dresses these issues from the perspective of the nonpsychiatrist, recognizing that the optimal management of most of these patients should involve psychiatrists and psychologists experienced with and interested in the geriatric population.

AGING AND DEPRESSION

Symptoms and signs of depression are common in the geriatric population (NIH Consensus Conference, 1991). The prevalence of major depression among community-dwelling older people is 1 to 2 percent, and an additional 2 percent suffer from dysthymia. The prevalence of subsyndromal depression (i.e., symptoms of depression that do not meet standard criteria for depression) approaches 25 percent (Lebowitz et al., 1997). The prevalence of these conditions is even higher among the geriatric patients in acute care hospitals and nursing homes. Major depression is found in up to 22 percent and other depressive syndromes in up to 28 percent of acutely hospitalized older patients (Koenig et al., 1988; Koenig, 1997). Among institutionalized older persons, major depression is found in close to 15 percent, with another 15 to 20 percent having depressive symptoms; incidence rates of these disorders in nursing homes are in a similar range (Rovner et al., 1991; Parmalee et al., 1989; Parmalee et al., 1992a). Depression is highly associated with mortality in the nursing home population (Rovner et al., 1991; Parmalee et al., 1992b). Suicide is disturbingly common in the geriatric population and its incidence continues to increase. Older white males have the highest rate of suicide—up to six times that in the general population (Osgood, 1985; Lebowitz et al., 1997). Several factors are associated with suicide in the geriatric population (Table 6-1).

Several biological, physical, psychological, and sociological factors predispose older persons to depression (Table 6-2). Aging changes in the central nervous system, such as increased monoamine oxidase activity and decreased neurotransmitter concentrations (especially catecholaminergic neurotransmitters), may play a role in the development of geriatric depression. Current research is focusing on the central nervous system effects of cytokines (particularly interleukin-1b), cortisol production, inflammation and other immune responses, and the role these effects may play in the genesis of depression among medically ill geriatric patients (Lebowitz et al., 1997).

Table 6-1 Factors associated with suicide in the geriatric population

Factor	High risk	Low risk
Sex	Male	Female
Religion	Protestant	Catholic or Jewish
Race	White	Nonwhite
Marital status	Widowed or divorced	Married
Occupational background	Blue-collar low-paying job	Professional or white-collar job
Current employment status	Retired or unemployed	Employed full or part time
Living environment	Urban Living alone Isolated Recent move	Rural Living with spouse or other relatives Living in close-knit neighborhood
Physical health	Poor health Terminal illness Pain and suffering	Good health
Mental health	Depression (current or previous) Alcoholism Low self-esteem Loneliness Feeling rejected, unloved	Happy and well adjusted Positive self-concept and outlook Sense of personal control over life
Personal background	Broken home Dependent personality History of poor interpersonal relationships Family history of mental illness Poor marital history Poor work record	Intact family of origin Independent, assertive, flexible personality History of close friendships No family history of mental illness No previous suicide attempts No history of suicide in family Good marital history Good work record

Source: From Osgood, 1985, with permission.

Table 6-2   Factors predisposing older people to depression

Biological
  Family history (genetic predisposition)
  Prior episode(s) of depression
  Aging changes in neurotransmission
  Effects of cytokines on central nervous system

Physical
  Specific diseases (see Table 6-5)
  Chronic medical conditions (especially with pain or loss of function)
  Exposure to drugs (see Table 6-6)
  Sensory deprivation (loss of vision or hearing)
  Loss of physical function

Psychological
  Unresolved conflicts (e.g., anger, guilt)
  Memory loss and dementia
  Personality disorders

Social
  Losses of family and friends (bereavement)
  Isolation
  Loss of job
  Loss of income

The incidence of several specific diseases associated with symptoms of depression, the prevalence of chronic medical conditions, and the frequency of medication usage increase with age. Each of these factors can predispose older people to depression. Vascular disease in particular may play an important role in geriatric depression. Depressed geriatric patients often have comorbid vascular disorders accompanied by lesions in the basal ganglia and prefrontal areas of the brain. These patients commonly display motor retardation, lack of insight, and impairment of executive functions (Lebowitz et al., 1997).

Other psychosocial factors also predispose older people to depression. Losses are common in the geriatric population. Physical losses can mean a reduction in the ability for self-care, often leading to loss of independence; markedly reduced sensory capacities (especially vision and hearing) can result in isolation and sensory deprivation. Both can play a role in the development of depression. Memory loss and loss of other intellectual functions (dementia) are commonly associated with depression (see Chap. 5). Losses of job, income, and

social supports (especially the death of family members and friends) increase with age and can predispose older people to bereavement and frank depression.

SYMPTOMS AND SIGNS OF DEPRESSION

Many common symptoms and signs can represent depression in geriatric patients. Several factors may make these difficult to interpret:

- Aging changes, as well as several common medical conditions, can lead to the physical appearance of depression, even when depression is not present.
- Nonspecific physical symptoms (such as fatigue, weakness, anorexia, diffuse pain) may represent a variety of treatable medical illnesses as well as depression.
- Specific physical symptoms, relating to every major organ system, can represent depression as well as physical illness in geriatric patients.
- Depression can exacerbate symptoms of coexisting physical illnesses.

The physical appearance of older patients suspected of being depressed should be interpreted cautiously. Aging changes such as graying and loss of hair, wrinkled skin, loss of teeth (with altered facial architecture), stooped posture, and slowed gait can present an image of depression. Several medical conditions can further emphasize the physical appearance of depression. Parkinson's disease, which manifests itself by masked facies, bradykinesia, and stooped posture, can be misinterpreted as depression. Patients with presbycusis may appear withdrawn and disinterested simply because they cannot hear enough of normal conversation to participate actively; therefore they withdraw out of frustration. The psychomotor retardation of hypothyroidism may offer the physical appearance of depression. Systemic illnesses—such as disseminated tuberculosis, malignancy, and malnutrition (alone or resulting from a medical condition)—can produce a depressed appearance. Moreover, true depression commonly accompanies many of these medical conditions in geriatric patients (Small et al., 1996; Koenig, 1997).

Symptoms must also be interpreted very cautiously. Many different symptoms can represent depression, physical illness, or a combination of both. Table 6-3 lists several examples of somatic symptoms that may actually represent, or be exacerbated by, depression in older patients. Depression presenting primarily with physical symptoms, termed *masked depression,* is especially common in the geriatric population for several reasons. Many of today's older generation were raised in an atmosphere that inhibited the expression of emotion. Finding direct expression of feelings of sadness, guilt, and anger difficult, they may somatasize these emotions and complain of physical symptoms. In addition, many older persons with diminished sensory input from losses of vision, hearing, or touch may overrespond to

Table 6-3 Examples of physical symptoms that can represent depression

System	Symptom
General	Fatigue
	Weakness
	Anorexia
	Weight loss
	Anxiety
	Insomnia (see Table 6-4)
	"Pain all over"
Cardiopulmonary	Chest pain
	Shortness of breath
	Palpitations
	Dizziness
Gastrointestinal	Abdominal pain
	Constipation
Genitourinary	Frequency
	Urgency
	Incontinence
Musculoskeletal	Diffuse pain
	Back pain
Neurologic	Headache
	Memory disturbance
	Dizziness
	Paresthesias

internal cues (such as their heartbeat and gastrointestinal motility) and focus on these concerns when they are feeling anxious and depressed.

Insomnia is an example of a very common yet nonspecific symptom in the geriatric population. Although it is one of the key symptoms in diagnosing different forms of depression, a variety of factors may underlie this complaint (Table 6-4). Persistent complaints of sleep disturbance are, in fact, associated with depression among community-dwelling older people (Newman et al., 1997). In addition to depression, insomnia may be caused by other psychiatric disorders as well as several types of medical problems. For example, orthopnea and noctu-

Table 6-4 Key factors in evaluating the complaint of insomnia

Sleep disturbance should be carefully characterized
    Delayed sleep onset
    Frequent awakenings
    Early-morning awakenings

Physical symptoms can underlie insomnia (from patient and bed partner)
    Symptoms of physical illnesses
        Pain from musculoskeletal disorders
        Orthopnea, paroxysmal nocturnal dyspnea or cough
        Nocturia
        Gastroesophageal reflux
    Symptoms suggestive of nocturnal myoclonus
        Periodic leg movements
    Symptoms suggestive of sleep apnea
        Loud or irregular snoring
        Awakening sweating, anxious, tachycardiac
        Excessive movement
        Morning drowsiness

Aging changes occurring in sleep patterns
    Increased sleep latency
    Decreased time in deeper stages of sleep
    Increased awakenings

Behavioral factors can affect sleep patterns
    Daytime naps
    Earlier bedtime

Medications can affect sleep
    Hypnotic withdrawal
    Alcohol (causes sleep fragmentation)

ria caused by congestive heart failure, abdominal discomfort from reflux esophagitis, or anxiety and restlessness from hyperthyroidism can underlie the complaint of insomnia. A careful history should help identify these and other medical conditions that might be contributing to the problem. Insomnia can also be caused by the effects of (or withdrawal from) several types of drugs and alcohol. As more older patients with sleep disturbances have undergone detailed analysis (including continuous observation during sleep and monitoring by polysomnography), other conditions have been detected, including sleep apnea and nocturnal myoclonus. As many as one-third of the geriatric population may have a specific sleep disorder (Dement et al., 1982). Obstructive sleep apnea is the most common of these disorders and results not only in complaints of insomnia but also in nighttime hypoxia with associated risks for cardiac arrhythmias and myocardial and cerebral infarction. Specific symptoms, which are often elicited from the bed partner, should prompt consideration for referral to a sleep center, because hypnotics may exacerbate the conditions. Other more specific treatments are available, including nasal continuous positive airway pressure and uvulopalatopharyngeoplasty. Aging itself is associated with changes in sleep patterns, such as daytime naps, early bedtime, increased time until onset of sleep, decreases in the absolute and relative amounts of the deeper stages of sleep, and increased periods of wakefulness, which could contribute to the complaint of insomnia. Thus there is a lengthy differential diagnosis of insomnia in the older patient; the complaint should not be attributed simply to aging or depression and treated with a sedating antidepressant or hypnotic before other potential causes are considered.

DEPRESSION ASSOCIATED WITH MEDICAL CONDITIONS

Symptoms and signs of depression are associated with medical conditions in the geriatric population in several ways:

- Some diseases can result in the physical appearance of depression, even when depression is not present (e.g., Parkinson's disease).

- Many diseases can either directly cause depression or elicit a reaction of depression. The latter is especially true of conditions that cause or produce fear of chronic pain, disability, and dependence.
- Drugs used to treat medical conditions can cause symptoms and signs of depression.
- The environment (factors such as isolation, sensory deprivation, forced dependency) in which medical conditions are treated can predispose to depression.

Depression among older patients with medical illnesses is associated with high levels of functional impairment (Covinsky et al., 1997) and health care costs (Unutzer et al., 1997). A wide variety of physical illnesses can present with or be accompanied by symptoms and signs of depression (Table 6-5). Any medical condition associated with systemic involvement and metabolic disturbances can have profound effects on mental function and affect. The most common among these are fever, dehydration, decreased cardiac output, electrolyte disturbances, and hypoxia. Hyponatremia (whether from disease process or drugs) and hypercalcemia (associated especially with malignancy) may also cause older patients to appear depressed. Systemic diseases, especially malignancies and endocrine disorders, are often associated with symptoms of depression. Depression—accompanied by anorexia, weight loss, and back pain—is commonly present in patients with cancer of the pancreas. These patients often lack the feelings of guilt, agitation, delusions, memory impairment, and suicidal thoughts that can accompany depression in later years. Among the endocrine disorders, thyroid and parathyroid conditions are most commonly accompanied by symptoms of depression. Most hypothyroid patients manifest psychomotor retardation, irritability, or depression. Hyperthyroidism may also present as withdrawal and depression in older patients—so-called apathetic thyrotoxicosis. Hyperparathyroidism, with attendant hypercalcemia, can simulate depression and is often manifest by apathy, fatigue, bone pain, and constipation. Other systemic physical conditions—such as infectious diseases, anemia, and nutritional deficiencies—can also have prominent manifestations of depression in the geriatric population.

Because cardiovascular and nervous system diseases are among the most threatening and potentially disabling, they can precipitate symptoms of depression. Myocardial infarction, with attendant fear

Table 6-5 Medical illnesses associated with depression

Metabolic disturbances
  Dehydration
  Azotemia, uremia
  Acid-base disturbances
  Hypoxia
  Hypo- and hypernatremia
  Hypo- and hyperglycemia
  Hypo- and hypercalcemia

Endocrine
  Hypo- and hyperthyroidism
  Hyperparathyroidism
  Diabetes mellitus
  Cushing's disease
  Addison's disease

Infections

Cardiovascular
  Congestive heart failure
  Myocardial infarction

Pulmonary
  Chronic obstructive lung disease
  Malignancy

Gastrointestinal
  Malignancy (especially pancreatic)
  Irritable bowel

Genitourinary
  Urinary incontinence

Musculoskeletal
  Degenerative arthritis
  Osteoporosis with vertebral compression or hip fracture
  Polymyalgia rheumatica
  Paget's disease

Neurologic
  Dementia (all types)
  Parkinson's disease
  Stroke
  Tumors

Other
  Anemia (of any cause)
  Vitamin deficiencies
  Hematologic or other systemic malignancy

Source: From Levenson and Hall, 1981, with permission.

of shortened life span and restricted lifestyle, commonly precipitates depression. Stroke is often accompanied by depression, but the depression may not always correlate with the extent of physical disability. Patients in whom stroke has produced substantial disability (e.g., hemiparesis, aphasia) can become depressed in response to their loss of function; others whose stroke has produced only minor degrees of physical disability (but in theory may have affected areas of the brain controlling emotion) can also become depressed. Other causes of brain damage, especially in the frontal lobes, such as tumors and subdural hematomas, can also be associated with depression. Older individuals with dementia, both Alzheimer's and multi-infarct dementia, may have prominent symptoms of depression (see Chap. 5). Patients with Parkinson's disease also have a high incidence of clinically diagnosed depression. Depression that develops in response to the chronic pain, loss of function and self-esteem, dependence, and fear of death that accompany physical illness can become severe. Many older individuals who commit suicide have an active physical illness at the time of death (Osgood, 1985).

Symptoms of depression are often caused not only by physical illness and in response to it but also by the treatment of medical conditions. A variety of psychological responses to hospitalization (including depression) have been observed in the older patients. Isolation, sensory deprivation, and immobilization, common in hospitalized patients with physical illness, can cause or contribute to depressive symptoms. Iatrogenic complications such as fecal impaction and urinary retention or incontinence can also cause psychological symptoms, including those of depression. Drugs are the most common cause of treatment-induced symptoms and signs of depression. Although a wide variety of pharmacologic agents can produce symptoms of depression (Table 6-6), antihypertensive agents and sedatives are probably the most common drugs that cause symptoms and signs of depression in the geriatric population. The mechanisms by which various drugs cause these effects differ and are poorly understood in many instances. Some drugs—such as alcohol, sedatives, antipsychotics, and antihypertensives—have direct effects on the central nervous system. Thus, depressive symptoms, especially new symptoms, should raise a high index of suspicion about the role of drug and/or alcohol abuse. Whenever possible, drugs that can potentially produce these symptoms should be discontinued.

Table 6-6 Drugs that can cause symptoms of depression

Antihypertensives	Psychotropic agents
Reserpine	Sedatives
Propranolol	Barbiturates
Clonidine	Benzodiazepines
Hydralazine	Meprobamate
Analgesics	Antipsychotics
Narcotics	Chlorpromazine
	Haloperidol
Antiparkinsonism drugs	Thiothixene
Levodopa	Hypnotics
Antimicrobials	Chloral hydrate
Sulfonamides	Benzodiazepines
Isoniazid	Steroids
Cardiovascular preparations	Corticosteroids
Digitalis	Estrogens
Diuretics	Others
Lidocaine	Cimetidine
Hypoglycemic agents	Cancer chemotherapeutic agents
	Alcohol

Source: From Levenson and Hall, 1981, with permission.

DIAGNOSING DEPRESSION

In view of the prevalence of symptoms and signs of depression in the geriatric population; aging changes that may complicate the diagnosis; and the interrelationship between depression and its signs and symptoms, medical illnesses, and treatment effects—how is the diagnosis of depression made?

Several general principles can be helpful:

- Questions that screen for depressive symptoms, or the use of a depression scale, may be helpful in identifying depressed geriatric patients. However, somatic components of many depression scales are less useful in older patients because of the high prevalence of physical symptoms and medical illnesses.
- Nonspecific or multiple somatic symptoms that are suggestive of depression should not be diagnosed as such until physical illnesses have been excluded.

- Somatic symptoms unexplained by physical findings or diagnostic studies, especially those of relatively sudden onset in an older person who is not usually hypochondriacal, should raise the suspicion of depression.
- Drugs used to treat medical illnesses (Table 6-6), sedatives, hypnotics, and alcohol abuse should be considered as potential causes for symptoms and signs of depression.
- Standard diagnostic criteria should be the basis for diagnosing various forms of depression in the geriatric population, but several differences may distinguish depressions in older as opposed to younger patients.
- Major depressive episodes should be differentiated from other diagnoses such as uncomplicated bereavement, bipolar disorder, dysthymic disorder, and adjustment disorders with a depressed mood.
- Consultation with experienced geriatric psychiatrists and/or psychologists should be obtained whenever possible to help diagnose and manage depressive disorders.
- Whenever there is uncertainty about the diagnosis, a judicious (but adequate) therapeutic trial of an antidepressant can be very helpful.

The *Diagnostic and Statistical Manual of Mental Disorders* of the American Psychiatric Association (DSM-IV) (American Psychiatric Association, 1994) lists several classifications and diagnoses that are useful to describe depressions in the geriatric population (Table 6-7). Several differences in the presentation of such depression can make the diagnosis much more challenging and difficult (Table 6-8). The most common clinical problem is differentiating major depressive episodes from other forms of depression. Some of the key features that can aid in this are shown in Table 6-9. In addition, as many as one-quarter of community-dwelling and one-half of medically ill older patients and nursing home residents suffer from "subsyndromal depressions" (Table 6-7). While the depressive symptoms may not be as severe as in major depression, they are associated with the development of major depression, physical disability, and heavy use of health services (Lebowitz et al., 1997).

Like the early stages of dementia, depression may go unrecognized unless specific questions are asked. It is well known that many older patients who commit suicide have been seen by their physicians

Table 6-7 Diagnostic criteria for depression

Major depressive episode
  A. At least five of the following symptoms have been present nearly every day, for most of the day, during the same 2-week period and represent a change from previous functioning; at least one of the symptoms is either (1) depressed mood or (2) loss of interest or pleasure.
     1. Depressed mood, as indicated by either subjective report or observations made by others
     2. Markedly diminished interest or pleasure in all or almost all activities
     3. Significant weight loss or gain when not dieting (e.g., more than 5% of body weight in a month) or decrease or increase of appetite
     4. Insomnia or hypersomnia
     5. Psychomotor agitation or retardation
     6. Fatigue or loss of energy
     7. Feelings of worthlessness or excessive or inappropriate guilt (which may be delusional; not merely self-reproach or guilt about being sick)
     8. Diminished ability to think or concentrate; indecisiveness
     9. Recurrent thoughts of death (not just fear of dying), recurrent suicidal ideation without a specific plan, or a suicide attempt, or a specific plan for committing suicide
  B. The symptoms cause clinically significant distress or impairment in daily activities, social life, or other important areas of functioning.
  C. The symptoms are not due to the direct effects of a substance (e.g., drugs of abuse, medication) or a general medical condition.

Dysthymic disorders
  A. Depressed or irritable mood present most of the day, more than half the time, for at least 2 years, associated with significant distress or impairment in important areas of functioning.
  B. Mood disturbance is accompanied by at least two other symptoms, including disturbed appetite or sleep, fatigue or low energy, low self-esteem, concentration problems, or hopelessness.
  C. Major depression is not present, and disturbance is not due to a major depression in partial remission.
  D. No history of mania or hypomania; psychosis is not present.
  E. Symptoms are not due to the direct physiologic effects of substance or general medical condition (e.g., hypothyroidism or cancer chemotherapy).

Depression not otherwise specified
DSM-IV recognizes several subsyndromal depressions, including the following:
  A. *Minor depressive disorder:* Episodes of 2 weeks or more of depressive symptoms, but with fewer than the five items required for major depressive disorder.
  B. *Recurrent brief depressive disorder:* Meets all criteria for major depression except duration. Episodes last from 2 days to 2 weeks and occur intermittently, but at least monthly for a year.
  C. *Other depressions:* The clinician cannot determine whether depression is primary or secondary (due to direct effects of a substance or medical illness).

Source: From the American Psychiatric Association, 1994, with permission.

Table 6-8 Some differences in the presentation of depression in the older compared with the younger population

1. Somatic complaints, rather than psychological symptoms, often predominate in the clinical picture.
2. Older patients often deny having a dysphoric mood.
3. Apathy and withdrawal are common.
4. Feelings of guilt are less common.
5. Loss of self-esteem is prominent.
6. Inability to concentrate, with resultant impairment of memory and other cognitive functions, is common (see Chap. 5).

Table 6-9 Major depression versus other forms of depression

Diagnostic classification	Key features distinguishing from major depression
Bipolar disorders	The patient may meet, or have met in the past, criteria for major depression but is having or has had one more manic episode; the latter are characterized by distinct periods of a relatively persistent elevated or irritable mood and other symptoms such as increased activity, restlessness, talkativeness, flight of ideas, inflated self-esteem, and distractibility.
Cyclothymic disorder	There are numerous periods during which symptoms of depression and mania are present but not of sufficient severity or duration to meet the criteria for a major depressive or manic episode; in addition to a loss of interest and pleasure in most activities, the periods of depression are accompanied by other symptoms such as fatigue, insomnia or hypersomnia, social withdrawal, pessimism, and tearfulness.
Dysthymic disorder	Patient usually exhibits a prominently depressed mood, marked loss of interest or pleasure in most activities, and other symptoms of depression; the symptoms are not of sufficient severity or duration to meet the criteria for a major depressive episode, and the periods of depression may be separated by up to a few months of normal mood.

Table 6-9 Major depression versus other forms of depression
(Continued)

Diagnostic classification	Key features distinguishing from major depression
Adjustment disorder with depressed mood	The patient exhibits a depressed mood, tearfulness, hopelessness, or other symptoms in excess of a normal response to an identifiable psychosocial or physical stressor; the response is not an exacerbation of another psychiatric condition, occurs within 3 months of the onset of the stressor, eventually remits after the stressor ceases (or the patient adapts to the stressor), and does not meet the criteria for other forms of depression or uncomplicated bereavement.
Uncomplicated bereavement	This is a depressive syndrome that arises in response to the death of a loved one—its onset is not more than 2 to 3 months after the death, and the symptoms last for variable periods of time; the patient generally regards the depression as a normal response—guilt and thoughts of death refer directly to the loved one; morbid preoccupation with worthlessness, marked or prolonged functional impairment, and marked psychomotor retardation are uncommon and suggest the development of major depression.

within the previous few weeks. At a minimum, all geriatric patients should periodically be asked such a screening question. Specific questions about other common depressive symptoms can also be added to the system review (e.g., sleep disturbance, appetite changes, trouble concentrating, lack of energy, loss of interest). Positive responses should be followed up by further questioning, especially about suicidal ideation. Examples of screening questions are shown in Table 6-10. A commonly used depression scale is provided in the Appendix.

Because of the overlap of symptoms and signs of depression and physical illness and the close association between many medical conditions and depression, older patients presenting with what appears to be a depression should have physical illnesses carefully excluded. This can almost always be accomplished by a thorough history,

Table 6-10   Examples of screening questions for depression

For each of the following questions, which description comes closest to the way you have been feeling *during the past month?*

	All the time	Most of the time	Some of the time	A little of the time	None of the time
a. How much of the time *during the past month* have you been a very nervous person?	1	2	3	4	5
b. *During the past month,* how much of the time have you felt calm and peaceful?	1	2	3	4	5
c. How much of the time *during the past month* have you felt downhearted and blue?	1	2	3	4	5
d. *During the past month,* how much of the time have you been a happy person?	1	2	3	4	5
e. How often *during the past month* have you felt so down in the dumps that nothing could cheer you up?	1	2	3	4	5
f. *During the past month,* how often did you feel like life isn't worth living anymore?	1	2	3	4	5

Source: Adapted from Stewart et al., 1988, with permission.

physical examination, and basic laboratory studies (Table 6-11). Other diagnostic studies can provide helpful objective data in patients with persistent somatic symptoms that are difficult to distinguish from psychosomatic complaints (e.g., masked depression). For example, echocardiography and radionuclide cardiac scans can help rule out organic heart disease as a basis for chest pain, fatigue, and dyspnea. Pulmonary function tests can exclude intrinsic lung disease as a cause for chronic shortness of breath. A new complaint of constipation may

Table 6-11 Diagnostic studies helpful in evaluating apparently depressed geriatric patients with somatic symptoms

Basic evaluation
History
Physical examination
Complete blood count
Erythrocyte sedimentation rate
Serum electrolytes, glucose, and calcium
Renal function tests
Liver function tests
Thyroid function tests

Examples of other potentially helpful studies	
Symptom or sign	Diagnostic study
Pain	Appropriate radiologic procedure (e.g., bone film, bone scan, GI series)
Chest pain	ECG, noninvasive cardiovascular studies (e.g., exercise stress test, echocardiography, radionuclide scans)
Shortness of breath	Chest films, pulmonary function tests, pulse oximetry arterial blood gases
Constipation	Test for occult blood in stool, barium enema, thyroid function tests
Focal neurologic signs or symptoms	CT or MRI scan EEG

be related to depression but may also be caused by hypothyroidism or colonic disease; thus a test for occult blood in the stool, barium enema or colonoscopy, and thyroid function tests can be helpful in the evaluation of this symptom.

MANAGEMENT

General Considerations

Several treatment modalities are available to manage depression in older persons (Table 6-12). Both pharmacologic treatment and psy-

Table 6-12 Treatment modalities for geriatric depression

Nonpharmacologic
Supportive measures
   Information and encouragement
   Environmental alterations
   Activities (physical and mental)
   Involvement of family and friends
   Ongoing interest and care

Psychotherapy
   Individual
   Group

Electroconvulsive

Pharmacologic

Antidepressants (see Table 6-12)

Sedatives for associated anxiety or agitation (see Chap. 13)

Antipsychotics for associated psychoses (see Chap. 13)

chotherapy have some effectiveness in mild to moderate depression in the outpatient geriatric population (McCusker et al., 1998). The choice of treatment(s) for an individual patient depends on many factors, including the primary disorder causing the depression, the severity of symptoms, the availability and practicality of the various treatment modalities, and underlying conditions that might contraindicate a specific form of treatment (e.g., disorders of vision and hearing that make psychotherapy difficult or severe cardiovascular disease that precludes the use of certain antidepressants).

When a specific active medical condition or drug is suspected as the cause of or contributor to the symptoms and signs of depression, these factors should be attended to before other therapies are initiated unless the depression is severe enough to warrant immediate treatment (e.g., the patient is delusional or suicidal). Treatment of the medical condition should be optimized and all drugs that could be worsening the depression should be discontinued if medically feasible.

Nonpharmacologic Management

Supportive measures, such as those listed in Table 6-12, and psychotherapy are often ignored, but they can be very helpful in manag-

ing mildly depressed patients; they may also be useful adjuncts to other treatments for patients with more severe depressions. Standard approaches to psychotherapy, such as cognitive-behavioral therapy and interpersonal therapy, have been shown to be effective in depressed geriatric patients. However, no single approach appears to be more effective than others (Lebowitz et al., 1997). Geriatric patients with depressions caused by uncomplicated bereavement, adjustment disorders related to a psychosocial stress (retirement, family conflicts, etc.) or physical conditions (myocardial infarction, stroke, hip fracture, etc.), dysthymic disorder, and subsyndromal depressions may respond well to supportive measures and psychotherapeutic approaches.

Many depressed patients have hearing impairments, other physical disabilities, or cognitive impairment that can make group and individual psychotherapy difficult. Behavioral treatment may be effective in some dementia patients who are depressed (Teri et al., 1997). Outpatient psychiatric "partial hospitalization" programs are available in many communities and may be especially helpful in managing frail depressed patients who are isolated during the day.

If pharmacologic treatment is contraindicated by medical conditions or fails or if rapid relief from depression is desired (as might be the case in delusional, suicidal, or extremely vegetative patients), electroconvulsive therapy (ECT) should be considered. ECT is relatively safe and can be highly effective in the geriatric population. Certain added precautions are necessary in older patients with hypertension and cardiac arrhythmias (such as close cardiac monitoring and diminished doses of pretreatment atropine), and cardiology consultation is advisable in these situations. Adequate pretreatment muscle relaxation will help avoid musculoskeletal complications, which are of special concern in those patients with osteoporosis. Posttreatment confusion and memory loss is usually mild and improves as the depression subsides. Many experts recommend unilateral ECT for the older depressed patients, feeling that it may cause fewer problems with memory and have the same clinical effectiveness.

Pharmacologic Treatment

When symptoms and signs of depression are of sufficient severity and duration to meet the criteria for major depression (Table 6-7), or if the depression is producing marked functional disability or interfering

with recovery from other illnesses, drug treatment should be considered. When pharmacologic treatment is initially considered, the patient and family should be educated to understand that an adequate therapeutic trial may take at least 4 to 6 weeks. If this is not discussed, patients may become discouraged by a lack of a rapid response to therapy.

Several types of drugs are available to treat depression in the geriatric population (Table 6-13). While many antidepressants have been studied in these patients, limitations in study designs, outcome measures, patient characteristics, and sample sizes make the clinical utility of several of these agents difficult to assess (Rigler et al., 1998). Experts recommend at least 6 months of therapy beyond recovery for patients with their first onset of depression in late life and at least 12 months for those with recurrent depression. Some older patients with recurrent depression may need to be treated indefinitely (Lebowitz et al., 1997).

The selective serotonin reuptake inhibitors (SSRIs) have largely replaced tricyclics as the first-line drug treatment for geriatric depression. Studies suggest that these agents are useful in treating depressed older people, but they have not been well studied in frail and medically ill geriatric patients. All SSRIs are metabolized by the liver and excreted by the kidney. Fluoxetine and its partially active metabolite have especially long half-lives. In addition, fluoxetine and paroxetine are potent inhibitors of the hepatic cytochrome P450 microsomal enzyme system. Toxicity can occur when these drugs are used concurrently with drugs that are metabolized by this system. Elevated levels or toxicity can occur with several drugs used relatively commonly in the geriatric population, including:

- Antiarrhythmics (type 1C)
- Anticonvulsants
- Antipsychotics
- Astemizole
- Benzodiazepines
- Beta blockers
- Calcium-channel blockers
- Carbamazepine
- Cisapride
- Codeine
- Erythromycin

- Oral hypoglycemics
- Terfenidine
- Theophylline
- Tricyclics
- Warfarin

The major side effects of SSRIs include gastrointestinal symptoms (nausea, vomiting, diarrhea), agitation, weight loss, sexual dysfunction, akathisia, and parkinsonian effects. These agents are also associated with the syndrome of inappropriate antidiuretic hormone (SIADH) and may thus cause or contribute to hyponatremia.

Tricyclic antidepressants are probably as effective as SSRIs, but they have anticholinergic and potential cardiovascular side effects. These include dry mouth, constipation, gastroesophageal reflux, blurred vision, cognitive impairment, tachycardia, and postural hypotension. In one study of older depressed patients with ischemic heart disease, paroxetine was associated with significantly fewer adverse cardiac events (2%) than nortriptyline (18%) (Roose et al., 1998). Postural hypotension is a special concern in frail geriatric patients already at risk for falls. Tricyclics, like SSRIs, are associated with SIADH.

Other new antidepressants—such as venlafaxine, buproprion, mirtazepine, and nefazadone—are available (Table 6-13). Early experience with these drugs suggest that they may be useful in geriatric depression. Both venlafaxine and mirtazepine should be used carefully in patients with underlying hypertension. Nefazadone may be useful in depressed older patients with prominent anxiety. This drug cannot, however, be used in conjunction with cisapride or the antihistamines terfenadine and astemizole, as it inhibits their metabolism and may thereby lead to life-threatening ventricular arrhythmias.

Methylphenidate (Ritalin) in small doses (10 mg one to three times a day) has been effective and safe in some geriatric patients with retarded depressions and cardiovascular disease (Katon and Raskind, 1980). Its effects may diminish over time, and anorexia can be a side effect. Monoamine oxidase inhibitors (such as isocarboxazid, phenelzine, and tranylcypromine) have been used in geriatric patients but necessitate a relatively strict diet (avoidance of tyramine-rich foods) and can cause prominent hypotension. SSRIs must be discontinued 2 weeks (6 weeks for fluoxetine) before initiating treatment with one of these drugs.

Table 6-13 Characteristics of selected antidepressants for geriatric patients

Drug*	Recommended starting daily dosage	Daily dosage range	Level of sedation	Elimination half-life[†]	Comments
Selective serotonin reuptake inhibitors					
Fluoxetine (Prozac)	5–10 mg	20–60 mg	Very low	Very long	Inhibits hepatic cytochrome P450[‡] Must be discontinued 6 weeks before initiating monamine oxidase inhibitor
Paroxetine (Paxil)	10 mg	10–50 mg	Very low	Long	Inhibits hepatic cytochrome P450[‡] Has anticholinergic side effects
Sertraline (Zoloft)	25 mg	50–200 mg	Very low	Very long	Less inhibition of cytochrome P450
Serotonin-norepinephrine reuptake blockers					
Venlafaxine (Effexor)	25 mg	75–225 mg	Very low	Intermediate	Reduced clearance with renal or hepatic impairment Can cause dose-related hypertension Must be tapered over 1–2 weeks when discontinuing

Tricyclic antidepressants				
Imipramine (Tofranil, others)	10–30 mg	25–150 mg	Mild–moderate	Long	Moderate anticholinergic side effects§ May be useful in treating urinary incontinence
Nortriptyline (Pamelor, others)	10–30	25–150 mg	Mild	Long	Lower but still substantial anticholinergic effects§ Blood levels can be monitored
Other agents†					
Buproprion (Wellbutrin)	50–100 mg	150–450 mg	Mild	Intermediate	
Mirtazepine (Remeron)	15 mg	15–45 mg	Mild	Long	Reduced clearance with renal impairment May cause or exacerbate hypertension
Nefazodone (Serzone)	100 mg	200–400 mg	Mild	Short	Can increase concentrations of terfenadine, astemizole, and cisapride Has antianxiety effects
Trazodone (Desyrel)	25–50 mg	75–400 mg	Moderate–high	Short	Can cause hypotension May be useful in low doses as a hypnotic

* Other less commonly used antidepressants are discussed in the text.
† Short = <8 h; intermediate = 8–20 h; long = 20–30 h; very long = >30 h. Half-lives may vary in older patients and some drugs have active metabolites.
‡ See text for drug interactions.
§ See text for anticholinergic side effects.

177

For patients with bipolar disorder, lithium is useful in treating the manic phase of the illness and in preventing recurrent depression. It may also enhance the effects of other antidepressants in treating unipolar depression. Lithium has a very narrow therapeutic-toxic ratio and must be used very carefully in the geriatric population. Its renal clearance is diminished, and blood levels can be influenced by diuretics and angiotensin converting enzyme (ACE) inhibitors. Blood levels should be monitored once or twice weekly until a stable dosage is achieved and then at least monthly. Dosages of 150 to 300 mg three times a day generally yield adequate blood levels in the elderly (0.3 to 0.6 meq/L for maintenance). Older patients are particularly susceptible to lithium toxicity, especially delirium. Hypothyroidism can occur in patients on lithium, and thyroid function tests should be monitored periodically in patients on chronic therapy.

Depressed geriatric patients with psychotic features (paranoid and other types of delusions, hallucinations) may also require antipsychotic drug treatment. These drugs, as well as sedative and hypnotic agents (which are also useful in some depressed older patients with prominent anxiety or psychomotor agitation), are discussed in Chap. 13. Further details on the drug treatment of depression in the elderly can be found in the Suggested Readings at the end of this chapter.

REFERENCES

American Psychiatric Association: *Diagnostic and Statistical Manual of Mental Disorders,* 4th ed, revised. Washington, DC, American Psychiatric Association, 1994.

Blazer D, Hughes DC, George LK: The epidemiology of depression in an elderly community population. *Gerontologist* 27:281–287, 1987.

Covinsky KE, Fortinsky RH, Palmer RM, et al: Relation between symptoms of depression and health status outcomes in acutely ill hospitalized older persons. *Ann Intern Med* 126:417–425, 1997.

Dement WC, Miles LE, Carkson MA: White paper on sleep and aging. *J Am Geriatr Soc* 30:25–50, 1982.

Katon W, Raskind M: Treatment of depression in the medically ill with methylphenidate. *Am J Psychiatry* 137:963–965, 1980.

Koenig HG: Differences in psychosocial and health correlates of major and minor depression in medically ill older adults. *J Am Geriatr Soc* 45:1487–1495, 1997.

Koenig HG, Meador KG, Cohen HJ, Blazer DG: Depression in elderly hospitalized patients with medical illness. *Arch Intern Med* 148:1929–1936, 1988.

Levenson AJ, Hall RCW (eds): *Neuropsychiatric Manifestations of Physical Disease in the Elderly.* New York, Raven Press, 1981.

Lebowitz BD, Pearson JL, Schneider LS, et al: Diagnosis and treatment of depression I late life. *JAMA* 278:1186–1190, 1997.

McCusker J, Cole M, Keller E, et al: Effectiveness of treatments of depression in older ambulatory patients. *Arch Intern Med* 158:705–712, 1998.

Newman AB, Enright PL, Manolio TA, et al: Sleep disturbance, psychosocial correlates, and cardiovascular disease in 5201 older adults: The Cardiovascular Health Study. *J Am Geriatr Soc* 45:1–7, 1997.

NIH Consensus Conference: *Diagnosis and Treatment of Depression in Late Life.* Washington, DC, National Institutes of Health, 1991.

Osgood NJ: *Suicide in the Elderly.* Rockville, MD, Aspen, 1985.

Parmelee PA, Katz IR, Lawton MP: Depression among institutionalized aged: Assessment and prevalence estimation. *J Gerontol* 44:M22–M29, 1989.

Parmelee PA, Katz IR, Lawton MP: Incidence of depression in long-term care settings. *J Gerontol* 47:M189–M196, 1992a.

Parmelee PA, Katz IR, Lawton MP: Depression and mortality among institutionalized aged. *J Gerontol* 47:P3–P10, 1992b.

Rigler SK, Studenski S, Duncan PW: Pharmacologic treatment of geriatric depression: Key issues in interpreting the evidence. *J Am Geriatr Soc* 46:106–110, 1998.

Roose SP, Laghriss-Thode F, Kennedy JS, et al: Comparison of paroxetine and nortriptyline in depressed patients with ischemic heart disease. *JAMA* 279:287–291, 1998.

Rovner BW, German PS, Brant LJ, et al: Depression and mortality in nursing homes. *JAMA* 265:993–996, 1991.

Small GW, Birkett M, Meyers BS, et al: Impact of physical illness on quality of life and antidepressant response in geriatric major depression. *J Am Geriatr Soc* 44:1220–1225, 1996.

Stewart AL, Hays RD, Ware JE: The MOS short-form general health survey: Reliability and validity in a patient population. *Med Care* 26:724–735, 1988.

Teri L, Logsdon RG, Uomoto J, et al: Behavioral treatment of depression in dementia patients: A controlled clinical trial. *J Gerontol Psychol Sci* 52(4):P159–P166, 1997.

Unutzer J, Patrick DL, Simon G, et al.: Depressive symptoms and the cost of health services in HMO patients aged 65 years and older. *JAMA* 277:1618–1623, 1997.

SUGGESTED READINGS

Alexopoulos GS (ed): Psychiatric disorders in late life. *Clin Geriatr Med* Volume 8, Number 2, 1992.

Blazer DG (ed): *Depression in Late Life.* St. Louis, Mosby, 1982.

Finkel SI: Efficacy and tolerability of antidepressant therapy in the old-old. *J Clin Psychiatry* 57:23–28, 1996.

Gordon WA, Hibbard MR: Poststroke depression: An examination of the literature. *Arch Phys Med Rehabil* 78:658–663, 1997.

Hay DP, Rodriguez MM, Franson KL: Treatment of depression in late life. *Clin Geriatr Med* 14:33–46, 1998.

Martin LM, Fleming KC, Evans JM: Recognition and management of anxiety and depression in elderly patients. *Mayo Clin Proc* 70:999–1006, 1995.

Small GW, Birkett M, Meyers BS, et al: Impact of physical illness on quality of life and antidepressant response in geriatric major depression. *J Am Geriatr Soc* 44:1220–1225, 1996.

Salzman C: Electroconvulsive therapy in the elderly patient. *Psychiatr Clin North Am* 5:191–197, 1982.

SEVEN

INCONTINENCE

Incontinence is a common, disruptive, and potentially disabling condition in the geriatric population. It is defined as the involuntary loss of urine or stool in sufficient amount or frequency to constitute a social and/or health problem. The prevalence of urinary incontinence is illustrated in Fig. 7-1. Incontinence is a heterogeneous condition, ranging in severity from occasional episodes of dribbling small amounts of urine to continuous urinary incontinence with concomitant fecal incontinence. Incontinent older persons are not always severely demented, bedridden, or in nursing homes. Many, both in institutions and in the community, are ambulatory and have good mental function. Approximately one-third of older women and 15 to 20 percent of older men have some degree of urinary incontinence. Between 5 and 10 percent of community-dwelling older adults have incontinence more often than weekly and/or use a pad for protection from urinary accidents. The prevalence is as high as 60 to 80 percent in many long-term-care institutions. In both community and institutional settings, incontinence is associated with both impaired mobility and poor cognition.

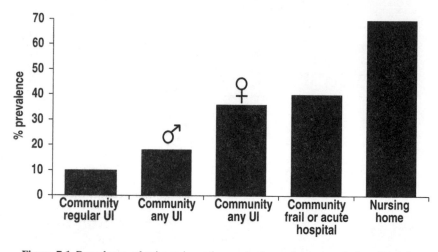

Figure 7-1 Prevalence of urinary incontinence in the geriatric population. "Regular UI" is more often than weekly and/or the use of a pad.

Physical health, psychological well-being, social status, and the costs of health care can all be adversely affected by incontinence (Table 7-1). Urinary incontinence is curable in many geriatric patients, especially those who have adequate mobility and mental functioning. Even when it is not curable, incontinence can always be managed in a manner that will keep patients comfortable, make life easier for caregivers, and minimize the costs of caring for the condition and its complications. Since many older patients are embarrassed and frustrated by their incontinence and either deny it or do not discuss it with a health professional, it is essential that specific questions about incontinence be included in periodic assessments and that incontinence be noted as a problem when it is detected in institutional settings. Examples of such questions include the following:

- "Do you have trouble with your bladder?"
- "Do you ever lose urine when you don't want to?"
- "Do you ever wear padding to protect yourself in case you lose urine?"

This chapter briefly reviews the pathophysiology of geriatric incontinence and provides detailed information on the evaluation and

**Table 7-1 Potential adverse effects
of urinary incontinence**

Physical heath
  Skin breakdown
  Recurrent urinary tract infections
  Falls (especially with nighttime incontinence)

Psychological health
  Isolation
  Depression
  Dependency

Social consequences
  Stress on family, friends, and caregivers
  Predisposition to institutionalization

Economic costs
  Supplies (padding, catheters, ect.)
  Laundry
  Labor (nurses, housekeepers)
  Management of complications

management of this condition. Although most of the chapter focuses on urinary incontinence, much of the pathophysiology also applies to fecal incontinence, which is briefly addressed at the end of the chapter.

NORMAL URINATION

Continence requires effective functioning of the lower urinary tract, adequate cognitive and physical functioning, motivation, and an appropriate environment (Table 7-2). Thus, the pathophysiology of geriatric incontinence can relate to the anatomy and physiology of the lower urinary tract as well as to functional psychological and environmental factors. Several anatomic components participate in normal urination (Fig. 7-2). At the most basic level, urination is governed by reflexes centered in the sacral micturition center. Afferent pathways (via somatic and autonomic nerves) carry information on bladder volume to the spinal cord as the bladder fills. Motor output is adjusted accordingly (Fig. 7-3). Thus, as the bladder fills, sympathetic tone closes the bladder neck, relaxes the dome of the bladder, and inhibits parasympathetic tone; somatic innervation maintains tone in the pelvic floor musculature (including striated muscle around the urethra).

Table 7-2 Requirements for continence

Effective lower urinary tract function
  Storage
    Accommodation by bladder of increasing volumes of urine under low pressure
      Closed bladder outlet
      Appropriate sensation of bladder fullness
      Absence of involuntary bladder contractions
  Emptying
      Bladder capable of contraction
      Lack of anatomic obstruction to urine flow
      Coordinated lowering of outlet resistance with bladder contractions

Adequate mobility and dexterity to use toilet or toilet substitute and to manage clothing

Adequate cognitive function to recognize toileting needs and to find a toilet or toilet substitute

Motivation to be continent

Absence of environmental and iatrogenic barriers such as inaccessible toilets or toilet substitutes, unavailable caregivers, or drug side effects

When urination occurs, sympathetic and somatic tones diminish, and parasympathetic cholinergically mediated impulses cause the bladder to contract. All these processes are under the influence of higher centers in the brainstem, cerebral cortex, and cerebellum. This is a simplified description of a very complex process, and the neurophysiology of urination remains incompletely understood. It appears, however, that the cerebral cortex exerts a predominantly inhibitory influence and the brainstem facilitates urination. Thus, loss of the central cortical inhibiting influences over the sacral micturition center from diseases such as dementia, stroke, and parkinsonism can produce incontinence in elderly patients. Disorders of the brainstem and suprasacral spinal cord can interfere with the coordination of bladder contractions and lowering of urethral resistance, and interruptions of the sacral innervation can cause impaired bladder contraction and problems with continence.

Normal urination is a dynamic process, requiring the coordination of several physiologic processes. Fig. 7-4 depicts a simplified schematic diagram of the pressure-volume relationships in the lower urinary tract, similar to measurements made in urodynamic studies. Under normal circumstances, as the bladder fills, bladder pressure remains low (e.g., $<115\,\mathrm{cmH_2O}$). The first urge to void is variable but generally

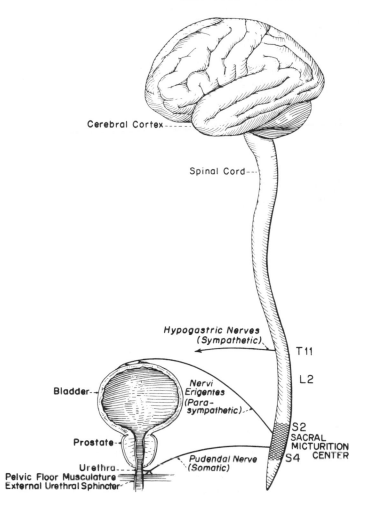

Figure 7-2 Structural components of normal micturition.

occurs between 150 and 300 mL, and normal bladder capacity is 300 to 600 mL. When normal urination is initiated, true detrusor pressure (bladder pressure minus intraabdominal pressure) increases, urethral resistance decreases, and urine flow occurs when detrusor pressure exceeds urethral resistance. If at any time during bladder filling total intravesicular pressure (which includes intraabdominal pressure) exceeds outlet resistance, urinary leakage will occur. This will happen

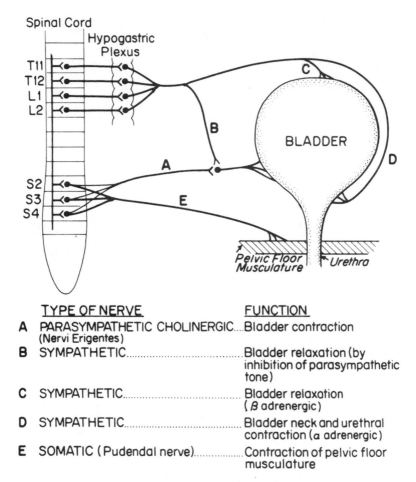

Figure 7-3 Peripheral nerves involved in micturition.

if, for example, intraabdominal pressure rises *without* a rise in true detrusor pressure when someone with low outlet or urethral sphincter weakness coughs or sneezes. This would be defined as *genuine stress incontinence* in urodynamic terminology. Alternatively, the bladder can contract involuntarily and cause urinary leakage. This would be defined as *detrusor motor instability* or *detrusor hyperreflexia* in patients with neurologic disorders.

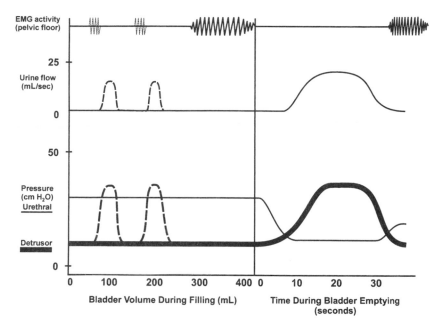

Figure 7-4 Schematic diagram of the dynamic function of the lower urinary tract during bladder filling (*left*) and emptying (*right*). As the bladder fills, true detrusor pressure (*thick line at bottom*) remains low (less than 5–10 cm H_2O) and does not exceed urethral resistance pressure (*thin line at bottom*). As the bladder fills to capacity (generally 300–600 mL), pelvic floor and sphincter activity increase as measured by electromyography (EMG, *top*). Involuntary detrusor contractions (illustrated by *dashed lines*) occur commonly among incontinent geriatric patients (see text). They may be accompanied by increased EMG activity in attempts to prevent leakage (*dashed lines at top*). If detrusor pressure exceeds urethral pressure during an involuntary contraction, as shown, urine will flow. During bladder emptying, detrusor pressure rises, urethral pressure falls, and EMG activity ceases in order for normal urine flow to occur.

CAUSES AND TYPES OF INCONTINENCE

Basic Causes

There are four basic categories of causes for geriatric urinary incontinence (Fig. 7-5). Determining the cause(s) is essential to proper management. It is very important to distinguish between urologic and neurologic disorders that cause incontinence and other problems (such as diminished mobility and/or mental function, inaccessible toilets, and psychological problems), which can cause or contribute to the

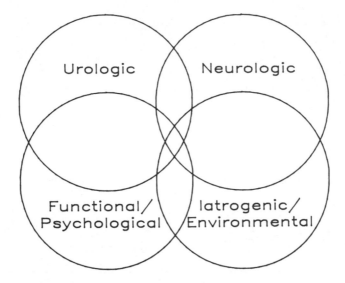

Figure 7-5 Basic underlying causes of geriatric urinary incontinence.

condition. As is the case for a number of other common geriatric problems discussed in this text, multiple disorders often interact to cause urinary incontinence, as depicted in Fig. 7-5.

Aging alone does *not* cause urinary incontinence. Several age-related changes can, however, contribute to its development.

In general, with age, bladder capacity declines, residual urine increases, and involuntary bladder contractions become more common (Fig. 7-4). These contractions are found in up to 80 percent of older incontinent patients as well as 5 to 10 percent of older women and one-third or more of older men with no or minimal urinary symptoms (Diokno et al., 1988; Elbawadi et al., 1993). Combined with impaired mobility, these contractions account for a substantial proportion of incontinence in frail geriatric patients.

Aging is associated with a decline in bladder outlet and urethral resistance pressure in women. This decline, which is related to diminished estrogen influence and laxity of pelvic structures associated with prior childbirths, surgeries, and deconditioned muscles, predisposes to the development of stress incontinence (Fig. 7-6). Decreased estrogen can also cause atrophic vaginitis and urethritis, which can, in turn, cause symptoms of dysuria and urgency and predispose to the

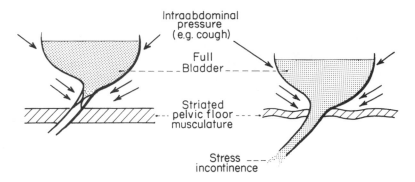

Figure 7-6 Simplified schematic diagram depicting age-associated changes in pelvic floor muscle, bladder, and urethra-vesicle position predisposing to stress incontinence. Normally (*left*), the bladder and outlet remain anatomically inside the intraabominal cavity, and rises in pressure contribute to bladder outlet closure. Age-associated changes (e.g., estrogen deficiency, surgeries, childbirth) can weaken the structures maintaining bladder position (*right*); in this situation, increases in intraabdominal pressure can cause urine loss (stress incontinence).

development of urinary infection and urge incontinence. In men, prostatic enlargement is associated with decreased urine flow rates and detrusor motor instability and can lead to urge and/or overflow types of incontinence (see below). Aging is also associated with abnormalities of arginine vasopressin (AVP) levels. Lack of the normal diurnal rhythm of AVP secretion may contribute to nocturnal polyuria, and predispose many older people to nighttime incontinence (Asplund and Aberg, 1991).

Reversible Factors Causing or Contributing to Incontinence

Numerous potentially reversible conditions and medications may cause or contribute to geriatric incontinence (Tables 7-3 and 7-4). The term *acute incontinence* refers to those situations in which the incontinence is of sudden onset, usually related to an acute illness or an iatrogenic problem, and subsides once the illness or medication problem has been resolved. *Persistent incontinence* refers to incontinence that is unrelated to an acute illness and persists over time. Potentially reversible conditions can play a role in *both* acute and persistent incontinence. A search for these factors should be undertaken in all incontinent geriatric patients.

Table 7-3 Reversible conditions that cause or contribute to geriatric urinary incontinence

Condition	Management
Conditions affecting the lower urinary tract	
Urinary tract infection (symptomatic with frequency, urgency, dysuria, etc.)	Antimicrobial therapy.
Atrophic vaginitis/urethritis	Oral or topical estrogen.
Postprostatectomy	Behavioral intervention. Avoid further surgical therapy until it is clear condition will not resolve.
Stool impaction	Disimpaction; appropriate use of stool softeners bulk-forming agents, and laxatives if necessary; implement high fiber intake, adequate mobility, and fluid intake.
Drug side effect (see Table 7-4)	Discontinue or change therapy if clinically appropriate. Dosage reduction or modification (e.g., flexible scheduling of rapid-acting diuretics) may also help.
Increased urine production	
Metabolic (hyperglycemia, hypercalcemia)	Better control of diabetes mellitus. Therapy for hypercalcemia depends on underlying cause.
Excess fluid intake	Reduction in intake of diuretic fluids (e.g., caffeinated beverages).
Volume overload	Support stockings.
Venous insufficiency with edema	Leg elevation. Sodium restriction. Diuretic therapy.
Congestive heart failure	Medical therapy.
Impaired ability or willingness to reach a toilet	
Delirium	Diagnosis and treatment of underlying cause(s) of acute confusional state.
Chronic illness, injury, or restraint that interferes with mobility	Regular toileting. Use of toilet substitutes. Environmental alterations (e.g., bedside commode, urinal).
Psychological	Remove restrains if possible. Appropriate pharmacologic and/or nonpharmacologic treatment.

Source: From Fantl et al., 1996, with permission.

Table 7-4 Medications that can affect continence

Type of medication	Potential effects on continence
Diuretics	Polyuria, frequency, urgency
Anticholinergics	Urinary retention, overflow incontinence, stool impaction
Psychotropics: Tricyclic Antidepressants	Anticholinergic actions, sedation
Antipsychotics	Anticholinergic actions, sedation, immobility
Sedative-hypnotics	Sedation, delirium, immobility, muscle relaxation
Narcotic analgesics	Urinary retention, fecal impaction, sedation, delirium
Alpha-adrenergic blockers	Urethral relaxation
Alpha-adrenergic agonists	Urinary retention
Angiotensin converting enzyme inhibitors	Cough precipitating stress incontinence
Beta-adrenergic agonists	Urinary retention
Calcium channel blockers	Urinary retention
Alcohol	Polyuria, frequency, urgency, sedation, delirium, immobility
Caffeine	Polyuria, bladder irritation

The causes of acute and reversible forms of urinary incontinence can be remembered by the acronym DRIP (Table 7-5). DIAPPERS is another, similar acronym for reversible causes of incontinence (Resnick, 1984).

Many older persons, because of urinary frequency and urgency, especially when they are limited in mobility, carefully arrange their schedules (and may even limit social activities) in order to be close to a toilet. Thus, an acute illness (e.g., pneumonia, cardiac decompensation, stroke, lower extremity or vertebral fracture) can precipitate incontinence by disrupting this delicate balance.

Hospitalization, with its attendant environmental barriers (such as bed rails, poorly lit rooms), and the immobility that often accompanies acute illnesses can contribute to acute incontinence. Acute incontinence in these situations is likely to resolve with resolution of the

**Table 7-5 Acronym for potentially
reversible conditions***

D	Delirium
R	Restricted mobility, retention
I	Infection, inflammation, impaction
P	Polyuria, pharmaceuticals

* See Tables 7-3 and 7-4.

underlying acute illness. Unless an indwelling or external catheter is necessary to record urine output accurately, this type of incontinence should be managed by environmental manipulations, scheduled toiletings, the appropriate use of toilet substitutes and pads, and careful attention to skin care. In a substantial proportion of patients, incontinence may persist for several weeks after hospitalization and should be evaluated as for persistent incontinence (see below) (Sier et al., 1987).

Fecal impaction is a common problem in both acutely and chronically ill geriatric patients. Large impactions may cause mechanical obstruction of the bladder outlet in women and may stimulate involuntary bladder contractions induced by sensory input related to rectal distention. Whatever the underlying mechanism, relief of fecal impaction can lead to improvement and sometimes resolution of the urinary incontinence.

Urinary retention with overflow incontinence should be considered in any patient who suddenly develops urinary incontinence. Immobility, anticholinergic and narcotic drugs, and fecal impaction can all precipitate overflow incontinence in geriatric patients. In addition, this condition may be a manifestation of an underlying process causing spinal cord compression and presenting acutely.

Any acute inflammatory condition in the lower urinary tract that causes frequency and urgency can precipitate incontinence. Treatment of an acute cystitis, vaginitis, or urethritis can restore continence.

Conditions that cause polyuria, including hyperglycemia and hypercalcemia, as well as diuretics (especially the rapid-acting loop diuretics), can precipitate acute incontinence. Patients with volume-expanded states, such as congestive heart failure and lower extremity venous insufficiency, may have polyuria at night, which can contribute to nocturia and nocturnal incontinence.

As in the case of many other conditions discussed throughout this text, a wide variety of medications can play a role in the develop-

ment of incontinence in elderly patients (Table 7-4). Whether the incontinence is acute or persistent, the potential role of these medications in causing or contributing to the patients' incontinence should be considered. Whenever feasible, stopping the medication, switching to an alternative, or modifying the dosage schedule can be an important component (and possibly the only one necessary) of the treatment for incontinence.

Persistent Incontinence

Persistent forms of incontinence can be classified clinically into four basic types (Fig. 7-7). As depicted, these types can overlap. Thus, an individual patient may have more than one type simultaneously. While this classification does not include all the neurophysiologic abnormalities associated with incontinence, it is helpful in approaching the clinical assessment and treatment of incontinence in the geriatric population.

Three of these types—stress, urge, and overflow—result from one or a combination of two basic abnormalities in lower genitourinary tract function:

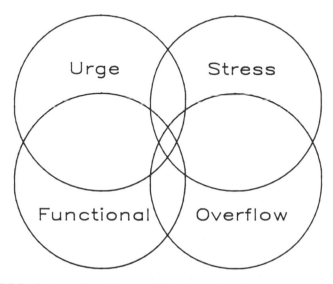

Figure 7-7 Basic types of persistent geriatric urinary incontinence.

1. Failure to store urine, caused by a hyperactive or poorly compliant bladder or by diminished outflow resistance
2. Failure to empty bladder, caused by a poorly contractile bladder or by increased outflow resistance

The clinical definitions and common causes of persistent urinary incontinence are shown in Table 7-6. *Stress incontinence* is common

Table 7-6 Basic types and causes of persistent urinary incontinence

Types	Definition	Common causes
Stress	Involuntary loss of urine (usually small amounts) with increases in intraabdominal pressure (e.g., cough, laugh, exercise)	Weakness of pelvic floor musculature and urethral hypermobility Bladder outlet or urethral sphincter weakness
Urge	Leakage of urine (variable but often larger volumes) because of inability to delay voiding after sensation of bladder fullness is perceived	Detrusor overactivity, isolated or associated with one or more of the following: Local genitourinary condition such as tumors, stones, diverticuli, or outflow obstruction CNS disorders such as stroke, dementia, parkinsonism, spinal cord injury
Overflow	Leakage of urine (usually small amounts) resulting from mechanical forces on an overdistended bladder or from other effects of urinary retention on bladder and sphincter function	Anatomic obstruction by prostate, stricture, cystocele Acontractile bladder associated with diabetes mellitus or spinal cord injury Neurogenic (detrusor-sphincter dyssynergy), associated with multiple sclerosis and other suprasacral spinal cord lesions
Functional	Urinary accidents associated with inability to toilet because of impairment of cognitive and/or physical functioning, psychological unwillingness, or environmental barriers	Severe dementia and other neurologic disorders Psychological factors such as depression and hostility

in older women, especially in ambulatory clinic settings. It may be infrequent and involve very small amounts of urine and need no specific treatment in women who are not bothered by it. On the other hand, it may be so severe and bothersome that it necessitates surgical correction. It is most often associated with weakened supporting tissues and consequent hypermobility of the bladder outlet and urethra caused by lack of estrogen and/or previous vaginal deliveries or surgery (Fig. 7-6). Obesity and chronic coughing can exacerbate this condition. Women who have had previous vaginal repair and/or surgical bladder neck suspension may develop a weak urethra (intrinsic sphincter deficiency, or ISD). These women generally present with severe incontinence and symptoms of constant wetting with any activity. This condition should be suspected during office evaluation if a woman loses urine with coughing in the supine position during a pelvic examination when her bladder is relatively empty. In general, women with ISD are less responsive to nonsurgical treatment but may benefit from periurethral injections or a surgical sling procedure (see below). Stress incontinence is unusual in men but can occur after transurethral surgery and/or radiation therapy for lower urinary tract malignancy when the anatomic sphincters are damaged.

Urge incontinence can be caused by a variety of lower genitourinary and neurologic disorders (Table 7-6). Patients with urge incontinence typically present with irritative symptoms of an overactive bladder, including frequency (voiding more than every 2 h), urgency, and nocturia (two or more voids during usual sleeping hours). Urge incontinence is most often but not always associated with detrusor motor instability or detrusor hyperreflexia (Fig. 7-4). Some patients have a poorly compliant bladder without involuntary contractions (e.g., radiation or interstitial cystitis, both relatively unusual conditions). Other patients have symptoms of an overactive bladder but do not exhibit detrusor motor instability on urodynamic testing. This is termed *sensory instability* or *hypersensitive bladder*; it is likely that some of these patients do have detrusor motor instability in their everyday lives, which is not documented at the time of the urodynamic study. On the other hand, there are some patients with neurologic disorders who do have detrusor hyperreflexia on urodynamic testing but do not have urgency and are incontinent without any warning symptoms ("unconscious incontinence"). The above-described patients are generally treated as if they had urge incontinence if they empty their bladders and do not have other correctable genitourinary

pathology. A subgroup of older incontinent patients with detrusor motor instability also have impaired bladder contractility—emptying less than one-third of their bladder volume with involuntary contractions on urodynamic testing (Resnick and Yalla, 1987; Elbawadi et al., 1993). This condition has been termed *detrusor hyperactivity with impaired contractility* (DHIC). Patients with DHIC may present with symptoms that are not typical of urge incontinence and may strain to complete voiding. These patients may be difficult to manage because of their urinary retention.

Urinary retention with *overflow incontinence* can result from anatomic or neurogenic outflow obstruction, a hypotonic or acontractile bladder, or both. The most common causes include prostatic enlargement, diabetic neuropathic bladder, and urethral stricture. Low spinal cord injury and anatomic obstruction in females (caused by pelvic prolapse and urethral distortion) are less common causes of overflow incontinence. Several types of drugs can also contribute to this type of persistent incontinence (Table 7-4). Some patients with suprasacral spinal cord lesions (e.g., multiple sclerosis) develop detrusor-sphincter dyssynergy and consequent urinary retention, which must be treated in a similar manner as overflow incontinence; in some instances a sphincterotomy is necessary. The symptoms of overflow incontinence are nonspecific and urinary retention is easily missed on physical examination. Thus a postvoid residual determination must be performed to exclude this condition.

The term *functional incontinence* refers to incontinence associated with the inability or lack of motivation to reach a toilet on time. Factors that contribute to functional incontinence (such as inaccessible toilets and psychological disorders) can also exacerbate other types of persistent incontinence. Patients with incontinence that appears to be predominantly related to functional factors may also have abnormalities of the lower genitourinary tract. In some patients, it can be very difficult to determine whether the functional factors or the genitourinary factors predominate without a trial of specific types of treatment. However, no matter what specific treatments are prescribed, patients with functional incontinence require systematic toileting assistance as a component of their management plan.

These basic types of incontinence may occur in combination, as depicted by the overlap in Fig. 7-7. Older women commonly have a combination of stress and urge incontinence (generally referred to as *mixed incontinence*). Frail geriatric patients often have urge incontinence with detrusor instability as well as functional disabilities that contribute to their incontinence.

EVALUATION

Basic Evaluation

In patients with the sudden onset of incontinence (especially when associated with an acute medical condition and hospitalization), the reversible factors that can cause acute incontinence (Tables 7-3, 7-4, and 7-5) can be ruled out by a brief history, physical examination, postvoid residual determination, and basic laboratory studies (urinalysis, culture, serum glucose or calcium). Table 7-7 shows the basic

Table 7-7 Components of the diagnostic evaluation of persistent urinary incontinence

All patients
    History, including bladder record
    Physical examination
    Urinalysis
    Postvoid residual determination

Selected patients*
    Laboratory studies
        Urine culture
        Urine cytology
        Blood glucose, calcium
        Renal function tests
        Renal ultrasound
    Gynecologic evaluation
    Urologic evaluation
    Cystourethroscopy
    Urodynamic tests
        Simple
            Observation of voiding
            Cough test for stress incontinence
            Simple (single channel) cystometry
        Complex
            Urine flowmetry
            Multichannel cystometrogram
            Pressure-flow study
            Leak-point pressure
            Urethral pressure profilometry
            Sphincter electromyography
            Videourodynamics

* See text and Table 7-9.

components of the evaluation of persistent urinary incontinence. Practice guidelines suggest that the basic evaluation should include a focused history, targeted physical examination, urinalysis, and post-void residual determination (PVR) (Fantl et al., 1996; American Medical Directors Association, 1996). The history should focus on the characteristics of the incontinence, current medical problems and medications, the most bothersome symptom(s), and the impact of the incontinence on the patient and caregivers (Table 7-8). Bladder records or voiding diaries such as those shown in Fig. 7-8 (for outpatients) and Fig. 7-9 (for institutionalized patients) can be helpful in initially characterizing symptoms as well as in following the response to treatment.

Table 7-8 Key aspects of an incontinent patient's history

Active medical conditions, especially neurologic disorders, diabetes mellitus, congestive heart failure, venous insufficiency

Medications (see Table 7-4)

Fluid intake pattern
Type and amount of fluid (especially before bedtime)

Past genitourinary history, especially childbirth, surgery, dilatations, urinary retention, recurrent urinary tract infections

Symptoms of incontinence
Onset and duration
Type—stress vs. urge vs. mixed vs. other
Frequency, timing, and amount of incontinence episodes and of continent voids (see Figs. 7-8 and 7-9)

Other lower urinary tract symptoms
Irritative—dysuria, frequency, urgency, nocturia
Voiding difficulty—hesitancy, slow or interrupted stream, straining, incomplete emptying
Other—hematuria, suprapubic discomfort

Other symptoms
Neurologic (indicative of stroke, dementia, parkinsonism, normal pressure hydrocephalus, spinal cord compression, multiple sclerosis)
Psychological (depression)
Bowel (constipation, stool incontinence)
Symptoms suggestive of volume-expanded state (e.g., lower extremity edema, shortness of breath while horizontal or with exertion)

(continued)

Table 7-8 Key aspects of an incontinent patient's history *(Continued)*

Environmental factors
  Location and structure of bathroom
  Availability of toilet substitutes

Perceptions of incontinence
  Patient's concerns or ideas about underlying cause(s)
  Most bothersome symptoms(s)
  Interference with daily life
  Severity (e.g., is it enough of a problem for you to consider surgery?)

BLADDER RECORD

Day:_____   Date:_____/_____.
                                              month   day

1NSTRUCTIONS:

1) In the 1st column make a mark every time during the 2—hour period you urinate into the toilet

2) Use the 2nd column to record the amount you urinate (if you are measuring amounts)

3) In the 3rd or 4th column, make a mark every time you accidentally leak urine

Time Interval	Urinated in Toilet	Amount	Leaking Accident	*or* Large Accident	Reason for Accident *
6—8 am					
8—10 am					
2—4 pm					
4—6 pm					
6—8 pm					
8—10 pm					
10—12 pm					
Overnight					

Number of pads used today: _____

* For example, if you coughed and have a leaking accident, write "cough".
If you had a large accident after a strong urge to urinate, write "urge".

Figure 7-8 Example of a bladder record for ambulatory care settings.

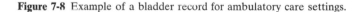

INCONTINENCE MONITORING RECORD

INSTRUCTIONS: EACH TIME THE PATIENT IS CHECKED:
1) Mark *one* of the circles in the BLADDER section at the hour closest to the time the patient is checked.
2) Make an X in the BOWEL section if the patient has had an incontinent or normal bowel movement.

🖊 = Incontinent, small amount	∅ = Dry	X = Incontinent BOWEL
● = Incontinent, large amount	⬭ = Voided correctly	X = Normal BOWEL

PATIENT NAME _____ ROOM # _____ DATE _____

	BLADDER			**BOWEL**			
	INCONTINENT OF URINE	DRY	VOIDED CORRECTLY	INCONTINENT X	NORMAL X	INITIALS	**COMMENTS**
12 am	● ●	○	△ cc ____				
1	● ●	○	△ cc ____				
2	● ●	○	△ cc ____				
3	● ●	○	△ cc ____.				
4	● ●	○	△ cc ____				
5	● ●	○	△ cc ____				
6	● ●	○	△ cc ____				
7	● ●	○	△ cc ____				
8	● ●	○	△ cc ____				
9	● ●	○	△ cc ____				
10	● ●	○	△ cc ____				
11	● ●	○	△ cc ____				
12 pm	● ●	○	△ cc ____				
1	● ●	○	△ cc ____				
2	● ●	○	△ cc ____				
3	● ●	○	△ cc ____				
4	● ●	○	△ cc ____				
5	● ●	○	△ cc ____				
6	● ●	○	△ cc ____				
7	● ●	○	△ cc ____				
8	● ●	○	△ cc ____				
9	● ●	○	△ cc ____				
10	● ●	○	△ cc ____				
11	● ●	○	△ cc ____				
TOTALS:							

Figure 7-9 Example of a record to monitor bladder and bowel functions in institutional settings. This type of record is expecially useful for implementing and following the results of various training procedures and other treatment protocols. *(From Ouslander et al., 1986a, with permission.)*

Physical examination should focus on abdominal, rectal, and genital examinations and an evaluation of lumbosacral innervation (Table 7-9). During the history and physical examination, special attention should be given to factors such as mobility, mental status, medications, and accessibility of toilets that may either be causing the incontinence or interacting with urologic and neurologic disorders to worsen the

Table 7-9 Key aspects of an incontinent patient's physical examination

Mobility and dexterity
    Functional status compatible with ability to self-toilet
    Gait disturbance (parkinsonism, normal-pressure hydrocephalus)

Mental status
    Cognitive function compatible with ability to self-toilet
    Motivation
    Mood and effect

Neurologic
    Focal signs (especially in lower extremities)
    Signs of parkinsonism
    Sacral arc reflexes

Abdominal
    Bladder distension
    Suprapubic tenderness
    Lower abdominal mass

Rectal
    Perianal sensation
    Sphincter tone (resting and active)
    Impaction
    Masses
    Size and contour of prostate

Pelvic
    Perineal skin condition
    Perineal sensation
    Atrophic vaginitis (friability, inflammation, bleeding)
    Pelvic prolapse (i.e., cystocele, rectocele; see Fig. 7-10)
    Pelvic mass
    Other anatomic abnormality

Other
    Lower extremity edema or signs of congestive heart failure
        (if nocturia is a prominent complaint)

condition. The pelvic examination in women should include careful inspections of the labia and vagina for signs of inflammation suggestive of atrophic vaginitis and for pelvic prolapse. Most older women have some degree of pelvic prolapse (e.g., grade 1 or 2 cystocele as depicted in Fig. 7-10). Not all incontinent older women with these degrees of prolapse need gynecologic evaluation (see below).

A clean urine should be collected for urinalysis. For men who are frequently incontinent, making a "clean catch" specimen difficult to obtain, a clean specimen can be obtained using a condom catheter after cleaning the penis (Ouslander et al., 1987b). For women, a clean specimen can be obtained by cleaning the urethral and perineal area and having the patient void into a disinfected bedpan (Ouslander

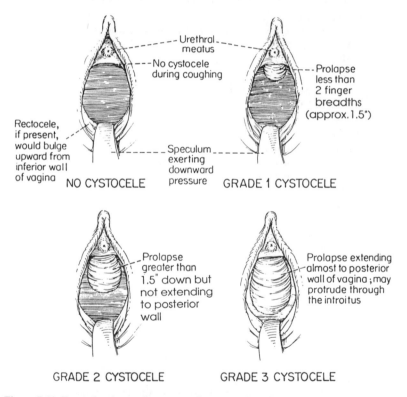

Figure 7-10 Example of a grading system for cystoceles. *(From Ouslander et al., 1989a, with permission.)*

et al., 1995d). Persistent microscopic hematuria (>5 red blood cells per high-power field) in the absence of infection is an indication for further evaluation to exclude a tumor or other urinary tract pathology.

Because the prevalence of "asymptomatic bacteriuria" roughly parallels the prevalence of incontinence, incontinent geriatric patients commonly have significant bacteriuria (Boscia et al., 1986a; Ouslander et al., 1996). Several studies have questioned the value of treating asymptomatic bacteriuria in geriatric patients (Nicolle et al., 1983, 1987; Boscia et al., 1987). In the initial evaluation of incontinent noninstitutionalized patients, especially those in whom the incontinence is new or worsening, otherwise asymptomatic bacteriuria should be treated before further evaluation is undertaken. In the nursing home population, we do not recommend eradicating bacteriuria unless symptoms of a urinary tract infection are present, because eradicating bacteriuria does not affect the severity of chronic, stable incontinence (Ouslander et al., 1995a). However, the new onset of incontinence, worsening incontinence, unexplained fever, and declines in mental and/or functional status may be the manifestations of a urinary tract infection in this population.

A PVR determination should be done either by catheterization or ultrasound to detect urinary retention, which cannot always be detected by physical examination. A portable ultrasound device that calculates residual urine is available (Diagnostic Ultrasound, Redmond, WA). Patients with residual volumes of more than 200 mL should be considered for further evaluation. The need for further evaluation in patients with lesser degrees of retention should be determined on an individual basis, considering the patient's symptoms and the degree to which they complain of straining or are observed to strain with voiding

Further Evaluation

The need for further evaluation and the specific diagnostic procedures listed in Table 7-7 should be determined on an individual basis. Clinical practice guidelines state that not all incontinent geriatric patients require further evaluation. Patients who have unexplained polyuria should have their blood glucose and calcium levels determined. Patients with significant urinary retention should have renal function tests and be considered for renal ultrasound and urodynamic testing to determine whether obstruction, impaired bladder contractility, or both are present. Persistent microscopic hematuria in the absence of infection

is an indication for urine cytology and urologic evaluation, including cystoscopy. Even in the absence of hematuria, patients with the recent and sudden onset of irritative urinary symptoms who have risk factors for bladder cancer (heavy smoking, industrial exposure to aniline dyes) should be considered for these evaluations. Women with marked pelvic prolapse (see Fig. 7-10) should be referred for gynecologic evaluation. Complex urodynamic testing is essential to determine the cause(s) of urinary retention and for any older patient for whom surgical intervention is being considered. Simple urodynamic tests, which can be performed without expensive equipment (including observation for straining during voiding, a cough test for stress incontinence with a comfortably full bladder, and simple cystometry) may be helpful in determining the cause(s) of incontinence in settings in which access to complex urodynamic testing is limited. Like complex urodynamic tests, these simple tests must be performed and interpreted very carefully in geriatric patients (Ouslander et al., 1989a, 1989b).

Table 7-10 summarizes criteria for referral for further evaluation, and Fig. 7-11 summarizes the overall approach to the evaluation of geriatric urinary incontinence.

Table 7-10 Criteria for referral of incontinent patients for urologic, gynecologic, or urodynamic evaluation

Criteria	Definition	Rationale
History		
Recent history of lower urinary tract or pelvic surgery or irradiation	Surgery or irradiation involving the pelvic area or lower urinary tract within the past 6 months.	A structural abnormality relating to the recent procedure should be sought.
Recurrent symptomatic urinary tract infections	Three or more symptomatic episodes in a 12-month period.	A structural abnormality or pathologic condition in the urinary tract predisposing to infection should be excluded.
Risk factors for bladder cancer	Recent or sudden onset of irritative symptoms, history of heavy smoking, or exposure to aniline dyes.	Urine for cytology and cystoscopy to exclude bladder cancer should be considered.

Table 7-10 Criteria for referral of incontinent patients for urologic, gynecologic, or urodynamic evaluation *(Continued)*

Criteria	Definition	Rationale
Physical examination		
Marked pelvic prolapse	A prominent cystocele that descends the entire height of the vaginal vault with coughing during speculum examination.	Anatomic abnormality may underlie the pathophysiology of the incontinence, and selected patients may benefit from surgical repair.
Marked prostatic enlargement and/ or suspicion of cancer	Gross enlargement of the prostate on digital exam; prominent induration or asymmetry of the lobes.	An evaluation to exclude prostate cancer may be appropriate and have therapeutic implications.
Postvoid residual		
Difficulty passing a 14-Fr straight catheter	Impossible catheter passage, or passage requiring considerable force, or a larger, more rigid catheter.	Anatomic blockage of the urethra or bladder neck may be present.
Postvoid residual volume >200	Volume of urine remaining in the bladder within a few minutes after the patient voids spontaneously in as normal a fashion as possible.	Anatomic or neurogenic obstruction or poor bladder contractility may be present.
Urinalysis		
Hematuria	Greater than five red blood cells per high-power field on repeated microscopic exams in the absence of infection.	A pathologic condition in the urinary tract should be excluded.
Therapeutic trial		
Failure to respond	Persistent symptoms that are bothersome to the patient after adequate trials of behavioral and/or drug therapy.	Urodynamic evaluation may help guide specific therapy

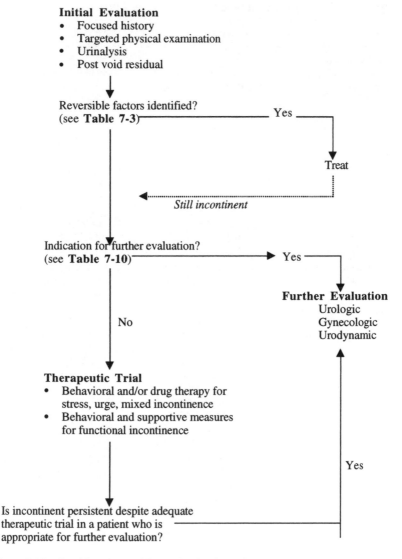

Initial Evaluation
- Focused history
- Targeted physical examination
- Urinalysis
- Post void residual

Reversible factors identified?
(see **Table 7-3**) ———————— Yes ————

Treat

Still incontinent

Indication for further evaluation?
(see **Table 7-10**) ————————————→ Yes ————

Further Evaluation
Urologic
Gynecologic
Urodynamic

No

Therapeutic Trial
- Behavioral and/or drug therapy for
  stress, urge, mixed incontinence
- Behavioral and supportive measures
  for functional incontinence

Yes

Is incontinent persistent despite adequate
therapeutic trial in a patient who is
appropriate for further evaluation?

Figure 7-11 Algorithm protocol for evaluating incontinence.

MANAGEMENT

General Principles

Several therapeutic modalities can be used in managing incontinent geriatric patients (Table 7-11). Treatment can be especially helpful if specific diagnoses are made and attention is paid to all factors that may be contributing to the incontinence in a given patient. Even when cure is not possible, the comfort and satisfaction of both patients and caregivers can almost always be enhanced.

Special attention should be given to the management of acute incontinence, which is most common among older patients in acute care hospitals. Acute incontinence may be transient if managed appropriately; on the other hand, inappropriate management may lead to a permanent problem. The most common approach to incontinent geriatric patients in acute care hospitals is indwelling catheterization. In some instances, this is justified by the necessity for accurate measurement of urine output during the acute phase of an illness. In many instances, however, it is unnecessary and poses a substantial and unwarranted risk of catheter-induced infection. Although it may be more difficult and time-consuming, making toilets and toilet substitutes accessible and combining this with some form of scheduled toileting is probably a more appropriate approach in patients who do not require indwelling catheterization. Newer launderable or disposable and highly absorbent bed pads and undergarments may also be helpful in managing these patients. These products may be more costly than catheters but probably result in less morbidity (and, therefore, overall cost) in the long run. All of the potential reversible factors that can cause or contribute to incontinence (Tables 7-3, 7-4, and 7-5) should be attended to in order to maximize the potential for regaining continence.

Supportive measures are critical in managing all forms of incontinence and should be used in conjunction with other, more specific treatment modalities. A positive attitude, education, environmental manipulations, the appropriate use of toilet substitutes, avoidance of iatrogenic contributions to incontinence, modifications of diuretic and fluid intake patterns, and good skin care are all important.

Specially designed incontinence undergarments and pads can be very helpful in many patients but must be used appropriately. They are now being marketed on television and are readily available in

Table 7-11 Treatment options for geriatric urinary incontinence

Nonspecific supportive measures
    Education
    Modifications of fluid and medication intake
    Use of toilet substitutes
    Environmental manipulations
    Garments and pads

Behavioral interventions (see Table 13)
    Patient-dependent
    Pelvic muscle exercises
    Bladder training

Bladder retraining (see Table 7-14)
    Adjunctive techniques
        Biofeedback
        Electrical stimulation
        Vaginal cones
    Caregiver-dependent
        Scheduled toileting
        Habit training
        Prompted voiding (see Table 7-15)

Drugs (see Table 7-16)
    Bladder relaxants
    Alpha agonists
    Alpha antagonists
    Estrogen

Periurethral injections
Surgery
    Bladder neck suspension or sling
    Removal of obstruction or pathologic lesion

Mechanical devices
    Urethral plugs
    Artificial sphincters

Catheters
    External
    Intermittent
    Indwelling

retail stores. Although they can be effective, several caveats should be noted:

1. Garments and pads are a nonspecific treatment. They should not be used as the first response to incontinence or before some type of diagnostic evaluation is done.
2. Many patients are curable if treated with specific therapies, and some have potentially serious factors underlying their incontinence that must be diagnosed and treated.
3. Pants and pads can interfere with attempts at behavioral intervention and thereby foster dependency.
4. Many disposable products are relatively expensive and are not covered by Medicare or other insurance.

To a large extent the optimal treatment of persistent incontinence depends on identifying the type(s). Table 7-12 outlines the primary treatments for the basic types of persistent incontinence in the geriatric

Table 7-12 Primary treatments for different types of geriatric urinary incontinence

Type of incontinence	Primary treatments
Stress	Pelvic muscle (Kegel) exercises Other behavioral interventions (see Table 7-13) Alpha-adrenergic agonists Estrogen Periurethral injections Surgical bladder neck suspension or sling
Urge	Bladder relaxants Estrogen (if atrophic vaginitis present) Bladder training (including pelvic muscle exercises)
Overflow	Surgical removal of obstruction Bladder retraining (see Table 7-14) Intermittent catheterization Indwelling catheterization
Functional	Behavioral interventions (caregiver-dependent; see Tables 7-13 and 7-15) Environmental manipulations Incontinence undergarments and pads

population. Each treatment modality is briefly discussed below. Behavioral interventions have been well studied in the geriatric population. These interventions are recommended by guidelines as an initial approach to therapy in many patients because they are generally noninvasive and nonspecific (i.e., patients with stress and/or urge incontinence respond equally well) (Fantl et al., 1991; Ouslander et al., 1996a).

Behavioral Interventions

Many types of behavioral interventions have been described for the management of urinary incontinence (Hadley, 1986). The nosology of these procedures has been somewhat confusing, and much of the literature has used the term *bladder training* to encompass a wide variety of techniques. It is very important to distinguish between procedures that are patient-dependent (i.e., necessitate adequate function, learning capability, and motivation of the patient), in which the goal is to restore a normal pattern of voiding and continence, and procedures that are caregiver-dependent and can be used for functionally disabled patients, in which the goal is to keep the patient and environment dry. Behavioral interventions are summarized in Table 7-13. All the patient-dependent procedures generally involve the patient's continuous self-monitoring, using a record such as the one depicted in Fig. 7-8, and the caregiver-dependent procedures usually involve a record such as the one shown in Fig. 7-9.

Pelvic muscle (Kegel) exercises are an essential component of patient-dependent behavioral interventions. These exercises consist of repetitive contractions and relaxations of the pelvic floor muscles. The exercises may be taught by having the patient interrupt voiding to get a sense of the muscles being used or by having women squeeze the examiner's fingers during a vaginal examination (without doing a Valsalva maneuver, which is the opposite of the intended effect). Many women, however, require biofeedback to help them identify the muscles and practice the exercises (see below). One exercise is a 10-s squeeze and a 10-s relaxation. Most older women will have to build endurance gradually to this level. Once learned, the exercises should be practiced many times throughout the day (up to 40 exercises per day) and, importantly, should be used in everyday life during situations (e.g., coughing, hearing running water) that might precipitate incontinence. Vaginal cones (weights) may be useful adjuncts to

pelvic muscle exercises in some patients. Electrical stimulation may also be used to help identify and train pelvic muscles. This technique (using a different frequency of stimulation) may also be useful in suppressing the involuntary bladder contractions associated with urge incontinence. Currently this intervention is not reimbursed by Medicare, and many patients are reluctant to purchase the devices for a therapeutic trial.

Biofeedback generally involves the use of vaginal (or rectal) pressure or electromyography (EMG) and abdominal muscle EMG recordings to train patients to contract pelvic floor muscles and relax the abdomen. Studies have shown that these techniques can be very effective for managing both stress and urge incontinence in the geriatric population (Burgio et al., 1985; Burns et al., 1993). The use of biofeedback techniques may be limited by their requirements for equipment and trained personnel. Some newer biofeedback techniques use surface electrodes and are less invasive. Numerous software packages are now available to assist with biofeedback training.

Other forms of patient-dependent interventions include bladder training and bladder retraining. Bladder training involves education, pelvic muscle exercises (with or without biofeedback), strategies to manage urgency, and the regular use of bladder records (Fig. 7-8). Bladder training is highly effective in selected community-dwelling patients, especially women (Burton et al., 1988; Fantl et al., 1991). Bladder retraining as described here is similar to "bladder drill," which has been used successfully to treat urge incontinence in young women. An example of a bladder retraining protocol is shown in Table 7-14. This protocol is also applicable to patients who have had indwelling catheterization for monitoring of urinary output during a period of acute illness or for treatment of urinary retention with overflow incontinence. Such catheters should always be removed as soon as possible, and this type of bladder retraining protocol should enable most indwelling catheters to be removed from patients in acute care hospitals as well as some in long-term-care settings. A patient who continues to have difficulty voiding after 1 to 2 weeks of bladder retraining should be examined for other potentially reversible causes of voiding difficulties, such as those mentioned in the preceding discussion of acute incontinence. When difficulties persist, a urologic referral should be considered in order to rule out correctable lower genitourinary pathology.

The goal of caregiver-dependent interventions is to prevent incontinence episodes rather than restore normal patterns of voiding and

Table 7-13 Examples of behavioral interventions for urinary incontinence

Procedure	Definition	Types of incontinence	Comments
Patient-dependent			
Pelvic muscle (Kegel) exercises	Repetitive contraction and relaxation of pelvic floor muscles	Stress and urge	Requires adequate function and motivation. May be done in conjunction with biofeedback and other adjunctive techniques.
Bladder training	Use of education, bladder records, pelvic muscle and other behavioral techniques	Stress and urge	Requires trained therpist, adequate cognitive and physical functioning, and motivation.
Bladder retraining	Progressive lengthening or shortening of intervoiding interval, with intermittent catheterization used in patients recovering from overdistention injuries with persistent retention (see Table 7-14)	Acute (e.g., postcatheterization with urge or overflow, poststroke)	Goal is to restore normal pattern of voiding and continence. Requires adequate cognitive and physical function and motivation.

Caregiver-dependent Scheduled toileting	Routine toileting at regular intervals (scheduled toileting)	Urge and functional	Goal is to prevent wetting episodes. Can be used in patients with impaired cognitive or physical functioning. Requires staff or caregiver availability and motivation.
Habit training	Variable toileting schedule based on patient's voiding patterns	Urge and functional	Goal is to prevent wetting episodes Can be used in patients with impaired cognitive or physical functioning. Requires staff or caregiver availability and motivation.
Prompted voiding	Offer opportunity to toilet every 2 h during the day; toilet only on request; social reinforcement; routine offering of fluids (see Table 7-5)	Urge, stress, mixed, functional	Same as above. 25–40% of nursing home residents respond well during the day and can be identified during a 3-day trial (see text and Table 7-15)

Table 7-14 Example of a bladder retraining protocol

Objective: To restore a normal pattern of voiding and continence after the removal of an indwelling catheter

1. Remove the indwelling catheter (clamping the catheter before removal is not necessary).
2. Treat urinary tract infection if present.
3. Initiate a toileting schedule. Begin by toileting the patient:
   a. Upon awakening
   b. Every 2 h during the day and evening
   c. Before getting into bed
   d. Every 4 h at night
4. Monitor the patient's voiding and continence pattern with a record that allows for the recording of:
   a. Frequency, timing, and amount of continent voids
   b. Frequency, timing, and amount of incontinence episodes
   c. Fluid intake pattern
   d. Postvoid catheter volume
5. If the patient is having difficulty voiding (complete urinary retention or very low urine outputs, e.g., <240 mL in an 8-h period while fluid intake is adequate):
   a. Perform in-an-out catheterization, recording volume obtained, every 6 to 8 h until residual values are <200 mL
   b. Instruct the patient on techniques to trigger voiding (e.g., running water, stroking inner thigh, suprapubic tapping) and to help completely empty bladder (e.g., bending forward, suprapubic pressure, double voiding)
   c. If the patient continues to have high residual volumes after 1–2 weeks, consider urodynamic evaluation
6. If the patient is voiding frequently (i.e., more often than every 2 h):
   a. Perform postvoid residual determination to ensure the patient is completely emptying the bladder
   b. Encourage the patient to delay voiding as long as possible and instruct him or her to use techniques to help completely empty bladder
   c. If the patient continues to have frequency and nocturia with or without urgency and incontinence:
      1. Rule out other reversible causes (e.g., urinary tract infection medication effects, hyperglycemia, and congestive heart failure)
      2. Consider urodynamic evaluation to rule out bladder instability (unstable bladder, detrusor hyperreflexia)

complete continence. Such procedures have been shown to be effective in reducing incontinence in selected nursing home residents (Hu et al., 1989; Colling et al., 1992; Ouslander et al., 1995b). In its simplest form, scheduled toileting involves toileting the patient at regular intervals, usually every 2 h during the day and every 4 h during

the evening and night. Habit training involves a schedule of toiletings or prompted voidings that is modified according to the patient's pattern of continent voids and incontinence episodes as demonstrated by a monitoring record such as that shown in Fig. 7-9. Adjunctive techniques to prompt voiding (e.g., running tap water, stroking the inner thigh, or suprapubic tapping) and to facilitate complete emptying of the bladder (e.g., bending forward after completion of voiding) may be helpful in some patients. Prompted voiding has been the best-studied of these procedures. An example of a prompted voiding protocol is outlined in Table 7-15. The success of these interventions is largely dependent on the knowledge and motivation of the caregivers who are implementing them rather than on the physical functional and mental status of the incontinent patient. Targeting of prompted voiding to selected patients, after a 3-day trial (see Table 7-15), may enhance its cost-effectiveness (Schnelle et al., 1988). Quality assurance methods, based on principles of industrial statistical quality control, have been shown to be helpful in maintaining the effectiveness of prompted voiding in nursing homes (Schnelle et al., 1993; Schnelle et al., 1995).

Drug Treatment

Table 7-16 lists the drugs used to treat various types of incontinence. The efficacy of drug treatment has not been as well studied in the geriatric population as it has in younger populations. However, for many patients, especially those with urge or stress incontinence, drug treatment may be very effective. Drug treatment can be prescribed in conjunction with various behavioral interventions. There are few data on the relative efficacy of drug versus behavioral versus combination treatment. Thus, until controlled trials are conducted, treatment decisions should be individualized and will depend in large part on the characteristics and preferences of the patient and the preference of the health care professional.

For urge incontinence, drugs with anticholinergic and relaxant effects on the bladder smooth muscle are used. All of them can have bothersome systemic anticholinergic side effects, especially dry mouth, and they can precipitate urinary retention in some patients. Men with some degree of outflow obstruction, diabetics, and patients with impaired bladder contractility are at the highest risk for

Table 7-15 Example of a prompted voiding protocol for a nursing home

Assessment period (3–5 days)

1. Contact resident every hour from 7 a.m. to 7 p.m. for 2–3 days, then every 2 h for 2–3 days
2. Focus attention on voiding by asking them whether he or she is wet or dry
3. Check residents for wetness, record on bladder record, and give feedback on whether response was correct or incorrect
4. Whether wet or dry, ask residents if they would like to use the toilet or urinal. If they say yes:
   • Offer assistance
   • Record results on bladder record
   • Give positive reinforcement by spending extra time talking with them
   If they say no:
   • Repeat the question once or twice
   • Inform them that you will be back in 1 h and request that they try to delay voiding until then
   • If there has been no attempt to void in the last 2–3 h, repeat the request to use the toilet at least twice more before leaving
5. Offer fluids

Targeting

1. Prompted voiding is more effective in some residents than others
2. The best candidates are residents who show the following characteristics during the assessment period:
   • Void in the toilet, commode, or urinal (as opposed to being incontinent in a pad or garment) more than two-thirds of the time
   • Wet on ≤20% of checks
   • Show substantial reduction in incontinence frequency on 2-h prompts
3. Residents who do not show any of these characteristics may be candidates for either:
   • Further evaluation to determine the specific type of incontinence if they attempt to toilet but remain frequently wet
   • Palliative management by containment devices and a checking-and-changing protocol if they do not cooperate with prompting

Prompted voiding (ongoing protocol)

1. Contact the resident every 2 h from 7 a.m. to 7 p.m.
2. Use same procedures as for the assessment period
3. For nighttime management, use either modified prompted voiding schedule or containment device, depending on resident's sleep pattern
4. If a resident who has been responding well has an increase in incontinence frequency despite adequate staff implementation of the protocol, he or she should be evaluated for reversible factors

developing urinary retention and should be followed carefully when these drugs are prescribed. Patients with Alzheimer's disease must be followed for the development of drug-induced delirium, which is, however, unusual. The newest bladder relaxant, tolterodine, appears to have an efficacy similar to that of other anticholinergics, with fewer systemic side effects (Appell, 1997). Oxybutynin, starting in half the usual recommended dose (i.e., 2.5 mg three times per day) does not have the potentially serious effects on blood pressure and cardiac conduction of imipramine (Ouslander et al., 1988b). Several studies suggest that cognitive and physical functional impairments are associated with poor responses to bladder-relaxant drug therapy (Zorzitto et al., 1986; Tobin and Brocklehurst, 1986a). The results of these studies should not, however, preclude a treatment trial in this patient population. Some patients may respond, especially in conjunction with prompted voiding (Ouslander et al., 1995c). The *goal* of treatment in these patients may not be to cure the incontinence but to reduce its severity and prevent discomfort and complications.

For stress incontinence, drug treatment involves a combination of an alpha agonist and estrogen. Drug treatment is appropriate for motivated patients who have mild to moderate degrees of stress incontinence, do not have a major anatomic abnormality (e.g., grade 3 cystocele or intrinsic sphincter deficiency), and do not have any contraindications to these drugs. These patients may also respond to concomitant behavioral interventions, as described above. For stress incontinence, estrogen alone is not as effective as it is in combination with an alpha agonist (Fantl et al., 1996). If oral estrogen is used for a prolonged period of time (more than a few months), cyclic administration and the addition of a progestational agent should be considered for women with a uterus. Estrogen is also used for the treatment of irritative voiding symptoms and urge incontinence in women with atrophic vaginitis and urethritis. Oral estrogen is probably not as effective as topical estrogen for these symptoms. Vaginal estrogen can be prescribed 5 nights per week for 1 to 2 months initially and then reduced to a maintenance dose of one to three times per week. A vaginal ring that which slowly releases estrogen is also available.

Drug treatment for chronic overflow incontinence using a cholinergic agonist or an alpha-adrenergic antagonist is rarely efficacious. Bethanechol may be helpful when given for a brief period subcutaneously in patients with persistent bladder contractility problems after

Table 7-16 Drugs used to treat urinary incontinence

Drugs	Dosages	Mechanisms of action	Type of incontinence	Potential adverse effects
Anticholinergic and antispasmodic agents:				
Dicyclomine (Bentyl, others)	10–20 mg tid	Increase bladder capacity		Dry mouth, blurry vision, elevated intraocular pressure, delirium, constipation
Hyoscamine (Levsin, others)	0.125 mg tid	Diminish involuntary bladder contractions		
Imipramine (Tofranil)	25–50 mg tid			
Oxybutynin (Ditropan)	2.5–5.0 mg tid		Urge or mixed with urge predominant	Above effects plus postural hypotension, cardiac conduction disturbances
Propantheline (Pro-Banthine)	15–30 mg tid			
Tolterodine (Detrol)	1–2 mg bid			
Alpha-adrenergic agonists:				
Imipramine (Tofranil)	25–50 mg tid	Increase urethral smooth muscle contraction		See above
Phenylpropanolamine (Entex, Ornade)	75 mg bid			Headache, tachycardia, elevation of blood pressure
Pseudoephedrine (Sudafed)	30–60 mg tid			

Drug	Dosage	Mechanism	Indication	Side effects
Conjugated estrogens:				
Oral (Premarin)	0.625 mg/day	Strengthen periurethral tissues	Urge associated with atrophic vaginitis	Endometrial cancer, elevated blood pressure, gallstones
Topical	0.5–1.0 g/application	Increase periurethral blood flow	Stress	
Vaginal ring (Estring)	One ring every 3 months			
Cholinergic agonists:				
Bethanechol (Urecholine)	10–30 mg tid	Stimulate bladder contraction	Overflow incontinence with atonic bladder	Bradycardia, hypotension, bronchoconstriction, gastric acid secretion
Alpha-adrenergic antagonist:				
Doxazosin (Cardura)	1–4 mg qhs	Relax smooth muscle of urethra and prostatic capsule	Urge incontinence and related irritative symptoms associated with benign prostatic enlargement	Postural hypotension
Tamsulosin (Flowmax)	0.4–0.8 mg/day			
Terazosin (Hytrin)	1–5 mg qhs			

an overdistension injury, but it is seldom effective when given over the long term orally (Finkbeiner, 1985). Alpha-adrenergic blockers may be helpful in relieving symptoms associated with outflow obstruction in some patients but are probably not efficacious for long-term treatment of overflow incontinence. These drugs are, however, effective in treating irritative voiding symptoms associated with urge incontinence in men with benign prostatic enlargement (Lepor et al., 1996).

Surgery

Surgery should be considered for older women with stress incontinence that continues to be bothersome after attempts at nonsurgical treatment and in women with a significant degree of pelvic prolapse or ISD. As with many other surgical procedures, patient selection and the experience of the surgeon are critical to success. All women being considered for surgical therapy should have a thorough evaluation, including urodynamic tests, before undergoing the procedure. Women with mixed stress incontinence and detrusor motor instability may also benefit from surgery, especially if the clinical history and urodynamic findings suggest that stress incontinence is the predominant problem. Many modified techniques of bladder neck suspension can be done with minimal risk and are highly successful in achieving continence over about a 5-year period. Urinary retention can occur after surgery, but it is usually transient and can be managed by a brief period of suprapubic catheterization. Periurethral injection of collagen and other materials is now available and may offer patients with ISD an alternative to surgery. Surgical intervention for patients with ISD involves a perivaginal sling procedure rather than bladder neck suspension.

Surgery may be indicated in men in whom incontinence is associated with anatomically and/or urodynamically documented outflow obstruction. Men who have experienced an episode of complete urinary retention are likely to have another episode within a short period of time and should have a prostatic resection, as should men with incontinence associated with a sufficient amount of residual urine to be causing recurrent symptomatic infections or hydronephrosis. The decision about surgery in men who do not meet these criteria must be an individual one, weighing carefully

the degree to which the symptoms bother the patient, the potential benefits of surgery (obstructive symptoms often respond better than irritative symptoms), and the risks of surgery (which may be minimal with newer prostate resection techniques). A small number of older patients, especially men who have stress incontinence related to sphincter damage due to previous transurethral surgery, may benefit from the surgical implantation of an artificial urinary sphincter.

Catheters and Catheter Care

Three basic types of catheters and catheterization procedures are used for the management of urinary incontinence: external catheters, intermittent straight catheterization, and chronic indwelling catheterization. External catheters generally consist of some type of condom connected to a drainage system. Improvements in design and observance of proper procedure and skin care when applying the catheter will decrease the risk of skin irritation as well as the frequency with which the catheter falls off. Data suggest that patients with external catheters are at increased risk of developing symptomatic infection (Ouslander et al., 1987a). External catheters should be used only to manage intractable incontinence in male patients who do not have urinary retention and who are extremely physically dependent. As with incontinence undergarments and padding, these devices should not be used as a matter of convenience, since they may foster dependency.

Intermittent catheterization can help in the management of patients with urinary retention and overflow incontinence due to an acontractile bladder or DIIIC. The procedure can be carried out by either the patient or a caregiver and involves straight catheterization two to four times daily, depending on residual urine volumes. In the home setting, the catheter should be kept clean (but not necessarily sterile). Studies conducted largely among younger paraplegics have shown that this technique is practical and reduces the risk of symptomatic infection as compared with chronic catheterization. Intermittent self-catheterization has also been shown to be feasible for older female outpatients who are functional, willing, and able to catheterize themselves. However, studies carried out in young paraplegics and elderly female outpatients cannot automatically be extrapolated to an elderly male or institutionalized popula-

tion. The technique may be useful for certain patients in acute care hospitals or nursing homes, as following removal of an indwelling catheter in a bladder retraining protocol (Table 7-14). Nursing home residents, however, may be difficult to catheterize, and the anatomic abnormalities commonly found in older patients' lower urinary tracts may increase the risk of infection due to repeated straight catheterizations. In addition, using this technique in an institutional setting (which may have an abundance of organisms that are relatively resistant to many commonly used antimicrobial agents) may yield an unacceptable risk of nosocomial infections, and using sterile catheter trays for these procedures would be very expensive; thus, it may be extremely difficult to implement such a program in a typical nursing home setting.

Chronic indwelling catheterization is overused in some settings and has been shown to increase the incidence of a number of complications, including chronic bacteriuria, bladder stones, periurethral abscesses, and even bladder cancer. Nursing home residents, especially men, managed by this technique are at relatively high risk of developing symptomatic infections (Warren et al., 1987; Ouslander et al., 1987c). Given these risks, it seems appropriate to recommend that the use of chronic indwelling catheters be limited to certain specific situations (Table 7-17). When indwelling catheterization is used, certain principles of catheter care should be observed in order to attempt to minimize complications (Table 7-18).

Table 7-17 Indications for chronic indwelling catheter use

Urinary retention that:
  Is causing persistent overflow incontinence, symptomatic infections, or renal dysfunction
  Cannot be corrected surgically or medically
  Cannot be managed practically with intermittent catheterization

Skin wounds, pressure sores, or irritations that are being contaminated by incontinent urine

Care of terminally ill or severely impaired patients for whom bed and clothing changes are uncomfortable or disruptive

Preference of patient when toileting or changing is cause excessive discomfort

Table 7-18   Key principles of chronic indwelling catheter care

1. Maintain sterile, closed gravity-drainage system.
2. Avoid breaking the closed system.
3. Use clean techniques in emptying and changing the drainage system; wash hands between patients in institutionalized setting.
4. Secure the catheter to the upper thigh or lower abdomen to avoid perineal contamination and urethral irritation due to movement of the catheter.
5. Avoid frequent and vigorous cleaning of the catheter entry site; washing with soapy water once per day is sufficient.
6. Do not routinely irrigate.
7. If bypassing occurs in the absence of obstruction, consider the possibility of a bladder spasm, which can be treated with a bladder relaxant.
8. If catheter obstruction occurs frequently, increase the patient's fluid intake and acidify the urine with dilute acetic acid irrigations.
9. Do not routinely use prophylactic or suppressive urinary antiseptics or antimicrobials.
10. Do not do surveillance cultures to guide management of individual patients because all chronically catheterized patients have bacteriuria (which is often polymicrobial) and the organisms change frequently.
11. Do not treat infection unless the patient develops symptoms; symptoms may be nonspecific and other possible sources of infection should be carefully excluded before attributing symptoms to the urinary tract.
12. If a patient develops frequent symptomatic urinary tract infections, a genitourinary evaluation should be considered to rule out pathology such as stones, periurethral or prostatic abscesses, and chronic pyelonephritis.

FECAL INCONTINENCE

Fecal incontinence is less common than urinary incontinence (Nelson et al., 1995). Its occurrence is relatively unusual in older patients who are continent with regard to urine; however, a large proportion (30 to 50 percent) of geriatric patients with frequent urinary incontinence also have episodes of fecal incontinence (Ouslander et al., 1982; Ouslander and Fowler, 1985; Tobin and Brocklehurst, 1986b). This coexistence suggests common pathophysiologic mechanisms.

Defecation, like urination, is a physiologic process that involves smooth and striated muscles, central and peripheral innervation, coordination of reflex responses, mental awareness, and physical ability to get to a toilet. Disruption of any of these factors can lead to fecal incontinence. The most common causes of fecal incontinence are problems with constipation and laxative use, neurologic disorders,

and colorectal disorders (Table 7-19). Constipation is extremely common in the geriatric population and, when chronic, can lead to fecal impaction and incontinence. The hard stool (or scybalum) of fecal impaction irritates the rectum and results in the production of mucus and fluid. This fluid leaks around the mass of impacted stool and precipitates incontinence. Constipation is difficult to define; technically it indicates less than three bowel movements per week, although many patients use the term to describe difficult passage of hard stools or a feeling of incomplete evacuation. Poor dietary and toilet habits, immobility, and chronic laxative abuse are the most common causes of constipation in geriatric patients (Table 7-20).

Appropriate management of constipation will prevent fecal impaction and resultant fecal incontinence. The first step in managing constipation is the identification of all possible contributory factors. If the constipation is a new complaint and represents a recent change in bowel habit, then colonic disease, endocrine or metabolic disorders, depression, or drug side effects should be considered (Table 7-19). Proper diet, including adequate fluid intake and bulk, is important in preventing constipation. Crude fiber in amounts of 4 to 6 g (equivalent to 3 or 4 tablespoons of bran) a day is generally recommended. Improving mobility, body positioning during toileting, and the timing and setting of toileting are all important in managing constipation. Defecation should optimally take place in a private, unrushed atmosphere and should take advantage of the gastrocolic reflex, which

Table 7-19 Causes of fecal incontinence

Fecal impaction

Laxative overuse or abuse

Neurologic disorders
  Dementia
  Stroke
  Spinal cord disease/injury

Colorectal disorders
  Diarrheal illness
  Diabetic autonomic neuropathy
  Rectal sphincter damage

Table 7-20 Causes of constipation

Diet low in bulk and fluid

Poor toilet habits

Immobility

Laxative abuse

Colorectal disorders
  Colonic tumor, stricture, volvulus
  Painful anal and rectal conditions
  (hemorrhoids, fissures)

Depression

Drugs
  Anticholinergic
  Narcotic

Diabetic autonomic neuropathy

Endocrine or metabolic
  Hypothyroidism
  Hypercalcemia
  Hypokalemia

---

occurs a few minutes after eating. These factors are often overlooked, especially in nursing home settings.

A variety of drugs can be used to treat constipation (Table 7-21). These drugs are often overused; in fact, their overuse may cause an atonic colon and contribute to chronic constipation ("cathartic colon"). Laxative drugs can also contribute to fecal incontinence. Rational use of these drugs necessitates knowing the nature of the constipation and quality of the stool. For example, stool softeners will not help a patient with a large mass of already soft stool in the rectum. These patients would benefit from a glycerin or irritant suppositories. The use of osmotic and irritant laxatives should be limited to no more than three or four times a week.

Fecal incontinence from neurologic disorders is sometimes amenable to biofeedback therapy, although most severely demented patients are unable to cooperate. For those patients with end-stage dementia who fail to respond to a regular toileting program and suppositories, a program of alternating constipating agents (if necessary) and laxatives on a routine schedule (such as giving laxatives or

Table 7-21 Drugs used to treat constipation

Type	Examples	Mechanism of action
Stool softeners and lubricants	Dioctyl sodium succinate Mineral oil	Soften and lubricate fecal mass
Bulk-forming agents	Bran Psyllium mucilloid	Increase fecal bulk and retain fluid in bowel lumen
Osmotic cathartics	Milk of magnesia Magnesium sulfate/ citrate Lactulose Sorbitol	Poorly absorbed and retain fluid in bowel lumen; increase net secretions of fluid in small intestine
Stimulants and irritants	Cascara Senna Bisacodyl Phyenolphthalein	Alter intestinal mucosal permeability; stimulate muscle activity and fluid secretions
Enemas	Tap water Saline Sodium phosphate Oil	Induce reflex evacuations
Suppositories	Glycerin Bisacodyl	Cause mucosal irritation

enemas three times a week) is often effective in controlling defecation. Experience suggests that these measures should permit management of even severely demented patients. As a last resort, specially designed incontinence undergarments are sometimes helpful in managing fecal incontinence and preventing complications. Frequent changing is essential, because fecal material, especially in the presence of incontinent urine, can cause skin irritation and predispose to pressure ulcers.

REFERENCES

American Medical Directors Association: *Urinary Incontinence: Clinical Practice Guideline.* Columbia, MD, AMDA, 1996.

Appell RA: Clinical efficacy and safety of tolterodine in the treatment of overactive bladder: a pooled analysis. *Urology* 50(suppl 6A):90–96, 1997.

Asplund R, Aberg H: Diurnal variation in the levels of antidiuretic hormone in the elderly. *J Intern Med* 229:131–134, 1991.

Boscia JA, Kobasa WD, Knight RA, et al: Epidemiology of bacteriuria in elderly ambulatory population. *Am J Med* 80:208–214, 1986a.

Boscia JA, Kobasa WD, Levison ME, et al: Lack of association between bacteriuria and symptoms in the elderly. *Am J Med* 81:979–982, 1986b.

Burgio KL, Whitehead WE, Engel BT: Urinary incontinence in elderly—Bladder-sphincter biofeedback and toilet skills training. *Ann Intern Med* 104:507–515, 1985.

Burns PA, Pranikoff K, Nochajski TH, et al: A comparison of effectiveness of biofeedback and pelvic muscle exercise treatment of stress incontinence in older community-dwelling women. *J Gerontol* 48(4):M167–M174, 1993.

Burton JR, Pearce KL, Burgio KL, et al: Behavioral training for urinary incontinence in elderly patients. *J Am Geriatr Soc* 36:693–698, 1988.

Colling J, Ouslander J, Hadley B, et al: The effects of patterned urge toileting on incontinence in nursing homes. *J Am Geriatr Soc* 39:135–141, 1992.

Diokno AC, Wells TJ, Brink CA: Urinary incontinence in elderly women: urodynamic evaluation. *J Am Geriatr Soc* 35:940–946, 1987.

Diokno AC, Brown MB, Brock BM, et al: Clinical and cystometric characteristics of continent and incontinent noninstitutionalized elderly. *J Urol* 140:567–571, 1988.

Elbadawi A, Yalla SV, Resnick N: Structural basis of geriatric voiding dysfunction: I. Methods of a prospective ultrastructural/urodynamic study and an overview of the findings. *J Urol* 150:1650–1656, 1993.

Elbadawi A, Hailemariam S, Yalla SV, et al: Structural basis of geriatric voiding dysfunction: VII. Prospective ultrastructural/urodynamic evaluation of its natural evolution. *J Urol* 157:1814–1822, 1997.

Fantl JA, Wyman FJ, McClish DK, et al: Efficacy of bladder training in older women with urinary incontinence. *JAMA* 265:609–613, 1991.

Fantl JA, Newman DK, Colling J, et al: *Urinary Incontinence in Adults: Acute and Chronic Management.* Clinical Practice Guideline No. 2, 1996, Update. U.S. Department of Health and Human Services. Public Health Service, Agency for Health Care Policy and Research. AHCPR Publication No. 96-0682: Rockville, MD, USDHHS, 1996.

Fantl JA, Bump RC, Robinson D, et al: Efficacy of estrogen supplementation in the treatment of urinary incontinence: The Continence Program for Women Research Group. *Obstet Gynecol* 88:745–749, 1996.

Finkbeiner AE: Is bethanechol chloride clinically effective in promoting bladder emptying? A literature review. *J Urol* 134:443–449, 1985.

Hadley E: Bladder training and related therapies for urinary incontinence in older people. *JAMA* 256:372–379, 1986.

Harris T: *Aging in the Eighties: Prevalence and Impact of Urinary Problems in Individuals Age 65 Years and Over.* National Center for Health Statistics, Advance Data No. 121, 1986.

Hu T-W, Igou JF, Kaltreider DL, et al: A clinical trial of a behavioral therapy to reduce urinary incontinence in nursing homes. *JAMA* 261:2656–2662, 1989.

Lepor H, Williford WO, Barry MJ, et al: The efficacy of terazosin, finasteride, or both in benign prostatic hyperplasia. Veterans Affairs Cooperative Studies Benign Prostatic Hyperplasia Study Group. *N Engl J Med* 335:533–539, 1996.

Nelson R, Norton N, Cautley E, Furner S: Community-based prevalence of anal incontinence. *JAMA* 274:559–561, 1995.

Nicolle LE, Bjornson J, Harding GMK, et al: Bacteriuria in elderly institutionalized men. *N Engl J Med* 309:1420–1425, 1983.

Nicolle LE, Mayhew JW, Bryan L, et al: Prospective randomized comparison of therapy and no therapy for asymptomatic bacteriuria in institutionalized elderly women. *JAMA* 83:27–33, 1987.

Ouslander JG, Kane RL, Abrass IB: Urinary incontinence in elderly nursing home patients. *JAMA* 248:1194–1198, 1982.

Ouslander JG, Fowler E: Incontinence in VA nursing home care units. *J Am Geriatr Soc* 33:33–40, 1985.

Ouslander JG, Raz S, Hepps K, et al: Genitourinary dysfunction in a geriatric outpatient population. *J Am Geriatr Soc* 34:507–514, 1986.

Ouslander JG, Uman GC, Urman HN: Development and testing of an incontinence monitoring record. *J Am Geriatr Soc* 34:83–90, 1986a.

Ouslander JG, Greengold BA, Chen S: External catheter use and urinary tract infections among male nursing home patients. *J Am Geriatr Soc* 35:1063–1070, 1987a.

Ouslander JG, Greengold BA, Silverblatt FJ, et al: An accurate method to obtain urine for culture in men with external catheters. *Arch Intern Med* 147:286–288, 1987b.

Ouslander JG, Greengold BA, Chen S: Complications of chronic indwelling urinary catheters among male nursing home patients: A prospective study. *J Urol* 138:1191–1195, 1987c.

Ouslander JG, Blaustein J, Connor A, et al: Pharmacokinetics and clinical effects of oxybutynin in geriatric patients. *J Urol* 140:47–50, 1988b.

Ouslander JG, Leach GE, Staskin DR: Simplified tests of lower urinary tract function in the evaluation of geriatric urinary incontinence. *J Am Geriatr Soc* 37:706–714, 1989a.

Ouslander JG, Leach G, Staskin D, et al: Prospective evaluation of an assessment strategy for geriatric urinary incontinence. *J Am Geriatr Soc* 37:715–724, 1989b.

Ouslander JG, Schapira M, Schnelle J, et al: Does eradicating bacteriuria affect the severity of chronic urinary incontinence among nursing home residents? *Ann Intern Med* 122:749–754, 1995a.

Ouslander JG, Schnelle JF, Uman G, et al: Predictors of successful prompted voiding among incontinent nursing home residents. *JAMA* 273:1366–1370, 1995b.

Ouslander JG, Schnelle JF, Uman G, et al: Does oxybutynin add to the effectiveness of prompted voiding for urinary incontinence among nursing home residents? A placebo-controlled trial. *J Am Geriatr Soc* 43:610–617, 1995c.

Ouslander JG, Schapira M, Schnelle JF: Urine specimen collection from incontinent female nursing home residents. *J Am Geriatr Soc* 43:279–281, 1995d.

Ouslander JG, Schapira M, Schnelle JF: Pyuria among chronically incontinent, otherwise asymptomatic nursing home residents. *J Am Geriatr Soc* 44:420–423, 1996.

Resnick NM: Urinary incontinence in the elderly. *Med Grand Rounds* 3:281–289, 1984.

Resnick NM, Yalla SV: Detrusor hyperactivity with impaired contractile function: an unrecognized but common cause of incontinence in elderly patients. *JAMA* 257:3076–3081, 1987.

Schnelle JF, Sowell VA, Hu TW, et al: Reduction of urinary incontinence in nursing homes: Does it reduce or increase costs? *J Am Geriatr Soc* 36:34–39, 1988.

Schnelle JF, Newman D, White W, et al: Maintaining continence in nursing home residents through the application of industrial quality control. *Gerontologist* 33:114–121, 1993.

Schnelle JF, McNees P, Crook V, et al: The use of a computer-based model to implement an incontinence management program. *Gerontologist* 35:656–665, 1995.

Sier H, Ouslander JG, Orzeck S: Urinary incontinence among geriatric patients in an acute care hospital. *JAMA* 257:1767–1771, 1987.

Tobin GW, Brocklehurst JC: The management of urinary incontinence in local authority residential homes for the elderly. *Age Ageing* 15:292–298, 1986a.

Tobin GW, Brocklehurst JC: Fecal incontinence in residential homes for the elderly: Prevalence, aetiology and management. *Age Ageing* 15:41–46, 1986b.

Warren JW, Damron D, Tenney JH, et al: Fever, bacteremia and death as complications of bacteriuria in women with long-term urethral catheters. *J Infect Dis* 155:1151–1158, 1987.

Wells TJ, Brink CA, Diokno AC, et al: Pelvic muscle exercises for stress urinary incontinence in elderly women. *J Am Geriatr Soc* 38:296–299, 1991.

Zorzitto ML, Jewett MAS, Fernie GR, et al: Effectiveness of propantheline bromide in the treatment of geriatric patients with detrusor instability. *Neurourol Urodynam* 5:133–140, 1986.

SUGGESTED READINGS

Abrams P, Wein AJ (eds): The overactive bladder: basic science to clinical management consensus conference. *Urology* 50(6A suppl), 1997.

Eastwood HDH, Smart CJ: Urinary incontinence in the disabled elderly male. *Age Ageing* 14:235–239, 1985.

Gartley C: *Managing Incontinence: A Guide to Living with the Loss of Bladder Control.* Ottowa, IL, Jameson Books, 1985.

Harari D, Gurwitz JH, Avorn J, et al: Bowel habit in relation to age and gender: findings from the National Health Interview Survey and clinical implications. *Arch Intern Med* 156:315–320, 1996.

Herzog AR, Fultz NH: Prevalence and incidence of urinary incontinence in community-dwelling populations. *J Am Geriatr Soc* 38:273–281, 1990.

Madoff RD, Williams JG, Caushaj PF: Fecal incontinence. *N Engl J Med* 326:1002–1007, 1992.

McCormick KA, Scheve AAS, Leahy E: Nursing management of urinary incontinence in geriatric inpatients. *Nurs Clin North Am* 23:231–264, 1988.

Ouslander JG (ed): Aging and the lower urinary tract. *Am J Med Sci,* 1997.

Ouslander JG, Schnelle JF: Incontinence in the nursing home. *Ann Intern Med* 122:438–449, 1995.

Resnick NM, Ouslander JG (eds): NIH Consensus Conference on Urinary Incontinence in Adults. *J Am Geriatr Soc* 38:263–386, 1990.

Resnick NM: An 89-year-old woman with urinary incontinence. *JAMA* 276:1832–1840, 1996.

Resnick NM, Brandeis GH, Baumann MM, et al: Misdiagnosis of urinary incontinence in nursing home women: prevalence and a proposed solution. *Neurourol Urodynam* 15:599–618, 1996.

Romero Y, Evans JM, Fleming KC, Phillip SF: Constipation and fecal incontinence in the elderly population. *Mayo Clin Proc* 71:81–92, 1996.

Skelly J, Flint AJ: Urinary incontinence associated with dementia. *J Am Geriatr Soc* 42:286–294, 1995.

Thom D: Variation in estimates of urinary incontinence prevalence in the community: effects of differences in definition, population characteristics, and study type. *J Am Geriatr Soc* 46:473–480, 1998.

Tramonte SM, Brand MB, Mulrow CD, et al: The treatment of chronic constipation in adults: a systematic review. *J Gen Intern Med* 12:15–24, 1997.

EIGHT

INSTABILITY AND FALLS

Unstable gait and falls are common among older people, and falls are among the major causes of morbidity in this population. Falling is often a marker for frailty, and falls may be predictors of death as well as indirect causes (usually through fractures). Close to one-third of those aged 65 and older living at home suffer a fall each year, and about one in 40 of those will be hospitalized. Only about half of the elderly patients hospitalized as the result of a fall will be alive a year later. Among geriatric nursing homes residents, as many as half suffer a fall each year; 10 to 25 percent have serious consequences. Accidents are the fifth leading cause of death in persons older than 65, and falls account for two-thirds of these accidental deaths. Of deaths from falls in the United States, over 70 percent occur in the 11 percent of the population over age 65 (Rubenstein et al., 1988; Sattin et al., 1990). Fear of falling can adversely affect older persons' functional status (Tinetti et al., 1994b).

Table 8-1 lists potential complications of falls. Fractures of the hip, femur, humerus, wrist, and ribs and painful soft tissue injuries are the most frequent physical complications. Many of these injuries will result in hospitalization, with the attendant risks of immobilization

Table 8-1 Complications of falls in elderly patients

Injuries
  Painful soft tissue injuries
  Fractures
    Hip
    Femur
    Humerus
    Wrist
    Ribs
  Subdural hematoma

Hospitalization
  Complications of immobilization (see Chap. 9)
  Risk of iatrogenic illnesses (see Chap. 4)

Disability
  Impaired mobility due to physical injury
  Impaired mobility from fear, loss of self-confidence,
    and restriction of ambulation

Risk of institutionalization

Death

and iatrogenic illnesses (see Chaps. 4 and 9). Fractures of the hip and lower extremities often lead to prolonged disability because of impaired mobility. A less common, but important, injury is subdural hematoma. Neurologic symptoms and signs that develop days to weeks after a fall should prompt consideration of this treatable problem. Even when the fall does not result in serious injury, substantial disability may result from fear of falling, loss of self-confidence, and restricted ambulation (either self-imposed or imposed by caregivers). Repeated falls and consequent injuries can be important factors in the decision to institutionalize an elderly person.

Falls and their attendant complications should be preventable, but it is easier to identify risk factors for falling than to prevent its occurrence. There is a growing body of studies that suggest that at least some types of falls can be prevented. Moreover, it is possible to prevent the untoward consequences of falls (i.e., fractures) by changing the way old people fall. The potential for prevention together with the use of falling as an indicator of underlying frailty combine to make an understanding of the causes of falls and a practical approach to the evaluation and management of patients with instability

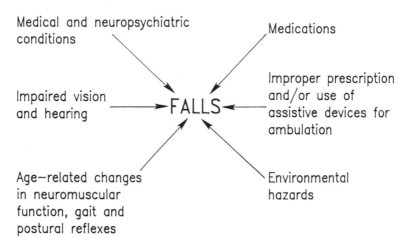

INTRINSIC FACTORS

Medical and neuropsychiatric
conditions

Impaired vision
and hearing

Age—related changes
in neuromuscular
function, gait and
postural reflexes

EXTRINSIC FACTORS

Medications

Improper prescription
and/or use of
assistive devices for
ambulation

Environmental
hazards

FALLS

Figure 8-1 Multifactorial causes and potential contributors to falls in older persons.

and falls important components of geriatric care. Similar to many other conditions described throughout this text, the factors that can contribute to or cause falls are multiple, and very often more than one of these factors plays an important role (Fig. 8-1).

Falling may be a useful indicator of frailty in general. Persons with a history of falling have higher levels of subsequent health care utilization and poor functional status (Kiel et al., 1991). Fallers who were thoroughly assessed showed a benefit in functional outcomes over those who were not, even when the cause of the fall could not be determined or treated (Rubenstein et al., 1990).

AGING AND INSTABILITY

Several age-related factors contribute to instability and falls (Table 8-2). Most "accidental" falls are caused by one or a combination of these factors interacting with environmental hazards.

Aging changes in postural control and gait probably play a major role in many falls among older persons. Increasing age is associated with diminished proprioceptive input, slower righting reflexes, di-

Table 8-2 Age-related factors contributing to instability and falls

Changes in postural control
  Decreased proprioception
  Slower righting reflexes
  Decreased muscle tone
  Increased postural sway
  Orthostatic hypotension

Changes in gait
  Feet not picked up as high
  Men: develop flexed posture and wide-based, short-stepped gait
  Women: develop narrow-based, waddling gait

Increased prevalence of pathologic conditions relative to stability
  Degenerative joint disease
  Fractures of hip and femur
  Stroke with residual deficits
  Muscle weakness from disuse and deconditioning
  Peripheral neuropathy
  Diseases or deformities of the feet
  Impaired vision
  Impaired hearing
  Forgetfulness and dementia
  Other specific disease processes (e.g., cardiovascular disease, Parkinsonism—see
    Table 8-3)

Increased prevalence of conditions causing nocturia (e.g., congestive heart failure,
  venous insufficiency)

Increased prevalence of dementia

minished strength of muscles important in maintaining posture, and increased postural sway. All these changes can contribute to falling—especially the ability to avoid a fall after encountering an environmental hazard or an unexpected trip. Changes in gait also occur with increasing age. Although these changes may not be sufficiently prominent to be labeled truly pathologic, they can increase susceptibility to falls. In general, elderly people do not pick their feet up as high, thus increasing the tendency to trip. Elderly men develop wide-based, short-stepped gaits; elderly women often walk with a narrow-based, waddling gait. Orthostatic hypotension (defined as a drop in systolic blood pressure of 20 mmHg or more when moving from a lying to a standing position) occurs in 11 to 30 percent of older persons (Mader et al., 1987). Although not all elderly individuals with

orthostatic hypotension are symptomatic, this impaired physiologic response could play a role in causing instability and precipitating falls in a substantial proportion of patients. Older people have been shown to experience a postprandial fall in blood pressure as well (Lipsitz et al., 1983; Jonsson et al., 1990).

Several pathologic conditions that increase in prevalence with increasing age can contribute to instability and falling. Degenerative joint disease (especially of the neck, the lumbosacral spine, and the lower extremities) can cause pain, unstable joints, muscle weakness, and neurologic disturbances. Healed fractures of the hip and femur can cause an abnormal and less steady gait. Residual muscle weakness or sensory deficits from a recent or remote stroke can cause instability. Muscle weakness as a result of disuse and deconditioning (caused by pain and/or lack of exercise) can contribute to an unsteady gait and impair the ability to right oneself after a loss of balance. Diminished sensory input, such as in diabetic and other peripheral neuropathies, visual disturbances, and impaired hearing diminish cues from the environment that normally contribute to stability and thus predispose one to falls (Dargent-Molina, 1996). Impaired cognitive function may result in the creation of, or wandering into, unsafe environments and may lead to falls. Podiatric problems (bunions, calluses, nail disease, joint deformities, etc.) that cause pain, deformities, and alterations in gait are common, correctable causes of instability. Other specific disease processes common in older people (such as Parkinson's disease and cardiovascular disorders) can cause instability and falls and are discussed further below.

Inability to get up after a fall can be an indication of a poor prognosis. In one study almost half those who fell at least once reported being unable to get up. These older persons had poorer functional outcomes (Tinetti et al., 1993).

CAUSES OF FALLS IN OLDER PERSONS

Table 8-3 outlines the multiple and often interacting causes of falls among older persons. Over half of all falls are related to medically diagnosed conditions (Rubenstein et al., 1988), emphasizing the importance of a careful medical assessment for patients who fall (see below). Several studies have examined risk factors for falls among older persons and have found a variety of these—including cognitive

Table 8-3 Causes of falls

Accidents
  True accidents (trips, slips, etc.)
  Interactions between environmental hazards and factors increasing susceptibility
    (Table 8-2)

Syncope (sudden loss of consciousness)

Drop attacks (sudden leg weaknesses without loss of consciousness)

Dizziness and/or vertigo
  Vestibular disease
  CNS disease

Orthostatic hypotension
  Hypovolemia or low cardiac output
  Autonomic dysfunction
  Impaired venous return
  Prolonged bed rest
  Drug-induced hypotension
  Postprandial hypotension

Drug-related causes
  Diuretics
  Antihypertensives
  Tricyclic antidepressants
  Sedatives
  Antipsychotics
  Hypoglycemics
  Alcohol

Specific disease processes
  Acute illness of any kind ("premonitory fall")
  Cardiovascular
    Arrhythmias
    Valvular heart disease (aortic stenosis)
    Carotid sinus syncope
  Neurologic causes
    Transient ischemic attack (TIA)
    Stroke (acute)
    Seizure disorder
    Parkinson's disease
    Cervical or lumbar spondylosis (with spinal cord or nerve root compression)
    Cerebellar disease
    Normal-pressure hydrocephalus (gait disorder)
    CNS lesions (e.g., tumor, subdural hematoma)

Idiopathic (no specific cause identifiable)

---

impairment, disabilities of the lower extremities, gait and balance abnormalities, nocturia, and the number and nature of medications being taken—as important risk factors (Tinetti et al., 1988; Robbins et al., 1991; Campbell et al., 1989; Cummings et al., 1991; Myers et al., 1991; Stewart et al., 1992). Frequently overlooked, environmental factors can increase susceptibility to falls and other accidents. Homes of elderly people are often full of environmental hazards (Table 8-4). Unstable furniture, rickety stairs with inadequate railings, throw rugs and frayed carpets, and poor lighting should be specifically sought on home visits. There are several factors associated with falls among older nursing home residents (Table 8-5). Awareness of these factors can help prevent morbidity and mortality in these settings. A checklist for the identification of hazards for falling is included in the Appendix.

Several factors can hinder precise identification of the specific causes for falls. These factors include lack of witnesses, inability of the elderly person to recall the circumstances surrounding the event, the transient nature of several causes [e.g., arrhythmia, transient ischemic attack (TIA), postural hypotension], and the fact that the majority of elderly people who fall do not seek medical attention. Somewhat more detailed information is available on the circumstances surrounding falls in nursing homes (Table 8-5), but these individuals represent a relatively low proportion and a highly select group among the total senior population.

Close to half of all falls can be classified as accidental. Usually an accidental trip or a slip can be precipitated by an environmental hazard, often in conjunction with factors listed in Table 8-2. Addressing the environmental hazards begins with a careful assessment of

Table 8-4 Common environmental hazards

Old, unstable, and low-lying furniture
Beds and toilets of inappropriate height
Unavailability of grab bars
Uneven stairs and inadequate railing
Throw rugs, frayed carpets, cords, wires
Slippery floors and bathtubs
Inadequate lighting or glaring
Cracked and uneven sidewalks

Table 8-5 Factors associated with falls among older nursing home residents

Recent admission
Dementia
Hip weakness
Certain activities (toileting, getting out of bed)
Psychotropic drugs causing daytime sedation
Cardiovascular medications (vasodilators, diuretics)
Polypharmacy
Low staff-patient ratio
Unsupervised activities
Unsafe furniture
Slippery floors

the patient's environment. Some older persons have developed a strong attachment to their cluttered surroundings and may need active encouragement to make the necessary changes, but many may simply take such environmental risks for granted until they are specifically identified.

Syncope, "drop attacks," and "dizziness" are commonly cited causes of falls in elderly persons. If there is a clear history of loss of consciousness, a cause for true syncope should be sought. Although the complete differential diagnosis of syncope is beyond the scope of this chapter, some of the more common causes of syncope in older people include vasovagal responses, cardiovascular disorders (such as brady- and tachyarrhythmias and aortic stenosis), acute neurological events (such as TIA, stroke, or seizure), pulmonary embolus, and metabolic disturbances (e.g., hypoxia, hypoglycemia). Cardiovascular causes for syncope are more common in the elderly than in younger populations (Kapoor, 1994). A precise cause for syncope may remain unidentified in 40 to 60 percent of elderly patients (Lipsitz et al., 1983).

Drop attacks, described as sudden leg weakness causing a fall without loss of consciousness, are probably overdiagnosed in elderly people who fall. They are often attributed to vertebrobasilar insufficiency, frequently precipitated by a change in head position. Although a small proportion of older people who fall have truly had a drop attack, the underlying pathophysiology is poorly understood, and care should be taken to rule out other causes (Rubenstein et al., 1988).

Dizziness and unsteadiness are extremely common complaints among elderly people who fall (as well as those who do not). A feeling

of light-headedness can be associated with several different disorders but is a nonspecific symptom and should be interpreted with caution. Patients complaining of light-headedness should be carefully evaluated for postural hypotension and intravascular volume depletion. Vertigo (a sensation of rotational movement), on the other hand, is a more specific symptom and is probably an uncommon precipitant of falls in the elderly. It is most commonly associated with disorders of the inner ear, such as acute labyrinthitis, Ménière's disease, and benign positional vertigo. Vertebrobasilar ischemia and infarction and cerebellar infarction can also cause vertigo. Patients with vertigo due to organic disorders often have nystagmus, which can be observed by having the patient quickly lie down and turning the patient's head to the side in one motion (Bérény's positional test). Many older patients with symptoms of dizziness and unsteadiness are anxious, depressed, and chronically afraid of falling, and the evaluation of their symptoms is quite difficult. Some patients, especially those with symptoms suggestive of vertigo, will benefit from a thorough otologic examination including auditory testing, which may help clarify the symptoms and differentiate inner-ear from CNS involvement.

As mentioned above, a substantial number (10 to 20 percent) of elderly persons have orthostatic hypotension. Orthostatic hypotension is best detected by taking the blood pressure and pulse in supine position, after 1 min in the sitting position, and after 1 and 3 min in the standing position. A drop of more than 20 mmHg in systolic blood pressure is generally considered to represent significant orthostatic hypotension. In many instances, this condition is asymptomatic; however, several conditions can cause orthostatic hypotension or worsen it to a severity sufficient to precipitate a fall (Mader et al., 1987). These conditions include low cardiac output from heart failure or hypovolemia, autonomic dysfunction (which can result from diabetes), impaired venous return (e.g., venous insufficiency), prolonged bed rest with deconditioning of muscles and reflexes, and several different drugs. Simply eating a full meal can precipitate a reduction in blood pressure in an older person that may be worsened and precipitate a fall when the person stands up (Lipsitz et al., 1983). The association of orthostatic hypotension with elevated blood pressure but not with the use of antihypertensive medication suggests that treatment of hypertension may improve this condition (Ooi et al., 1997).

Drugs that should be suspected of playing a role in falls include diuretics (hypovolemia), antihypertensives (hypotension), tricyclic an-

tidepressants (postural hypotension), sedatives (excessive sedation), antipsychotics (sedation, muscle rigidity, postural hypotension), hypoglycemics (acute hypoglycemia), and alcohol (intoxication). Combinations of these drug types may greatly increase the risk of a fall. Psychotropic drugs are commonly prescribed and appear to substantially increase the risk of falls and hip fractures, especially in patients prescribed tricyclic antidepressants (Ray et al., 1987, 1989; Ray, 1992).

Many disease processes, especially of the cardiovascular and neurologic systems, can be associated with falls. Cardiac arrhythmias are common in ambulatory elderly persons and may be difficult to associate directly with a fall or syncope (Gibson et al., 1984; Rosado et al., 1989). In general, cardiac monitoring should document a temporal association between a specific arrhythmia and symptoms (or a fall) before the arrhythmia is diagnosed (and treated) as the cause of falls. Syncope can be a symptom of aortic stenosis and is an indication of the need to evaluate a patient suspected of having significant aortic stenosis for valve replacement. Aortic stenosis is difficult to diagnose by physical examination alone, and all patients suspected of having this condition should have appropriate diagnostic tests (see below). Some elderly individuals have sensitive carotid baroreceptors and are susceptible to syncope resulting from reflex increase in vagal tone (caused by cough, straining at stool, micturition, etc.), which leads to bradycardia and hypotension. Carotid sinus sensitivity can be detected by bedside maneuvers (see below).

Cerebrovascular disease is often implicated as a cause or contributing factor for falls in older patients. Although cerebral blood flow and cerebrovascular autoregulation may be diminished, these aging changes alone are not enough to cause unsteadiness or falls. They may, however, render the elderly person more susceptible to stresses such as diminished cardiac output, which will more easily precipitate symptoms. Acute strokes (caused by thrombosis, hemorrhage, or embolus) can cause and may initially manifest themselves in falls. TIAs of both the anterior and posterior circulations frequently last only minutes and are often poorly described. Thus, care must be taken in making these diagnoses. Anterior circulation TIAs may cause unilateral weakness and thus precipitate a fall. Vertebrobasilar (posterior circulation) TIAs may cause vertigo, but a history of transient vertigo alone is not a sufficient basis for the diagnosis of a TIA. The diagnosis of posterior circulation TIA necessitates that one or more other symptoms (visual field cuts, dysarthria, ataxia, or limb weakness—which

can be bilateral) be associated with vertigo. Vertebrobasilar insuffi-ciency, as mentioned above, is often cited as a cause of drop attacks; in addition, mechanical compression of the vertebral arteries by osteo-phytes of the cervical spine when the head is turned has also been proposed as a cause of unsteadiness and falling. Both of these condi-tions have been poorly documented, are probably overdiagnosed, and should not be used as causes of a fall simply because nothing else can be found.

Other diseases of the brain and central nervous system can also cause falls. Parkinson's disease and normal-pressure hydrocephalus (Fisher, 1982) cause disturbances of gait, which lead to instability and falls. Cerebellar disorders, intracranial tumors, and subdural hemato-mas can cause unsteadiness, with a tendency to fall. A slowly progres-sive gait disability with a tendency to fall, especially in the presence of spasticity or hyperactive reflexes in the lower extremities, should prompt consideration of cervical spondylosis and spinal cord compres-sion. It is especially important to consider these diagnoses because treatment may improve the condition before permanent disability ensues.

Despite this long list, the precise causes of many falls will remain unknown—even after a thorough evaluation. The ultimate test of the etiology for falls is its reversibility. As noted earlier, we are better at finding putative causes than in correcting them.

EVIDENCE OF FALLS PREVENTION

The intense effort to identify risk factors for falls has been matched more recently with interventive efforts. Although the results of clinical trials do not yet provide strong evidence of clearly effective ap-proaches, good clinical sense still dictates active efforts to identify remediable risk factors. A randomized trial by Tinetti showed that targeted intervention to reduce the rate of falls did lower the overall rate (as compared with a control group) but there was no significant difference in the rate of serious falls (Tinetti et al., 1994a). A metanal-ysis of the several studies conducted under the auspices of the FICSIT project showed only modest results. In only two cases did an interven-tion lead to a significant reduction in falls; exercise and balance were associated with fewer falls but not with falls with injuries (Province et al., 1995). Tai Chi training was shown to increase the time to a fall

but not to a serious fall compared with an educational control group (Wolf et al., 1996). When a specific fall prevention program was compared with a more general chronic disease prevention program, the falls program achieved lower rates of falls and serious falls at the end of the first year, but by year 2 the differences disappeared (Wagner et al., 1994). A study directed specifically at older persons with osteoarthritis showed that both simple exercise and resistance exercise led to significant functional benefits (Ettinger et al., 1997). A New Zealand study showed that elderly patients could be taught at home to perform exercises that reduced the rate of falls (Campbell et al., 1997). A successful multifactorial approach to reducing falls among nursing home patients employed training in environmental and personal safety, wheelchair use, psychotropic drug management, and transferring and ambulation (Ray et al., 1997). Although not immediately connected to reducing fall risks, a study directed at frail nursing home patients showed that moderate exercise improved gait and stair-climbing ability (Fiatarone et al., 1994). If the falls per se cannot be prevented, the risk of fractures can be reduced by having those at high risk wear external hip protectors (Lauritzen et al., 1993).

EVALUATING THE ELDERLY PATIENT WHO FALLS

Older patients who report a fall (or recurrent falls) that is not clearly due to an accidental trip or slip should be carefully evaluated, even if the falls have not resulted in serious physical injury. A thorough evaluation consists of a detailed history, physical examination, gait and balance assessment, and, in certain instances, selected laboratory studies.

The history should focus on the general medical history and medications, the patient's thoughts about what caused the fall, the circumstances surrounding it, any premonitory or associated symptoms (such as palpitations caused by a transient arrhythmia or focal neurologic symptoms caused by a TIA), and whether there was loss of consciousness (Table 8-6). A history of loss of consciousness after the fall (which is often difficult to document) is important information and should raise the suspicion of a cardiac event (transient arrhythmia or heart block) or a seizure (especially if there has been incontinence). Falls are often unwitnessed, and elderly patients may not recall any details of the circumstances surrounding the event. Detailed questioning can

Table 8-6 Evaluating the elderly patient who falls: Key points in the history

General medical history

History of previous falls

Medications (especially antihypertensive and psychotropic agents)

Patient's thoughts on the cause of the fall
  Was patient aware of impending fall?
  Was it totally unexpected?
  Did patient trip or slip?

Circumstances surrounding the fall
  Location and time of day
  Witnesses
  Relationship to changes in posture, turning of head,
    cough, urination

Premonitory or associated symptoms
  Light-headedness, dizziness, vertigo
  Palpitations, chest pain, shortness of breath
  Sudden focal neurologic symptoms (weakness, sensory disturbance,
    dysarthria, ataxia, confusion, asphasia)
  Aura
  Incontinence of urine or stool

Loss of consciousness
  What is remembered immediately after the fall?
  Could the patient get up and, if so, how long did it take?
  Can loss of consciousness be verified by a witness?

sometimes lead to identification of environmental factors that may have played a role in the fall and to symptoms that may lead to a specific diagnosis. Many elderly patients will not be able to give details about an unwitnessed fall and will simply report "I just fell down, I don't know what happened."

The skin, extremities, and painful soft tissue areas should be assessed to detect any injury that may have resulted from a fall. Several other aspects of the physical examination can be helpful in determining the cause(s) (Table 8-7). Because a fall can herald the onset of a variety of acute illnesses ("premonitory" falls), careful attention should be given to vital signs. Fever, tachypnea, tachycardia, and hypotension should prompt a search for an acute illness (such as pneumonia or sepsis, myocardial infarction, pulmonary embolus,

Table 8-7 Evaluating the elderly patient who falls: Key aspects of the physical examination

Vital signs
    Fever, hypothermia
    Respiratory rate
    Pulse and blood pressure (lying, sitting, standing)

Skin
    Turgor
    Pallor
    Trauma

Eyes
    Visual acuity

Cardiovascular
    Arrhythmias
    Carotid bruits
    Signs of aortic stenosis
    Carotid sinus sensitivity

Extremities
    Degenerative joint disease
    Range of motion
    Deformities
    Fractures
    Podiatric problems (calluses; bunions; ulcerations; poorly fitted,
        inappropriate, or worn-out shoes)

Neurologic
    Mental status
    Focal signs
    Muscles (weakness, rigidity, spasticity)
    Peripheral innervation (especially position sense)
    Cerebellar (especially heel-to-shin testing)
    Resting tremor, bradykinesia, other involuntary movements
    Observing the patient stand up and walk (the "get up and go" test)

gastrointestinal bleeding). Postural blood pressure and pulse determinations taken supine, sitting, and standing (after 1 and 3 min) are critical in the diagnosis and management of falls in older patients. As noted earlier, postural hypotension occurs in a substantial number of healthy, asymptomatic elderly persons as well as in those who are deconditioned from immobility or have venous insufficiency. This finding can also be a sign of dehydration, acute blood loss (occult gastrointestinal bleeding), or a drug side effect. Visual acuity should

be assessed for any possible contribution to instability and falls. The cardiovascular examination should focus on the presence of arrhythmias (many of which are easily missed during a brief examination) and signs of aortic stenosis. Since both of these conditions are potentially serious and treatable yet difficult to diagnose by physical examination, the patient should be referred for continuous monitoring and echocardiography if they are suspected. If the history suggests carotid sinus sensitivity, the carotid can be gently massaged for 5 s to observe whether this precipitates a profound bradycardia (0.50 percent reduction in heart rate) or a long pause (0.2 s). The extremities should be examined for evidence of deformities, limits to range of motion, or active inflammation that might underlie instability and cause a fall. Special attention should be given to the feet because deformities, painful lesions (calluses, bunions, ulcers), and poorly fitted, inappropriate, or worn-out shoes are common and can contribute to instability and falls.

Neurologic examination is also an important aspect of this physical assessment. Mental status should be assessed (see Chap. 5), with a careful search for focal neurologic signs. Evidence of muscle weakness, rigidity, or spasticity should be noted, and signs of peripheral neuropathy (especially posterior column signs such as loss of position or vibratory sensation) should be ruled out. Abnormalities in cerebellar function (especially heel-to-shin testing) and signs of Parkinson's disease (such as resting tremor, muscle rigidity, and bradykinesia) should be sought.

Gait and balance assessments are a critical component of the examination and are probably more useful in identifying remediable problems than is the standard neuromuscular exam (Tinetti et al., 1988). Although sophisticated techniques have been developed to assess gait and balance, careful observation of a series of maneuvers is the most practical and useful assessment technique. The "get up and go" test and other practical performance-based balance and gait assessments have been developed (Mathias et al., 1986; Tinetti, 1986; Wolfson et al., 1990). Tables 8-8 and 8-9 provide examples of these types of assessment. A copy of the "get up and go" test is reproduced in the Appendix. Abnormalities on these assessments may be helpful in identifying patients who are likely to fall again and potentially remediable problems that might prevent future falls (Tinetti, 1986, 1989).

There is no specific laboratory workup for an elderly patient who falls (Rubenstein et al., 1990). Laboratory studies should be ordered

(Text continues on page 250.)

Table 8-8 Example of a performance-based assessment of gait

Components	Observation	
	Normal	Abnormal
Initiation of gait (patient asked to begin walking down hallway at a normal pace using any assistive device they normally walk with)	Begins walking immediately without observable hesitation; initiation of gait is single, smooth motion	Hesitates; multiple attempts; initiation of gait not a smooth motion
Step height (begin observing after first few steps: observe one foot, then the other; observe from side)	Swing foot completely clears floor but by no more than 1–2 in.	Swing foot is not completely raised off floor (may hear scraping) or is raised too high (<1–2 in.)
Step length (observe distance between toe of stance foot and heel of swing foot; observe from side; do not judge first few or last few steps; observe one side at a time)	At least the length of individual's foot between the stance toe and swing heel (step length usually longer but foot length provides basis for observation)	Step length less than described under "normal"
Step symmetry (observe the middle part of the path, not the first or last steps; observe distance between heel of each swing foot and toe of each stance foot)	Step length same or nearly same on both sides for most step cycles	Step length varies between sides, or patient advances with same foot every step

Step continuity	Begins raising heel of one foot (toe off) as heel of other foot touches the floor (heel strike); no breaks or stops in stride; step lengths equal over most cycles	Places entire foot (heel and toe) on floor before beginning to raise other foot; or stops completely between steps; or step length varies over cycles
Path deviation [observe from behind; observe one foot over several strides; observe in relation to line on floor (e.g., tiles) if possible; difficult to assess if patient uses a walker]	Foot follows close to straight line as patient advances	Foot deviates from side to side or toward one direction
Trunk stability (observe from behind; side-to-side motion of trunk may be a normal gait pattern; need to differentiate this from instability)	Trunk does not sway; knees or back are not flexed; arms are not abducted in effort to maintain stability	Any of preceding features present
Walk stance (observe from behind)	Feet should almost touch as one passes other	Feet apart with stepping
Turning while walking	No staggering; turning continuous with walking; steps are continuous while walking; steps are continuous while turning	Staggers; stops before initiating turn; or steps are discontinuous

Source: From Tinetti, 1986, with permission.

Table 8-9 Example of a performance-based assessment of balance

Maneuver	Normal	Adaptive	Abnormal
Sitting balance	Steady, stable	Holds onto chair to keep upright	Leans, slides down in chair
Arising from chair	Able to arise in a single movement without using arms	Uses arms (on chair or walking aid) to pull or push up and/or moves forward in chair before attempting to rise	Multiple attempts required or unable without human assistance
Immediate standing balance (first 325 s)	Steady without holding onto walking aid or other object for support	Steady, but uses walking aid or support grabbing objects for support	Any sign of unsteadiness (e.g., other object for staggering, more than minimal trunk sway)
Standing balance	Steady, able to stand with feet together without holding onto an object for support	Steady, but cannot put feet together	
Balance with eyes closed (with feet as close together as possible)	Steady without holding onto any object with feet together	Steady with feet apart	Any sign of unsteadiness or needs to hold onto an object
Turning balance (360°)	No grabbing or staggering; no need to hold onto any objects; steps are continuous (turn is a flowing movement)	Steps are discontinuous (patient puts one foot completely on floor before raising other foot)	Any sign of unsteadiness or holds onto an object
Nudge on sternum (patient standing with feet as close together as possible; examiner pushes with light, even pressure over sternum three times; reflects ability to withstand displacement)	Steady, able to withstand pressure	Needs to move feet, but able to maintain balance	Begins to fall, or examiner has to help maintain balance

Maneuver		
Neck turning (patient asked to turn head side to side and look up while standing with feet as close together as possible)	Able to turn head at least halfway side to side and able to bend head back to look at ceiling; no staggering, grabbing, or symptoms of light-headedness, unsteadiness, or pain	Decreased ability to turn side to side to extend neck, but no staggering, grabbing, or symptoms of light-headedness, unsteadiness, or pain	Any sign of unsteadiness or symptoms when turning head or extending neck
One-leg standing balance	Able to stand on one leg for 5 s without holding onto object for support		Unable
Back extension (ask patient to lean back as far as possible, without holding onto object if possible)	Good extension without holding object or staggering	Tries to extend, but range of motion is decreased or needs to hold object to attempt extension	Will not attempt, no extension seen, or staggers
Reaching up (have patient attempt to remove an object from a shelf high enough to necessitate stretching or standing on toes)	Able to take down object without needing to hold onto other object for support and without becoming unsteady	Able to get object but needs to steady self by holding onto something for support	Unable or unsteady
Bending down (patient is asked to pick up small objects, such as pen, from the floor)	Able to bend down and pick up the object and able to get up easily in single attempt without needing to pull self up with arms	Able to get object and get upright in single attempt but needs to pull self up with arms or hold onto something for support	Unable to bend down or unable to get upright after bending down or takes multiple attempts to upright self
Sitting down	Able to sit down in one smooth movement	Needs to use arms to guide self into chair or not a smooth movement	Falls into chair, misjudges distances (lands off center)

based on information gleaned from the history and physical examination. If the cause of the fall is obvious (such as a slip or a trip) and no suspicious symptoms or signs are detected, laboratory studies are unwarranted. If the history or physical examination (especially vital signs) suggests an acute illness, appropriate laboratory studies (such as complete blood count, electrolytes, blood urea nitrogen, chest films, electrocardiogram) should be ordered. If a transient arrhythmia or heart block is suspected, ambulatory electrocardiographic monitoring should be done. Although the sensitivity and specificity of this procedure for determining the cause of falls in the elderly is unknown, and many elderly people have asymptomatic ectopy (Gibson et al., 1984; Rosado et al., 1989), cardiac abnormalities detected on continuous monitoring that are clearly related to symptoms should be treated. Because it is difficult to diagnose aortic stenosis on physical examination, echocardiography should be considered in all patients with suggestive histories and louder than a grade 2 systolic heart murmur or those who have a delay in the carotid upstroke. If the history suggests anterior circulation TIA, noninvasive vascular studies should be considered to rule out treatable vascular lesions. CT scans and electroencephalograms should be reserved for those patients in whom there is a high suspicion of an intracranial lesion or seizure disorder.

MANAGEMENT

The basic principles of managing elderly patients with instability problems and a history of falls are outlined in Table 8-10. Assessment and treatment of physical injury should not be overlooked because it may be helpful in preventing recurrent falls.

When specific conditions are identified by history, physical examination, and laboratory studies, they should be treated in order to minimize the risk of subsequent falls, morbidity, and mortality. Examples of treatments for some of the more common conditions are outlined in Table 8-11. This table is meant only as a general outline; most of these topics are discussed in detail in general textbooks of medicine.

Physical therapy and patient education are important aspects of the management of these elderly patients. Gait training, muscle strengthening, the use of assistive devices, and adaptive behaviors (such as rising slowly, using rails or furniture for balance, and

Table 8-10 Principles of management for elderly patients with complaints of instability and/or falls

Assess and treat physical injury

Treat underlying conditions (Table 8–11)

Provide physical therapy and education
Gait retraining
Muscle strengthening
Aids to ambulation
Properly fitted shoes
Adaptive behaviors

Alter the environment*
Safe and proper-size furniture
Elimination of obstacles (loose rugs, etc.)
Proper lighting
Rails (stairs, bathroom)

---

* See Appendix for checklist.

Table 8-11 Examples of treatment for underlying causes of falls

Condition and cause	Potential treatment
Cardiovascular	
Tachyarrhythmias	Antiarrhythmics*
Bradyarrhythmias	Pacemaker*
Aortic stenosis	Valve surgery (for syncope)
Postural hypotension	
Drug-related	Elimination of drugs(s)
With venous insufficiency	Support stockings
	Leg elevation
	Adaptive behaviors
Autonomic dysfunction or idiopathic	Support stockings
	Mineralocorticoids
	ProAmatine (Midodrine
	hydrochloride)
	Adaptive behaviors

(continued)

Table 8-11 Examples of treatment for underlying causes of falls *(Continued)*

Condition and cause	Potential treatment
Neurologic	
Anterior circulation transient ischemic attack (TIA)	Aspirin and/or surgery[†]
Posterior circulation TIA	Aspirin
Cervical spondylosis (with spinal cord compression)	Physical therapy
	Neck brace
	Surgery
Parkinson's disease	Antiparkinsonian drugs
Visual impairment	Ophthalmologic evaluation and specific treatment
Seizure disorder	Anticonvulsants
Normal-pressure hydrocephalus	Surgery (shunt)[†]
Dementia	Supervised activities
	Hazard-free environment
Benign positional vertigo	Habituation exercises
	Antivertiginous medication
Others	
Foot disorders	Podiatric evaluation and treatment
Gait disorders (miscellaneous)	Properly fitted shoes
	Physical therapy
Drug overuse (e.g., sedatives, alcohol, other psychotropic drugs, antihypertensives)	Elimination of drug(s)

* These treatments may be indicated only if the cardiac disturbance is clearly related to symptoms.

† Risk-benefit ratio must be carefully assessed.

techniques of getting up after a fall) are all helpful in preventing subsequent morbidity from instability and falls.

Environmental manipulations can be critical in preventing further falls. The environments of the elderly are often unsafe (Table 8-4), and appropriate interventions can often be instituted to improve safety (Table 8-10). Physical restraints (vests, belts, mittens, geri-chairs, etc.) have been commonly used in institutional settings for those felt to be at high risk of falling. Nursing home regulations in the Omnibus

Budget Reconciliation Act of 1987 (OBRA '87) and the increasing recognition that physical restraints probably do not decrease and may in fact increase falls and injuries (Tinetti et al., 1992) have led to the reduced and more appropriate use of these devices in many institutional settings.

The Appendix contains an assessment form for patients who fall as well as a Fall Hazard Checklist.

ACKNOWLEDGMENT

The authors wish to acknowledge Dr. Laurence Rubenstein for his assistance in preparing this chapter.

REFERENCES

Campbell A, Robertson M, Gardner M, et al: Randomised controlled trial of a general practice programme of home based exercise to prevent falls in elderly. *BMJ* 315:1065–1069, 1997.

Campbell JA, Borrie JJ, Spears GF: Risk factors for falls in a community-based prospective study of people 70 years and older. *J Gerontol Med Sci* 44:M112–M117, 1989.

Cummings RG, Miller PJ, Kelsy JL, et al: Medications and multiple falls in elderly people: The St. Louis OASIS study. *Age Ageing* 20:455–461, 1991.

Dargent-Molina P: Fall-related factors and risk of hip fracture: The EPIDOS prospective study. *Lancet* 384:145–149, 1996.

Ettinger WH, Burns R, Messler SP, et al: A randomized trial comparing aerobic exercise and resistance exercise with a health education program in older adults with knee osteoarthritis: The fitness arthritis and seniors trial (FAST). *JAMA* 277:25–31, 1997.

Fiatarone MA, O'Neill EF, Ryan ND, et al: Exercise training and nutritional supplementation for physical frailty in very elderly people. *N Engl J Med* 330:1769–1775, 1994.

Fisher CM: Hydrocephalus as a cause of disturbances of gait in the elderly. *Neurology* 32:1358–1363, 1982.

Gibson TC, Heitzman MR: Diagnostic efficacy of 24-hour electrocardiographic monitoring for syncope. *Am J Cardiol* 53:1013–1017, 1984.

Jonsson PV, Lipsitz LA, Kelley M, et al: Hypotensive responses to common daily activities in institutionalized elderly: A potential risk for recurrent falls. *Arch Intern Med* 150:1518–1524, 1990.

Kapoor W: Syncope in older persons. *J Am Geriatr Soc* 42:426–436, 1994.

Kiel DP, O'Sullivan P, Teno JM, et al: Health care utilization and functional status in the aged following a fall. *Med Care* 29:221–228, 1991.

Lauritzen JB, Petersen MM, Lund B: Effect of external hip protectors on hip fractures. *Lancet* 341:11–13, 1993.

Lipsitz LA, Nyquist RP, Wei JY, et al: Postprandial reduction in blood pressure in the elderly. *N Engl J Med* 309:81–83, 1983.

Mader SC, Josephson KR, Rubenstein LZ: Low prevalence of postural hypotension among community-dwelling elderly. *JAMA* 258:1511–1514, 1987.

Mathias SN, Nayak USL, Isaacs B: Balance in elderly patients: The "get up and go" test. *Arch Phys Med Rehabil* 67:387–389, 1986.

Myers AH, Baker SP, Van Natta ML, et al: Risk factors associated with falls and injuries among elderly institutionalized persons. *Am J Epidemiol* 133:1179–1190, 1991.

Ooi WL, Barrett S, Hossain M, et al: Patterns of orthostatic blood pressure change and their clinical correlates in a frail, elderly population. *JAMA* 277:1299–1304, 1997.

Province MA, Hadley EC, Hornbrook MC, et al: The effects of exercise on falls in elderly patients: A preplanned metanalysis of the FICSIT trials. *JAMA* 273: 1341–1347, 1995.

Ray WA: Psychotropic drugs and injuries among the elderly: A review. *J Clin Psychopharmacol* 12:386–396, 1992.

Ray WA, Griffin MR, Schaffner W, et al: Psychotropic drug use and the risk of hip fracture. *N Engl J Med* 316:363–369, 1987.

Ray WA, Griffin MR, Downey W: Benzodiazepines of long and short elimination half-life and the risk of hip fracture. *JAMA* 262:3303–3307, 1989.

Ray WA, Taylor JA, Meador KG, et al: A randomized trial of a consultation service to reduce falls in nursing homes. *JAMA* 278:557–562, 1997.

Robbins AS, LZ Rubenstein, KR Josephson, et al: Predictors of falls among elderly people: Results of two population-based studies. *Arch Intern Med* 149:1628–1633, 1991.

Rosado JA, Rubenstein LZ, Robbin AS, et al: The value of Holter monitoring in evaluating the elderly patient who falls. *J Am Geriatr Soc* 37:430–434, 1989.

Rubenstein LZ, Robbins AS, Schulman BL, et al: Falls and instability in the elderly. *J Am Geriatr Soc* 36:266–278, 1988.

Rubenstein LZ, Robbins AS, Josephson KR, et al: The value of assessing falls in an elderly population. *Ann Intern Med* 113:308–316, 1990.

Sattin RW, Lambert Huber DA, DeVito C, et al: The incidence of fall injury events among the elderly in a defined population. *Am J Epidemiol* 131:1028–1037, 1990.

Stewart RB, Moore MT, May FE, et al: Nocturia: A risk factor for falls in the elderly *J Am Geriatr Soc* 40:1217–1220, 1992.

Tinetti ME: Performance-oriented assessment of mobility problems in elderly patients. *J Am Geriatr Soc* 34:119–126, 1986.

Tinetti ME, Ginter SF: Identifying mobility dysfunctions in elderly patients. *JAMA* 259:1190–1193, 1988.

Tinetti ME, Spechley M: Prevention of falls among the elderly. *Med Intell* 320:1055–1059, 1989.

Tinetti ME, Liu W, Ginter SF: Mechanical restraint use and fall-related injuries among residents of skilled nursing facilities: *Ann Intern Med* 116:369–374, 1992.

Tinetti ME, Liu W-L, Claus EB: Predictors and prognosis of inability to get up after falls among elderly persons. *JAMA* 269:65–70, 1993.

Tinetti ME, Mendes de Leon CF, Doucette JT, ct al: Fear of falling and fall-related efficacy in relationship to functioning among community-living elders. *J Gerontol Med Sci* 49:M140–M147, 1994b.

Tinetti M, Baker D, McAvay G, et al: A multifactorial intervention to reduce the risk of falling among elderly people living in the community. *N Engl J Med* 331:821–827, 1994a.

Wagner EH, LaCroix AZ, Grothaus L, et al: Preventing disability and falls in older adults: A population-based randomized trial. *Am J Public Health* 84:1800–1806, 1994.

Wolf SL, Barnhart HX, Kutner NG, et al: Reducing frailty and falls in older persons: An investigation of Tai Chi and computerized balance training. *J Am Geriatr Soc* 44:489–497, 1996.

Wolfson L, Whipple R, Amerman P, et al: Gait assessment in the elderly: A gait abnormality rating scale and its relation to falls. *J Gerontol Med Sci* 45:M12–M19, 1990.

SUGGESTED READINGS

Alexander N: Gait disorders in older adults. *J Am Geriatr Soc* 44:434–451, 1996.

Connell B: Role of the environment in falls prevention. *Clin Geriatr Med* 12:859–880, 1996.

King MB, Tinetti ME: Falls in community-dwelling older persons. *J Am Geriatr Soc* 43:1146–1154, 1995.

Luukinen H, Koski K, Konkanen R: Incidence of injury-causing falls among older adults by place of residence: A population-based study. *J Am Geriatr Soc* 43:871–876, 1995.

Rubenstein L, Josephson K, Robbins A: Falls in nursing homes. *Ann Intern Med:* 121:442–451, 1994.

Thapa PB, Brockman KG, Gideon P, Fought RL, Ray WA: Injurious falls in nonambulatory nursing home residents: A comparative study of circumstances, incidence, and risk factors. *J Am Geriatr Soc* 44:273–278, 1996.

NINE

IMMOBILITY

Immobility is a common pathway by which a host of diseases and problems in older individuals produce further disability. Immobility often cannot be prevented, but many of its adverse effects can be. Improvements in mobility are possible, even in the most immobile older patients. Relatively small improvements in mobility can decrease the incidence and severity of complications, improve the patient's well-being, and make life easier for caregivers.

This chapter outlines the common causes and complications of immobility and reviews the principles of management for some of the more common problems associated with immobility in the older population.

CAUSES

Many physical, psychological, and environmental factors can cause immobility in older persons (Table 9-1). The most common causes are musculoskeletal, neurologic, and cardiovascular disorders.

Table 9-1 Common causes of immobility in older adults

Musculoskeletal disorders
  Arthritides
  Osteoporosis
  Fractures (especially hip and femur)
  Podiatric problems
  Other (e.g., Paget's disease)

Neurologic disorders
  Stroke
  Parkinson's disease
  Other (cerebellar dysfunction, neuropathies)

Cardiovascular disease
  CHF (severe)
  Coronary artery disease (frequent angina)
  Peripheral vascular disease (frequent claudication)

Pulmonary disease
  Chronic obstructive lung disease (severe)

Sensory factors
  Impairment of vision
  Fear (from instability and fear of falling)

Environmental causes
  Forced immobility (in hospitals and nursing homes)
  Inadequate aids for mobility

Other
  Deconditioning (after prolonged bed rest from acute illness)
  Malnutrition
  Severe systemic illness (e.g., widespread malignancy)
  Pain
  Depression
  Drug side effects (e.g., antipsychotic-induced rigidity)

Degenerative joint disease (especially that involving the weight-bearing joints), osteoporosis, and hip fractures are probably the most prevalent conditions that predispose to immobility among older adults. Podiatric problems such as bunions, calluses, and onychomycoses frequently cause pain and reluctance or inability to walk.

The incidence of several neurologic disorders that can cause immobility increases with age. About half of the individuals who suffer a stroke have residual deficits for which they require assistance; most

of these deficits involve immobility. Parkinson's disease, especially in its later stages, causes severe limitations in mobility. Early and active management of these patients can improve their mobility and help to avoid complications.

Severe congestive heart failure, coronary artery disease with frequent angina, peripheral vascular disease with frequent claudication, and severe chronic lung disease can restrict activity and mobility in many elderly patients. Peripheral vascular disease, especially in older diabetics, can cause claudication, limit ambulation, and eventually result in lower extremity amputations, which can restrict mobility further.

Psychological and environmental factors can play an important role in immobility. Decreased mobility (i.e., taking to bed) is a common manifestation of depression. Fear of falling, especially among those with a history of instability problems and previous falls or with impaired vision, can lead to a bed-and-chair existence. Older patients with instability problems, impaired vision, and acute illnesses are often inappropriately restricted to bed or chair in acute care hospitals and nursing homes. Lack of mobility aids (e.g., canes, walkers, and appropriately placed railings) also contributes to immobility in acute care hospitals and home settings.

Drug side effects may cause immobility. Sedatives and hypnotics, by causing drowsiness and ataxia, can impair mobility. Antipsychotic drugs (especially the phenothiazine-like agents) have prominent extrapyramidal effects and can cause muscle rigidity and diminished mobility (see Chap. 13).

COMPLICATIONS

Immobility can lead to complications in almost every major organ system (Table 9-2). Prolonged inactivity or bed rest has adverse physical and psychological consequences. Metabolic effects include negative nitrogen and calcium balance and impaired glucose tolerance; diminished plasma volume and altered drug pharmacokinetics can result. Immobilized older patients often become depressed, are deprived of environmental stimulation, and, in some instances become delirious and appear demented.

The skin and musculoskeletal system often bear the brunt of immobility. Pressure sores are all too common. Muscle weakness,

Table 9-2 Complications of immobility

Skin
  Pressure sores

Musculoskeletal
  Muscular deconditioning and atrophy
  Contractures
  Bone loss (osteoporosis)

Cardiovascular
  Deconditioning
  Orthostatic hypotension
  Venous thrombosis, embolism

Pulmonary
  Decreased ventilation
  Atelectasis
  Aspiration pneumonia

Gastrointestinal
  Anorexia
  Constipation
  Fecal impaction, incontinence

Genitourinary
  Urinary infection
  Urinary retention
  Bladder calculi
  Incontinence

Metabolic
  Altered body composition (e.g., decreased plasma volume)
  Negative nitrogen balance
  Impaired glucose tolerance
  Altered drug pharmacokinetics

Psychological
  Sensory deprivation
  Dementia, delirium
  Depression

atrophy, and contractures can lead to prolonged disability and dysfunction. Bone density decreases in immobile patients, predisposing to fractures when the patient is mobilized. Cardiopulmonary complications of immobility are probably the most serious and life-threatening. Prolonged immobility results in cardiovascular deconditioning; the combination of deconditioned cardiovascular reflexes and

diminished plasma volume can lead to postural hypotension. Postural hypotension may not only impair rehabilitative efforts but also predispose to serious cardiovascular events such as stroke and myocardial infarction. Deep venous thrombosis and pulmonary embolism are well-known complications. Immobility, especially bed rest, also impairs pulmonary function. Tidal volume is diminished; atelectasis may occur, and, when combined with the supine position, predisposes to the development of aspiration pneumonia.

Gastrointestinal and genitourinary problems are among the most bothersome consequences of immobility to the patient and can lead to further complications. Immobility slows down both the gastrointestinal tract and urine flow. This predisposes to constipation, fecal impaction, urinary tract stones and infection, and fecal and urinary incontinence. These conditions and their management are discussed in Chap. 7.

ASSESSING IMMOBILE PATIENTS

Several aspects of the history and physical examination are important in the assessment of immobile patients (Table 9-3). Useful historical information includes the extent and duration of disabilities causing immobility, the underlying medical conditions that influence mobility, and a review of medications in order to eliminate iatrogenic problems contributing to immobility. Psychological factors such as depression and fear may contribute to immobility and may make recovery difficult. They should therefore receive special attention. An assessment of the environment is important in determining measures that may improve the patient's mobility, such as an overhead triangle, bedside commode, railing, and other environmental manipulations.

When immobile patients are being examined, the skin should be inspected repeatedly to identify early pressure sores. Cardiopulmonary status, especially intravascular volume, and postural changes in blood pressure and pulse are important to the process of treatment. A detailed musculoskeletal examination—including evaluation of muscle tone and strength and testing of joint range of motion—and a search for potentially remediable podiatric problems should be carried out. Standardized and repeated measures of muscle strength (performed by rehabilitation therapists) can be helpful in gauging a patient's progress (Table 9-4). The neurologic examination should

Table 9-3 Assessment of immobile older patients

History
  Nature and duration of disabilities causing immobility
  Medical conditions contributing to immobility
  Drugs that can affect mobility
  Motivation and other psychological factors
  Environment

Physical examination
  Skin
  Cardiopulmonary status

Musculoskeletal assessment
  Muscle tone and strength (Table 9-4)
  Joint range of motion
  Foot deformities and lesions

Neurologic deficits
  Focal weakness
  Sensory and perceptual evaluation

Levels of mobility
  Bed mobility
  Ability to transfer (bed to chair)
  Wheelchair mobility
  Standing balance
  Gait (see Chap. 8)

Table 9-4 Example of a grading system for muscle strength in immobile older patients

	Grade	Observed strength
Normal	5	
Good	4	Muscle produces movements against gravity and can overcome some resistance
Fair	3	Muscle produces movements against gravity but cannot overcome any resistance
Poor	2	Muscle produces movements but not against gravity
Trace	1	Muscle tightens but cannot produce movement, even after gravity is eliminated
None	0	Muscle does not contract at all

identify focal weakness as well as sensory and perceptual problems that can impair mobility and frustrate rehabilitative efforts. Hemianopsia, or neglect of and inattention to one side of the body (usually the left side is ignored in patients with nondominant hemisphere lesions), and various apraxias are common after strokes.

Most importantly, the patient's mobility should be assessed and reassessed on an ongoing basis. There are several levels of mobility (Table 9-3) as well as important distinctions within each level. For example, a patient may be bed-bound but may be able to sit up without help, or he or she may be able to transfer independently into a wheelchair but may be unable to propel the wheelchair. Rehabilitation therapists are skilled in making these detailed evaluations of mobility and should be involved in the care of immobile patients.

MANAGEMENT OF IMMOBILITY

Optimal management of immobile older patients necessitates a thorough assessment, specific diagnoses, and multimodal treatment directed at specific diseases and disabilities. This process most often involves a team of health professionals. Physical and occupational therapists can be especially helpful in the assessment and management of immobility and associated functional disabilities, and they should be consulted as early as possible when the problem of an immobile patient presents itself. In many patients, mobility cannot be completely restored and intensive rehabilitative efforts will not be cost-effective. Specific goals must be individualized, and in some patients these goals will involve preventing complications of immobility and adapting the environment to the individual (and vice versa).

It is beyond the scope of this text to detail the management of all conditions associated with immobility in older adults; important general principles of the management of some of the most common of these conditions are reviewed. A brief section at the end of the chapter provides an overview of key principles in the rehabilitation of geriatric patients. The Suggested Readings at the end of this chapter provide more detailed discussions of management for these conditions.

Arthritis

Several different rheumatologic disorders occur in the older persons. They can usually be distinguished from each other by clinical features,

radiographic abnormalities, synovial fluid analysis, and selected laboratory studies (see Table 9-5).

It is important to make specific diagnoses for these conditions whenever possible, because the most appropriate treatment(s) of the primary disorders, as well as associated abnormalities, may differ. For example, polymyalgia rheumatica is a common condition in elderly women; its clinical features are often nonspecific—fatigue, malaise, muscle aches. Because this disorder necessitates treatment with systemic steroids and is highly associated with temporal arteritis (a disease that can rapidly lead to blindness if appropriate treatment is not instituted), it is essential to make this diagnosis. Older patients with fatigue and symmetrical muscle aches (especially in the shoulders) should be tested for sedimentation rate, which will generally be markedly elevated (about three-quarters of patients have values greater than 40 mm/h) in polymyalgia rheumatica (Chuang et al., 1982; Goodwin, 1992). The sedimentation rate does increase with age in some people, but elevations above normal are usually associated with a clinical disorder (Tinetti et al., 1986; Crawford et al., 1987). Any symptoms suggestive of involvement of the temporal artery—headache, recent changes in vision—especially when the sedimentation rate is very high (over 75 mm/h) should prompt consideration of temporal artery biopsy because treatment of temporal arteritis requires higher doses of steroids than does the treatment of polymyalgia alone. Patients with polymyalgia are generally treated with 10 to 20 mg of prednisone in a single dose, whereas patients with temporal arteritis are treated with 40 to 80 mg of prednisone daily in divided doses (Goodwin, 1992).

Another example of the importance of making a specific diagnosis is the carpal tunnel syndrome. This disorder may be overlooked when symptoms of pain, weakness, and paresthesias in the hand are mistaken for osteoarthritis. Objective weakness, sensory deficit, and atrophy of intrinsic musculature of the hand should prompt consideration of performing nerve conduction studies and surgical therapy to relieve symptoms and prevent progressive disability. Wrist splints, generally provided by occupational therapists, are sometimes effective in relieving the discomfort of this syndrome.

History and physical examination can be helpful in differentiating osteoarthritis from inflammatory arthritides (Table 9-6); however, other procedures are often essential. Osteoarthritis itself may be inflammatory in some instances.

Table 9-5 Clinical aspects of common rheumatologic disorders in older patients

Disorder	Osteoarthritis	Rheumatoid arthritis	Polymyalgia rheumatica	Gout	Pseudogout	Carpal tunnel syndrome	Drug-induced disorder
Gradual onset	+++	+++	+++	0	+	+++	+++
Joint swelling or effusion	+++	++++	+	++++	++++	+	++
Joint pain	++++	++++	+	++++	++++	+	+++
Symmetrical involvement	+	+++	++++	+	+	++	+++
Muscle pain	+	+	+++	+	+	+	+++
Radiographic abnormalities	++++	+++	0	+	+++	0	0
Synovial fluid crystals	+	+	0	+++	+++	0	0
Elevated sedimentation rate	+	+++	++++	+	+	+	+++
Anemia	0	++	+++	0	0	0	++
Positive antinuclear antibody	0	+	+	0	0	+	++++
Positive rheumatoid factor	0	+++	+	0	0	0	+

Key: 0, does not occur; +, occurs occasionally; ++, occurs frequently; +++, almost always occurs; ++++, difficult to make diagnosis without it.

Source: After Reich, 1982.

Table 9-6 Clinical features of osteoarthritis versus inflammatory arthritides

Clinical feature	Osteoarthritis	Inflammatory arthritides
Duration of stiffness	Minutes	Hours
Pain	Usually with activity	Occurs even at rest and at night
Fatigue	Unusual	Common
Swelling	Common but little synovial reaction	Very common, with synovial proliferation and thickening
Erythema and warmth	Unusual	Common

Synovial fluid analysis can be especially helpful in differentiating osteoarthritis from crystal-induced arthritides such as gout and pseudogout (Table 9-5). Because clinical examination alone cannot determine whether an inflamed joint is infected and joint infections can occur in conjunction with other inflammatory joint diseases, all newly inflamed joints should be tapped, Gram stained, and cultured to rule out infection. Failure to diagnose and treat joint infections can lead to osteomyelitis, joint destruction, and permanent disability.

In addition to making specific diagnoses of rheumatologic disorders whenever possible, careful physical examination can detect treatable nonarticular conditions such as tendinitis and bursitis. For example, bicipital tendinitis and trochanteric bursitis are reasonably common in geriatric patients. Dramatic relief from pain and disability from these conditions can be achieved by local treatments such as the injection of steroids.

Osteoarthritis is by far the most common rheumatologic disorder afflicting older adults. A wide variety of modalities can be used to treat osteoarthritis as well as other painful musculoskeletal conditions. Optimal management often involves the use of multiple treatment modalities, and the best combination of treatments will vary from patient to patient.

In general, patients with osteoarthritis and pain from inflammatory musculoskeletal conditions should be treated with an anti-inflammatory agent unless they respond to local measures alone. Some older patients with chronic pain due to osteoarthritis will respond to acetaminophen; however, when inflammation is present, nonsteroidal anti-inflammatory drugs are generally appropriate. There are many

such drugs; their side effects and prices vary. In general, aspirin is the least expensive; enteric-coated preparations can diminish gastrointestinal irritation and still yield adequate absorption. The half-life of aspirin may be prolonged in older patients on higher doses; thus, less frequent administration may provide adequate analgesia. Salicylate blood levels can be used to monitor treatment. When compliance is a problem or when aspirin cannot be tolerated or is ineffective, other nonsteroidal drugs can be tried. These drugs can also cause gastrointestinal upset and bleeding and are associated with an increased risk of peptic ulcer disease (Griffin et al., 1991; Soll et al., 1991). Although the absolute risk of a significant gastrointestinal bleed may be small (Beard et al., 1987), monitoring of patients on chronic nonsteroidal therapy for bleeding with periodic hemoglobin levels and/or stools for occult blood is advisable. Ibuprofen appears to be associated with the lowest risk for gastrointestinal bleeding. Although drug-induced gastric ulcers can be prevented by misoprostol, the risks and costs of adding another drug must be weighed carefully. Nonsteroidal agents can also cause sodium retention and impair renal function, especially in patients with already compromised renal function and those on loop diuretics (Gurwitz et al., 1990). Nonsteroidal agents can also interfere with the efficacy of antihypertensive therapy. Although sulindac (Clinoril) has been reported to have less effect on renal function, blood urea nitrogen and creatinine should be monitored in older patients on all nonsteroidal agents. Combining lower doses of these drugs with acetaminophen can sometimes improve pain relief and minimize side effects. There is no place for systemic steroids in the treatment of osteoarthritis in older patients. Guidelines for the management of chronic pain in older persons have recently been published (AGS Panel, 1998).

Osteoporosis

Osteoporosis is a common disorder in the elderly and frequently leads to complications that result in pain, disability, and immobility. Approximately one-third of women older than 65 have suffered either a vertebral or hip fracture related to osteoporosis; by age 80, approximately half of women have evidence of vertebral fractures and close to 30 percent will have suffered a hip fracture. Thus, osteoporosis is a major health problem in the older adult population, resulting in substantial morbidity and cost.

Osteoporosis is a generalized bone disorder in which bone mass is diminished but the relative composition (i.e., the ratio of mineral to organic matrix content) is not changed. This is in contrast to osteomalacia, in which the ratio of mineral to matrix is diminished. Aging is associated with a decrease in bone mass. White women lose the greatest proportion of bone mass with increasing age; the bone loss accelerates after menopause, and as much as 40 percent of bone mass may be lost by age 90.

A working group of the World Health Organization has defined osteoporosis as a bone mineral density that is 2.5 SD below the mean peak value in young adults. Values between 1.0 and 2.5 SD below the mean are defined as osteopenia. The diagnosis of osteoporosis no longer requires the presence of a low impact fracture.

Two major types of age-related osteoporosis have been defined (Table 9-7). Type I or postmenopausal osteoporosis affects mainly trabecular bone and is related to accelerated bone loss in women during the first two decades after menopause. Type II or senile osteoporosis affects both trabecular and cortical bone and is related to impaired production of 1,25-dihydroxy vitamin D (Riggs and Melton, 1986). Several factors have been associated with increased risk of osteoporosis among women (Table 9-8); many of them (e.g., gastric resection, steroid or anticonvulsant use, immobility) are also risk factors among men.

Table 9-7 Two basic types of age-related osteoporosis

	Type I (postmenopausal)	Type II (senile)
Age (years)	51–75	>70
Sex ratio (F:M)	6:1	2:1
Type of bone loss	Mainly trabecular	Trabecular and cortical
Rate of bone loss	Accelerated	Not accelerated
Fracture sites	Vertebrae (crush) and distal radius	Vertebrae (multiple wedge) and hip
Parathyroid function	Decreased	Increased
Calcium absorption	Decreased	Decreased
Metabolism of 25-OH-D to 1,25-dihydroxy vitamin D	Secondary decrease	Primary decrease

Source: After Riggs and Melton, 1986.

Table 9-8 Factors associated with an increased risk of osteoporosis among women*

Postmenopausal (within 20 years after menopause)
White or Asian
Premature menopause
Positive family history
Short stature and small bones
Leanness
Low calcium intake
Inactivity or immobility
Early menopause (before age 45)
Previous amenorrhea
Malabsorption syndromes
Long-term glucocorticoid therapy
Long-term use of anticonvulsants
Hyperparathyroidism
Thyrotoxicosis
Cushing's syndrome
Smoking
Heavy alcohol use

* Several of these factors also increase risk among men.
Source: After Riggs and Melton, 1986.

Because routine radiographs are relatively insensitive in detecting significant bone loss (20 to 30 percent of bone mass must be lost before the radiograph appears abnormal), the prevalence of osteoporosis in older adults is probably underestimated. Even with the use of this insensitive measure, close to 30 percent of elderly women and 20 percent of elderly men have osteoporosis. Lateral radiographs of the thoracolumbar vertebrae can show loss of horizontal trabeculation, prominent end plates, and anterior wedging, and radiographs of the upper femur can reveal loss of the trabecular pattern that normally traverses the greater trochanter. Techniques such as computed tomography and single- or dual-photon absorptiometry are more sensitive than routine radiographs but are expensive. Patients with a bone mineral density of less than 1 g/cm^3 are at higher risk for all types of fractures. Although many centers are now using the latter techniques to screen for osteoporosis, data documenting the cost-effectiveness

of screening bone mass measurements for reducing the incidence of subsequent fractures are not yet available. Thus the cost-effectiveness of these techniques as screening tools remains unproven (American College of Physicians, 1987; Melton et al., 1990). Bone biopsy may be necessary in certain patients to help distinguish osteoporosis from other disorders such as osteomalacia, metastatic carcinoma, and multiple myeloma.

The clinically most useful technique for measuring bone density is dual-energy x-ray absorptiometry (DEXA). It is most useful in assisting physicians and patients on decisions for treatment when therapy, such as postmenopausal estrogens, might not otherwise be started, and in monitoring therapeutic response. Bone density of the hip is most helpful in predicting fractures, and bone density of the spine is most helpful for monitoring therapy (Eastell, 1998).

Laboratory studies in uncomplicated osteoporosis should be normal, including serum calcium, phosphorus, magnesium, alkaline phosphatase, and parathyroid and thyroid hormones, although some older patients with senile osteoporosis have elevated parathyroid hormone, presumably related to a primary decrease in 1,25-dihydroxy vitamin D levels. Vitamin D blood levels and 24-h urinary calcium excretion (which should be greater than 100 mg/24 h) should be measured if malabsorption is suspected.

Osteoporosis in older adults is commonly asymptomatic and discovered on routine radiographs. The presenting manifestations most often relate to a fracture of the hip (discussed below), the wrist (Colles' fracture), or the lower thoracic and upper lumbar vertebrae. Vertebral compression fractures can be asymptomatic and cause progressive kyphosis and loss of height. They may also be excruciatingly painful and be precipitated by relatively minor stress, such as sitting down quickly. The pain is exacerbated by twisting and increases in intraabdominal pressure (e.g., from coughing or straining to have a bowel movement). The pain can radiate around the thoracic cavity and mimic cardiac pain. Diagnosing a new compression fracture can be difficult, especially when old radiographs are not available. The combination of the new onset of characteristic pain and radiographic evidence of a compression fracture in a compatible location should be treated with bed rest (for as short a period as possible), heat, and analgesics. Posterior wedging of the fracture, fractures above the midthoracic vertebrae, and irregular-appearing vertebral bodies should raise the suspicion of a metastatic malignancy or plasmacytoma.

Several treatments are available for osteoporosis, including exercise, supplemental dietary calcium, vitamin D, bisphosphonates, fluoride, calcitonin, estrogen, and selective estrogen-receptor modulators (for recent review see Eastell, 1998). The most effective treatment for the different types of osteoporosis remains somewhat controversial and is influenced by a number of patient-related factors. Preventive approaches are clearly the most effective; but to be effective in preventing fractures and associated morbidity later in life, treatment should be initiated soon after the menopause and continued for 10 to 20 years. Exercise probably has modest beneficial effects on bone mass (Chow et al., 1987; Prince et al., 1991) and has other potential beneficial effects on muscle strength and agility (which may help prevent falls) and cardiovascular status. Thus, prescribing an exercise program suitable to the individual's preferences is certainly reasonable. Calcium supplementation of 1000 to 1500 mg/day is now recommended as a preventive measure (Dawson-Hughes et al., 1990; Reid et al., 1993). Routine vitamin D supplementation of 400 to 800 IU per day is also recommended because it may help reduce the incidence of vertebral and hip fractures (Tilyard et al., 1992; Chapuy et al., 1992). Sodium fluoride can increase bone mass, particularly vertebral bone mass, but data on its effectiveness in preventing vertebral and hip fractures are conflicting. Although a few studies have reported a decrease in new vertebral fractures without an increase in hip fractures when low-dose or slow-release sodium fluoride was used (Pak et al., 1995), most studies have demonstrated no decrease in vertebral fracture rate, and some have noted an increase in nonvertebral fractures. There is also a high incidence of gastrointestinal toxicity from fluoride, which is reduced with lower doses and simultaneous ingestion of calcium. Sodium fluoride is not routinely recommended for the prevention or treatment of osteoporosis. Calcitonin therapy results in an increase in bone mineral density and a decrease in the rate of vertebral fractures. It is less effective at preventing cortical bone loss than cancellous bone loss, is expensive, and can cause nausea, diarrhea, and flushing. Patients may become resistant to calcitonin after long-term use. Nasal calcitonin may be more acceptable and has fewer side effects but may not be effective in early postmenopausal women. It has a small effect on reducing vertebral fractures in older women. Both forms of calcitonin have analgesic effects on bone pain of new vertebral fractures. Calcitonin is generally reserved for high-risk patients with contraindications for other therapy.

Biophosphonate therapy results in increased bone mineral density and a decreased fracture rate. The two forms presently available in the United States are etidronate and alendronate. To avoid impaired mineralization, etidronate is given by low-dose intermittent therapy— 400 mg/day for 2 weeks, followed by daily calcium and vitamin D supplementation for 11 weeks (Storm et al., 1990). Alendronate is given at a dose of 10 mg/day and is associated with a decrease in vertebral fractures, nearly 50 percent reduction in two studies. Alendronate is associated with esophagitis. To minimize risk of esophagitis and improve absorption, the patient should take it with a glass of water while upright at least 30 min before breakfast.

Estrogen is the most effective treatment for preventing postmenopausal bone loss and subsequent fractures. Despite the benefits of estrogens, side effects and risks of its use must be considered in deciding whether to choose estrogen as therapy for osteoporosis in a postmenopausal woman (Table 9-9). In women who are at high risk for osteoporosis (Table 9-8) and who do not have a uterus, contraindications to estrogen treatment would be a history of breast cancer or recurrent thromboembolic disease. In women who have a uterus, the risk of endometrial cancer is reduced by the addition of a progestational agent to the estrogen. Although progestogen therapy may help to increase bone formation, it may also reverse some of the changes in lipid metabolism that may be responsible for the positive effects of estrogen on coronary heart disease. Cyclical estrogen-progestogen treatment results in withdrawal bleeding, which some postmenopausal

Table 9-9 Benefits and risk of estrogen therapy in postmenopausal women

Benefits	Risks and side effects
Relief of menopausal symptoms	Return of menstrual bleeding
Prevention of fractures	Breast tenderness
Prevention of ischemic heart disease	Exacerbation of migraine headaches
Delay in onset of Alzheimer's disease	Risk of endometrial carcinomas
	Risk of breast cancer
	Risk of deep vein thrombosis and pulmonary embolism

Source: Modified from Eastell, 1998.

women may find unacceptable. Continuous estrogen-progestogen therapy is associated with irregular menstrual bleeding for 9 to 12 months, a bothersome symptom; but by 1 year of therapy, the majority of treated women will stop menstruating completely. The best estrogen treatment regimen has not been defined. Several are listed in Table 9-10. Physician and patient together need to decide about initiation of therapy and the regimen to be used.

Recently, a new group of compounds have been developed to take advantage of estrogen's benefits and to minimize the side effects and risks. These mixed agonists/antagonists are known as selective estrogen-receptor modulators (SERMs). One, raloxifene, has recently been approved for clinical use in the United States. Raloxifene increases bone density without stimulating the endometrium (Delmas et al., 1997). It also decreases total and low-density lipoprotein cholesterol, but its effect on reducing ischemic heart disease is not known. In short-term studies, it is also reported to decrease the incidence of breast cancer. Its beneficial effect on bone density is less than that of estrogen, and results of studies on reduction of fractures are still awaited. New SERMs will likely take greater advantage of estrogen's benefits and further lower the risks.

Table 9-10 Hormonal regimens

Cycle	Conjugated estrogen 0.625 mg qd
	Medroxyprogesterone 10 mg/day, days 1–10; 5 mg may be protective
	Bleeding after day 15 requires evaluation
Continuous	Conjugated estrogens 0.625 mg qd
	Medroxyprogesterone 2.5–5 mg qd
	Irregular bleeding for 3–6 months
	Atrophic endometrium in 90% by 1 year
Other	Medroxyprogesterone every 3 months
	No data on endometrial cancer
	Estrogen patch
	Estrogen cream for vaginal symptoms
Surveillance	Unopposed estrogen
	Baseline and yearly endometrial biopsy
	Estrogen/progestins
	Biopsy for unexpected bleeding
	Annual mammography

Hip Fracture

Fractures of the hip and femoral neck, especially when associated with osteoporosis, are among the major causes of immobility, disability, and health care expenditures in older adults. Fear of hip fracture because of a prior fracture or its occurrence in a friend or relative is a common concern that contributes to limitation of mobility in many elderly persons. This fear is realistic: there are over 250,000 hip fractures in the United States every year, with the incidence increasing dramatically with advanced age. The mortality rate in the year after hip fracture has been reported in recent studies to be 12 to 29 percent (Jette et al., 1987; Fitzgerald et al., 1988; Marotolli et al., 1992), and as many as one-third of hip fracture patients remain in a nursing home 1 year after the fracture. These studies also document a high rate of decline in ability to ambulate and perform activities of daily living in the 6 to 12 months after fracture. Thus the prevention and optimal management of hip fractures are critical to the health of our older population.

The degree of immobility and disability caused by a hip fracture depends on several factors, including coexisting medical conditions, patient motivation, the nature of the fracture, and the techniques of management. Many older patients with hip fracture already have impaired mobility, and there is a high incidence of medical illnesses that necessitate treatment (e.g., infection, heart failure, anemia, dehydration) at the time of hip fracture. Patients with these underlying conditions and those with dementia are at especially high risk for poor functional recovery. The location of the fracture is especially important in determining the most appropriate management and the outcome of treatment (Table 9-11, Fig. 9-1). Subcapital fractures (which are inside the joint capsule) disrupt the blood supply to the proximal femoral head, thus resulting in a higher probability of necrosis of the femoral head and nonunion of the fracture. Replacement of the femoral head is often warranted in these cases. Inter- and subtrochanteric fractures generally do not disrupt the blood supply to the femoral head; open reduction and pinning are usually successful (for a review see Zuckerman, 1996).

In general, it takes 12 weeks for a hip fracture to heal. Surgical techniques such as the Austin-Moore prosthesis and Richard's compression screw allow for almost immediate ambulation in many patients. Like almost all acute conditions in elderly patients, early

Table 9-11 Characteristics of selected treatments for hip fracture

Type of fracture	Surgical technique	Comments
Displaced subcapital	Femoral head endoprosthesis (e.g., Austin-Moore)	Allows almost immediate ambulation
Non- or minimally displaced subcapital	Closed reduction with multiple pinnings	Protected weight bearing for 8–12 weeks or until fracture heals
Intertrochanteric and low subcapital	Open reduction with compression screw and side plate	Allows early ambulation
Subtrochanteric	Open reduction with Zickel nail and intramedullary rod	Protected weight bearing until fracture heals

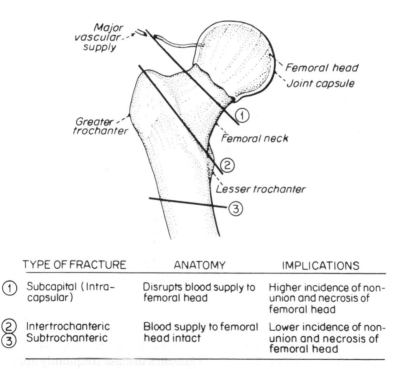

TYPE OF FRACTURE	ANATOMY	IMPLICATIONS
① Subcapital (Intra-capsular)	Disrupts blood supply to femoral head	Higher incidence of non-union and necrosis of femoral head
② Intertrochanteric ③ Subtrochanteric	Blood supply to femoral head intact	Lower incidence of non-union and necrosis of femoral head

Figure 9-1 Characteristics of different types of hip fractures.

mobilization is critical to the outcome. When combined with good rehabilitation and patient motivation, early mobilization can minimize disability and immobility from hip fracture. The current standard of care is for patients to receive prophylactic anticoagulation to prevent thromboembolic complications. The regimens differ. Aspirin is inexpensive and easy to administer, but its effectiveness is variable. Warfarin is effective but is associated with an increased incidence of bleeding complications. Low-dose intravenous heparin is effective, but low-dose subcutaneous heparin has not been shown to be effective. More recently, subcutaneous injection of low-molecular-weight heparin has been shown to be an effective method of prophylaxis in patients with hip fractures (Gerhart et al., 1991). Intermittent pneumatic compression is of value, but the equipment is costly and the need to apply and remove the device limits its usefulness. The long-term outcome of older patients with hip fracture depends, however, on many other factors besides the type of fracture and patient motivation. Many hip fracture patients have functional disabilities prior to the fracture as well as active medical conditions at the time of the fracture, and they may suffer complications while in the acute care hospital (Campion et al., 1987). An intensive interdisciplinary rehabilitation program may improve outcome in this patient population (Zuckerman et al., 1992).

Parkinson's Disease

The first step in successful management of Parkinson's disease is to recognize its presence. Although many parkinsonian patients have the classic triad of resting tremor, rigidity, and bradykinesia, many others do not. Early in the disease, the symptoms and signs can be subtle and sometimes unilateral. Many elderly patients, especially in institutions, carry a diagnosis of chronic brain syndrome (or other similar diagnoses) and actually have undiagnosed and treatable forms of parkinsonism. Many patients have drug-induced parkinsonism resulting from the extrapyramidal side effects of antipsychotics (see Chap. 13). Left untreated, these patients eventually become highly immobile; develop flexion contractures, pressure sores, and malnutrition; and often die of aspiration pneumonia.

Because Parkinson's disease often responds to treatment, especially early in its course, there should be a high index of suspicion for this diagnosis. Patients with Parkinson's disease frequently appear depressed or demented (sometimes both); in fact, many parkinsonian

Table 9-12 Drugs used to treat Parkinson's disease

Drug (brand name)	Usual dosages	Mechanism of action	Potential side effects
Levodopa (Dopar, Larodopa)	2000–5000 mg/day in divided doses	Increases availability of dopamine by providing metabolic precursor	Nausea, vomiting, anorexia Dyskinesias Orthostatic hypotension Behavioral disturbances Vivid dreams and hallucinations
Carbidopa (Lydosyn)	Up to 100 mg/day in divided doses	Decreases peripheral dopamine metabolism	May enhance toxicity of levodopa
Carbidopa, levodopa (Sinemet)	40/400 to 200/2000* mg/day in divided doses	Increases dopamine availability (both above mechanisms)	As above
Amantadine (Symmetrel)	100–300 mg/day†	Increases dopamine release	Delirium and hallucinations
Bromocriptine (Parlodel)	1–1.5 mg tid or qid (initial); gradually increase to maximum of 100–200 mg in divided doses	Directly activates dopaminergic receptors	Behavioral changes Hypotension Nausea
Pramipexole (Mirapex)	0.5–1.5 mg tid	Dopamine agonist	Hallucinations Nausea Somnolence

Drug	Dosage	Action	Side effects
Ropinirole (Requip)	3–5 mg tid	Dopamine agonist	Orthostasis Syncope Nausea Somnolence
Anticholinergic agents,‡ trihexyphenidyl (Artane, Tremin)	2–20 mg/day in divided doses	Decreases effects of acetylcholine and helps to restore balance between cholinergic and dopaminergic systems	Dry mouth Constipation Urinary retention Blurred vision Exacerbation of glaucoma Tachycardia Confusion Behavioral changes
Benztropine mesylate (Cogentin)	0.5–8 mg/day in divided doses		As above
Selegiline (Eldepryl)	10 mg/day in one dose	Inhibits type B monoamine oxidase Delays onset of disability, especially during first 12 months	Nausea Confusion Agitation Insomnia Involuntary movements

* Top number represents carbidopa; bottom number, levodopa.
† Eliminated by kidney; dosages should be adjusted when renal function is diminished.
‡ Several other anticholinergic agents are available.

patients become depressed and develop cognitive dysfunction. Experienced neurologists or psychiatrists should be consulted when the diagnosis is in question and when the clinical picture is complicated by dementia and/or depression.

Pharmacologic treatment of Parkinson's disease is based on an attempt to increase the ratio of dopamine to acetylcholine in the central nervous system, specifically the nigrostriatal system. Several drugs can be used, sometimes in combination (Table 9-12). Selegiline has recently been shown to delay the progression of disability in early Parkinson's disease, especially during the first 12 months of therapy (Parkinson Study Group, 1993). Thus, drug treatment can be initiated with selegiline, leaving other drugs for later when signs and disability progress. The choice of drugs may be based in part on the most prominent clinical manifestations; resting tremor may respond better to anticholinergics, whereas bradykinesia and rigidity may respond better to dopaminergic agents. Carbidopa/levodopa remains the mainstay of therapy. Whatever approach is used, all the drugs must be used carefully; treatment should begin with small doses that are gradually increased. Clinical response may take several weeks. Side effects from these drugs are common and often limit pharmacologic treatment. Wide variations in response can also occur, including morning akinesia, peak dose dyskinesias, and freezing episodes (sometimes referred to as the "on-off phenomenon"). There is some evidence that these variations may be due in part to dietary amino acids competing with dopamine for transport into the central nervous system (Nutt et al., 1984), but diets containing the recommended daily allowance do not appear to have a significant effect (Juncos et al., 1987). One- to two-week periods off drug therapy, so-called drug holidays, which were frequently recommended in the past, are not beneficial in the vast majority of patients (Mayeux et al., 1985).

The FDA has recently approved two new dopamine agonists, pramipexole (Miropex) and ropinirole (Requip) for treatment of both early (without levodopa) and advanced (with levodopa) Parkinson's disease (Medical Letter, 1997). These agents appear to be useful additions to the treatment of early and advanced Parkinson's disease, but more studies are needed to determine how they compare with bromocriptine and pergolide and to each other.

Patients who are difficult to manage or who do not respond should be referred to an experienced neurologist. Parkinsonian patients, especially those with more advanced disease, will also benefit from

rehabilitation therapy and an ongoing program of exercise and activity in order to maintain strength and functional capabilities and to prevent complications of immobility.

Stroke

To prevent disability from immobility and its complications, patients with completed strokes should receive prompt and intensive rehabilitative therapy. In many elderly patients, coexisting medical conditions (e.g., cardiovascular disease) limit the intensity of rehabilitation treatment; however, all patients should be evaluated and managed as actively as possible during the first several weeks after a stroke. Although all stroke patients deserve an assessment and consideration for intensive rehabilitation, the cost-effectiveness of various approaches to stroke rehabilitation is controversial. Whether the rehabilitative efforts occur in the acute care hospital, special rehabilitation unit, or nursing home, these efforts should involve a multidisciplinary team, and the basic principles remain the same (see below).

Despite the lack of data from controlled trials, even some of the most severely affected stroke patients can achieve meaningful improvements in functional status by early rehabilitative efforts. Although complete functional recovery occurs in less than half of stroke patients (Silliman et al., 1987), immobility and its attendant complications can almost always be prevented or minimized. Here again, development of realistic goals for individual patients is essential. Intensive efforts directed at functional recovery are probably not appropriate for patients with large or bilateral strokes causing flaccid paralysis or severe perceptual deficits or for patients with severe underlying medical conditions or dementia. The goals in these latter patients should be to prevent complications and adapt the environment.

The management of older patients with cerebrovascular disease is discussed further in Chap. 10. The Suggested Readings section at the end of this chapter lists comprehensive reviews of stroke management.

Pressure Sores

Pressure sores are among the most common, preventable, and treatable conditions associated with immobility in older adults. There are four factors that contribute to the development of pressure sores: pressure, shearing forces, friction, and moisture.

As the name implies, pressure sores develop because areas of the body (most often overlying bony prominences) are exposed to prolonged pressure. The amount of pressure necessary to occlude blood supply to the skin (and thus predispose to irreversible tissue damage) is small and is generated in normal sitting and supine positions. Irreversible tissue damage can occur (especially in aging skin) after only 2 h of continuous pressure that exceeds capillary pressure.

Shearing forces (such as those created when the head of a bed is elevated and the torso slides down and transmits pressure to the sacral area) contribute to the stretching and angulation of subcutaneous tissues. Friction, caused by the repeated movement of skin across surfaces such as bed sheets or clothing, increases the shearing force. This can eventually lead to thrombosis of small blood vessels, thus undermining and then destroying skin. Shearing forces and friction are worsened by loose, folded skin, which is common in the elderly because of loss of subcutaneous tissue and/or dehydration. Moisture from bathing, sweat, urine, and feces compounds the damage. Other risk factors for pressure sores include those that exacerbate oxygen transport (e.g., anemia) or impede healing (e.g., malnutrition) (Bergstrom and Braden, 1992). Hospitalized patients with fractures, fecal incontinence, and hypoalbuminemia are at especially high risk (Allman et al., 1986). The Agency for Health Care Policy and Research has published clinical practice guidelines for the prevention of pressure ulcers (AHCPR, 1992).

Pressure sores can be classified into four stages, depending on their clinical appearance and extent (Table 9-13). It is important to note that the area of damage below the pressure sore is much larger than the sore itself. (This is caused by the manner in which pressure and shearing forces are transmitted to subcutaneous tissues.) Over 90 percent of pressure sores occur in the lower body—mainly in the sacral and coccygeal areas, at the ischial tuberosities, and in the greater trochanter area.

The cornerstone of management of the skin in immobile patients is prevention of pressure sores (Table 9-14). Once a stage I or II pressure sore develops, all preventive measures listed in Table 9-13 should be used to avoid progression of the sore, and intensive local skin care must be instituted. A myriad of techniques have been advocated for local skin care; none have been proved to be more successful than others. The most important factor in all these techniques is the attention (and thus the relief from pressure) that the skin gets. Almost

Table 9-13 Clinical characteristics of pressure sores

Stage I
    Acute inflammatory response limited to epidermis
    Presents as irregular area of erythema, induration, and/or superficial ulceration
    Often over a bony prominence

Stage II
    Extension of acute inflammatory response through dermis to the junction of
        subcutaneous fat
    Appears as a blister, abrasion, or shallow ulcer with more distinct edges
    Early fibrosis and pigment changes occur

Stage III
    Full-thickness skin ulcer extending through subcutaneous fat, limited by deep
        fascia
    Skin undermined
    Base of ulcer infected, often with necrotic, foul-smelling tissue

Stage IV
    Extension of ulcer through deep fascia, so that bone is visible at base of ulcer
    Osteomyelitis and septic arthritis can be present

any technique that involves removing pressure from the area and regularly cleansing and drying the skin will work.

The management of stages III and IV pressure sores is somewhat more complicated. Debridement of necrotic tissue and frequent irrigation (two to three times daily), cleansing (with saline or peroxide), and dressing of the wound are essential. Eschars should be undermined and removed if they are suspected of hiding large amounts of necrotic and infected tissue. Some of the newer chemical debriding agents can be helpful. The role of wound cultures and antimicrobials in the management of stage III pressure sores is controversial. Topical antimicrobials may be useful, especially when bacterial colony counts are high, but they are generally not recommended. Systemic antimicrobials should not be used because they do not reach sufficient concentrations in the area of the sore; local therapy will be more effective unless cellulitis is present. Routine wound cultures are probably not warranted for stage III lesions because they almost always grow several different organisms and do not detect anaerobic bacteria, which are often pathogenic. Results of such cultures generally reflect colonization rather than infection. Once a lesion has progressed to stage IV, systemic antimicrobials are often necessary. Routine and

Table 9-14 Principles of skin care in immobile older patients

Preventive
  Identify patients at risk
  Decrease pressure, friction, and skin folding
  Keep skin clean and dry
  Avoid excessive bed rest
  Avoid oversedation
  Provide adequate nutrition and hydration

Stages I and II pressure sores
  Avoid pressure and moisture
  Prevent further injury
  Provide intensive local skin care*

Stage III pressure sores
  Debride necrotic tissue
  Cleanse and dress wound*
  Culture wound[†]
  Use topical antimicrobials[†]

Stage IV pressure sores
  Take tissue biopsy for culture
  Use systemic antimicrobials for cellulitis and/or osteomyelitis
  Have surgical consultation to consider surgical repair

---

* Many techniques are effective (see text).
[†] Cultures and topical antimicrobials should not be used routinely (see text).

anaerobic cultures of tissue or bone are most helpful in directing antimicrobial therapy. Patients with large pressure sores who become septic should be treated with broad-spectrum antimicrobials that will cover anaerobes, gram-negative organisms, and *Staphylococcus aureus*. In selected instances, consideration of plastic surgery for stage IV lesions is warranted. Air-fluidized and low-airloss beds are being used with increasing frequency for the management of patients with stage III and IV pressure sores as well as to prevent deep sores in high-risk patients. Although these beds are expensive, they may be helpful in accelerating the healing of pressure sores in selected patients in hospital and nursing home settings (Allman et al., 1987; Ferrel et al. 1993).

EXERCISE

The development of musculoskeletal disability with age frequently decreases quality of life. Musculoskeletal disability among older adults is commonly linked to osteoarthritis, soft tissue changes including deconditioning, and other chronic diseases. Smoking, body-mass index, and exercise patterns in midlife and late adulthood are predictors of subsequent disability (Fried et al., 1998; Vita et al., 1998). Persons with better health habits not only survive longer but their disability is postponed. In a longitudinal study, older persons who engaged in vigorous running had slower development of disability than the general population (Fries et al., 1994). Maximal cardiac output and aerobic exercise capacity decline with advancing age and physical inactivity. Endurance exercise training induces adaptations that can counteract some of the deleterious effects of aging, including an increase in maximal O_2 uptake and enhancement of cardiac function (Stratton et al., 1992). As another benefit of exercise, a recent met-analysis suggests that aerobic exercise helps maintain the bone mineral density of the lumbar spine in postmenopausal women (Kelley, 1998).

Strength training, too, has been shown to be feasible and effective in both community-dwelling older adults and frail nursing home residents (Ades et al., 1996; Fiatarone et al., 1994; Hunter et al., 1995). Training improves strength, walking endurance, and ability to carry out daily tasks.

These studies have demonstrated that exercise programs, both for endurance and strength, can be initiated in older adults with safety and with resultant benefit in delaying disability and improving function. Walking is cheap and safe, and strength training can be done with inexpensive devices. The program should be tailored with specific goals for the exercise and outcomes.

REHABILITATION

The goal of rehabilitation is to restore function and prevent further disability. It is therefore a core element of geriatric practice, especially for immobile elderly patients, and usually necessitates a team effort. It is beyond the scope of this text to provide a detailed discussion of

rehabilitation in the older adult. Table 9-15 outlines some of the key principles. Careful assessment of a patient's function, the setting of realistic goals, prevention of secondary disabilities and complications of immobility, repeated measures of functional abilities that are relevant to the patient's environment, and adapting the environment to the patients' abilities (and vice versa) are all essential elements of the rehabilitation process.

Physical and occupational therapists can be extremely valuable in assessing, treating, motivating, and monitoring patients whose mobility is impaired. Physical therapists generally attend to the relief of pain, muscle strength and endurance, joint range of motion, and gait. They use a variety of treatment modalities (Table 9-16). Occupational therapists focus on functional abilities, especially as they relate to activities of daily living. They make detailed assessments of mobility and help patients improve or adapt to their abilities to perform basic and instrumental activities of daily living. Even when mobility and function remain impaired, occupational therapists can make life easier for these patients by performing environmental assessments and recommending modifications and assistive devices that will improve the patient's ability to function independently (Table 9-17). Speech therapists are helpful in assessing and implementing rehabilitation for disorders of communication and swallowing.

Although these basic principles of geriatric rehabilitation are essential in providing optimal care for the growing populations of geriat-

Table 9-15 Basic principles of rehabilitation in older patients

Optimize the treatment of underlying diseases

Prevent secondary disabilities and complications of immobility

Treat primary disabilities

Set realistic, individualized goals

Emphasize functional independence
  Set measurable goals related to functional performance
  Enhance residual functional capacities
  Provide adaptive tools to maximize function
  Adapt the environment to the patient's functional disabilities when feasible

Attend to motivation and other psychological factors of both patients and caregivers

Utilize a team approach

Table 9-16 Physical therapy in the management of immobile older patients

Objectives
  Relieve pain
  Evaluate, maintain, and improve joint range of motion
  Evaluate and improve strength, endurance, motor skills, and coordination
  Evaluate and improve gait and stability
  Assess the need for and teach the use of assistive devices for ambulation
    (wheelchairs, walkers, canes)

Treatment modalities

Exercise
  Active (isometric and isotonic)
  Passive

Heat
  Hot packs
  Paraffin
  Diathermy

Hydrotherapy

Ultrasound

Transcutaneous electrical nerve stimulation

ric patients who may need rehabilitation, the cost-effectiveness of various approaches to rehabilitation in the elderly remains controversial. Most of the data on the effectiveness of rehabilitation for older adults come from studies of geriatric assessment units, where short-term rehabilitation is a major component of the intervention. Most geriatric assessment units described to date have been in either acute care hospitals or ambulatory settings, although some have been located in nursing homes (Schuman et al., 1980; Adelman et al., 1987). The effectiveness of such units has been summarized in Chap. 3 and elsewhere (Rubenstein et al., 1991). It is clear that targeting rehabilitative efforts to patients who are most likely to benefit is critical to cost-effectiveness. Unfortunately, much more data are needed to accurately predict which geriatric patients will benefit most from specific types of rehabilitative efforts. Until these data are available, geriatricians should work closely with experienced rehabilitation therapists in setting *realistic* and *individualized* goals for their patients. The goals should be compatible with the patients' preferences and socioeco-

Table 9-17 Occupational therapy in the management of immobile older patients

Objectives
Restore, maintain, and improve ability to function independently
Evaluate and improve sensory and perceptual motor function
Evaluate and improve ability to perform activities of daily living (ADL)
Fabricate and fit splints for upper extremities
Improve coping and problem-solving skills
Improve use of leisure time

Modalities
Assessment of mobility
  Bed mobility
  Transfers
  Wheelchair propulsion
Assessment of other ADL using actual or simulated environments
  Dressing
  Toileting
  Bathing and personal hygiene
  Cooking and cleaning
Visit home for environmental assessment and recommendations for adaptation
Provide task-oriented activities (e.g., crafts, projects)
Recommend and teach use of assistive devices (e.g., long-handled reachers, special eating and cooking utensils, sock aids)
Recommend and teach use of safety devices (e.g., grab bars and railing, raised toilet seats, shower chairs)

nomic environment and should be directed toward the maximum functional outcome realistic for that patient. Ongoing assessment of progress and the prevention of medical and psychological complications are also fundamental to the rehabilitative process.

REFERENCES

Adelman RD, Marron K, Libow LS, et al: A community-oriented geriatric rehabilitation unit in a nursing home. *Gerontologist* 27:143–146, 1987.
Ades PA, Ballor DL, Ashikaga T, et al: Weight training improves walking endurance in healthy elderly persons. *Ann Intern Med* 124:568–572, 1996.
AGS Panel on Chronic Pain in Older Persons: The management of chronic pain in older persons. *J Am Geriatr Soc* 46:635–651, 1998.

AHCPR: *Pressure Ulcers in Adults: Prediction and Prevention.* AHCPR Publication No. 92-0047. Rockville, MD: Agency for Health Care Policy and Research, 1992.

Allman RM, Laprade CA, Noel LB, et al: Pressure sores among hospitalized patients. *Ann Intern Med* 105:337–342, 1986.

Allman RM, Walker JM, Hart MK, et al: Air-fluidized beds or conventional therapy for pressure sores: A randomized trial. *Ann Intern Med* 107:641–648, 1987.

Aloia JF, Cohn SH, Ostuni A, et al: Prevention of involutional bone loss by exercise. *Ann Intern Med* 80:356–358, 1978.

American College of Physicians Health and Public Policy Committee: Bone mineral densitometry. *Ann Intern Med* 107:932–936, 1987.

Beard K, Walker AM, Perera DR, et al: Nonsteroidal anti-inflammatory drugs and hospitalization for gastroesophageal bleeding in the elderly. *Arch Intern Med* 147:1621–1623, 1987.

Bergstrom N, Braden B: A prospective study of pressure sore risk among institutionalized elderly. *J Am Geriatr Soc* 40:747–758, 1992.

Campion EW, Jette AM, Cleary PD, et al: Hip fracture: A prospective study of hospital course, complications, and costs. *J Gen Intern Med* 2:78–82, 1987.

Chow R, Harrison JE, Notarius C: Effect of two randomised exercise programmes on bone mass of healthy postmenopausal women. *BMJ* 295:1441–1444, 1987.

Chapuy MC, Arlot ME, Duboeuf F, et al: Vitamin D_3 and calcium to prevent hip fractures in elderly women. *N Engl J Med* 327:1637–1642, 1992.

Chuang T, Wunder GG, Istrup DM, et al: Polymyalgia rheumatica: A 10-year epidemiologic and clinical study. *Ann Intern Med* 97:672–680, 1982.

Crawford J, Eye-Boland MK, Cohen HJ: Clinical utility of erythrocyte sedimentation rate and plasma protein analysis in the elderly. *Am J Med* 82:239–246, 1987.

Dawson-Hughes B, Dallai GE, Drall EA, et al: A controlled trial of the effect of calcium supplementation on bone density in postmenopausal women. *N Engl J Med* 323:878–883, 1990.

Delmas PD, Bjarnason NH, Mitlak BH, et al: Effects of raloxifene on bone mineral density, serum cholesterol concentrations, and uterine endometrium in postmenopausal women. *N Engl J Med* 337:1641–1674, 1997.

Duvoisin R: To treat early or to treat late? *Ann Neurol* 22:2–3, 1987.

Eastell R: Treatment of postmenopausal osteoporosis. *N Engl J Med* 338:736–746, 1998.

Ferrell BA, Osterweil D, Christenson P: A randomized trial of low-air-loss beds for treatment of pressure ulcers. *JAMA* 269:494–497, 1992.

Fiatarone MA, O'Neill EF, Ryan ND, et al: Exercise training and nutritional supplementation for physical frailty in very elderly people. *N Engl J Med* 330:1769–1775, 1994.

Fitzgerald JF, Moore PS, Dittus RS: The care of elderly patients with hip fracture: Changes since implementation of the prospective payment system. *N Engl J Med* 319:1392–1397, 1988.

Fried LP, Kronmal RA, Newman AB, et al: Risk factor for 5-year mortality in older adults: The cardiovascular health study. *JAMA* 279:585–592, 1998.

Fries JF, Singh G, Morfeld D, et al: Running and the development of disability with age. *Ann Intern Med* 121:502–509, 1994.

Frost R: To treat early or to treat late? *Ann Neurol* 22:2–3, 1987.

Gerhart TN, Yett HS, Robertson LK, et al: Low-molecular-weight heparinoid compared with warfarin for prophylaxis of deep vein thrombosis in patients who are operated

on for fracture of the hip: a prospective, randomized trial. *J Bone Joint Surg Am* 73:494-502, 1991.

Goodwin JS: Progress in gerontology: Polymyalgia rheumatica and temporal arteritis. *J Am Geriatr Soc* 40:515-525, 1992.

Griffin MR, Piper JM, Daugherty JR, et al: Nonsteroidal anti-inflammatory drug use and increased risk for peptic ulcer disease in elderly persons. *Ann Intern Med* 114:257-263, 1991.

Gurwitz JH, Avorn J, Ross-Degnan D, Lipsitz LA: Nonsteroidal anti-inflammatory drug-associated azotemia in the very old. *JAMA* 264:471-475, 1990.

Hunter GR, Treuth MS, Weinsier RL, et al: The effects of strength conditioning on older women's ability to perform daily tasks. *J Am Geriatr Soc* 43:756-760, 1995.

Jette AM, Harris BA, Cleary PD, et al: Functional recovery after hip fracture. *Arch Phys Med Rehabil* 68:735-740, 1987.

Juncos JL, Fabbrini G, Mouradian MM, et al: Dietary influences on the antiparkinsonian response to levodopa. *Arch Neurol* 44:1003-1005, 1987.

Kelley G: Aerobic exercise and lumbar spine bone mineral density in postmenopausal women: A meta-analysis. *J Am Geriatr Soc* 46:143-152, 1998.

Mayeux R, Stern Y, Mulvey K, et al: Reappraisal of temporary levodopa withdrawal ("drug holiday") in Parkinson's disease. *N Engl J Med* 313:724-728, 1985.

Marottoli RA, Berkman LF, Cooney Jr., LM: Decline in physical function following hip fracture. *J Am Geriatr Soc* 40:861-866, 1992.

Medical Letter: Pramipexole and ropinirole for Parkinson's disease. *Med Lett* 39(1014):109-110, 1997.

Melton LJ III, Eddy DM, Johnston CC Jr: Screening for osteoporosis. *Ann Intern Med* 112:516-528, 1990.

Nutt JG, Woodward WR, Hammerstad JP, et al: The "on-off" phenomenon in Parkinson's disease. *N Engl J Med* 310:483-488, 1984.

Pak CYC, Sakhaee K, Adams-Huet B, et al: Treatment of postmenopausal osteoporosis with slow-release sodium fluoride: Final reprot of a randomized controlled trial. *Ann Intern Med* 123:401-408, 1995.

Parkinson Study Group: Effects of tocopherol and deprenyl on the progression of disability in early Parkinson's disease. *N Engl J Med* 328:176-183, 1993.

Powers PJ, Gent M, Jay RM, et al: A randomized trial of less intense postoperative warfarin or aspirin therapy in the prevention of venous thromboembolism after surgery for fractured hip. *Arch Intern Med* 149:771-774, 1989.

Prince RL, Smith M, Dick IM, et al: Prevention of postmenopausal osteoporosis: A comparative study of exercise, calcium supplementation, and hormone-replacement therapy. *N Engl J Med* 325:1189-1195, 1991.

Reich ML: Arthritis: Avoiding diagnostic pitfalls. *Geriatrics* 37:46-54, 1982.

Reid IR, Ames RW, Evans MC, et al: Effect of calcium supplementation on bone loss in postmenopausal women. *N Engl J Med* 328:460-464, 1993.

Riggs BL, Melton JL: Involutional osteoporosis. *N Engl J Med* 314:1676-1684, 1986.

Rubenstein LZ, Stuck AE, Siu AL, Wieland D: Impacts of geriatric evaluation and management programs on defined outcomes: Overview of the evidence. *J Am Geriatr Soc* 39(suppl):85-165, 1991.

Schuman JE, Beattie EJ, Steed DA, et al: Rehabilitative and geriatric teaching programs: Clinical efficacy in a skilled nursing facility. *Arch Phys Med Rehabil* 61:310-315, 1980.

Silliman RA, Wagner EH, Fletcher RH: The social and functional consequences of stroke for elderly patients. *Stroke* 18:200–203, 1987.

Soll AH, Weinstein WM, Kurata J, McCarthy D: Nonsteroidal anti-inflammatory drugs and peptic ulcer disease. *Ann Intern Med* 114:307–319, 1991.

Storm T, Thamsborg G, Steiniche T, et al: Effect of intermittent cyclical etidronate therapy on bone mass and fracture rate in women with postmenopausal osteoporosis. *N Engl J Med* 322:1265–1271, 1990.

Stratton JR, Cerqueira MD, Schwartz RS, et al: Differences in cardiovascular responses to isoproterenol in relation to age and exercise training in healthy men. *Circulation* 86:504–512, 1992.

Tilyard MW, Spears GFS, Com B, et al: Treatment of postmenopausal osteoporosis with calcitriol or calcium. *N Engl J Med* 326:357–362, 1992.

Tinetti ME, Schmidt A, Baum J: Use of the erythrocyte sedimentation rate in chronically ill, elderly patients with a decline in health status. *Am J Med* 80:844–848, 1986.

Vita AJ, Terry RB, Hubert HB, Fries JF: Aging, health risks, and cumulative disability. *N Engl J Med* 338:1035–1041, 1998.

Zuckerman JD: Hip fracture. *N Engl J Med* 334:1519–1525, 1996.

Zuckerman JD, Sakales SR, Fabian DR, Frankel VH: Hip fractures in geriatric patients: results of an interdisciplinary hospital care program. *Clin Orthop Rel Res* 274:213–225, 1992.

SUGGESTED READINGS

Immobility, General

Bortz WM: Disuse and aging. *JAMA* 248:1203–1208, 1982.

Harper CM, Lyles YM: Physiology and complications of bed rest. *J Am Geriatr Soc* 36:1047–1054, 1988.

Musculoskeletal Disorders

Borenstein DG, Burton JR: Lumbar spine disease in the elderly. *J Am Geriatr Soc* 41:167–175, 1993.

Davis MA: Epidemiology of osteoarthritis. *Clin Geriatr Med* 4:241–256, 1988.

Ferrell BA: Pain management in elderly people. *J Am Geriatr Soc* 39:64–73, 1991.

Frymoyer JW: Back pain and sciatica. *N Engl J Med* 318:291–300, 1988.

Gall EP, Higbee M: Pharmacologic therapy of rheumatic diseases, in Bressler R, Katz MD (eds): *Geriatric Pharmacology.* McGraw-Hill, New York, 1993, pp. 467–506.

Roth SH: Pharmacologic approaches to musculoskeletal disorders. *Clin Geriatr Med* 4:441–461, 1988.

Osteoporosis

American College of Physicians: Guidelines for counseling postmenopausal women about preventive hormone therapy. *Ann Intern Med* 117:1038–1041, 1992.

Kaplan FS: Osteoporosis. *Ciba Clin Symp* 35(5), 1983.

Manolagas SC, Jilka RL: Bone marrow, cytokines, and bone remodeling: Emerging insights into the pathophysiology of osteoporosis. *N Engl J Med* 33:305–311, 1995.

Marottoli RA, Berkman LF, Leo-Summers L, Cooney LM Jr: Predictors of mortality and institutionalization after hip fracture: The New Haven EPESE cohort. *Am J Public Health* 84:1807–1812, 1994.

Morley JE, Mooradian AD, Brickman AS, Kaiser FE: UCLA geriatric grand rounds: Osteoporosis. *J Am Geriatr Soc* 36:845–859, 1988.

Resnick NM, Greenspan SL: Senile osteoporosis reconsidered. *JAMA* 261:1025–1029, 1989.

Riggs BL, Melton LJ: Involutional osteoporosis. *N Engl J Med* 314:1676–1684, 1986.

Parkinson's Disease

Boshes B: Sinemet and the treatment of parkinsonism. *Ann Intern Med* 94:364–370, 1981.

Duvoisin R: Parkinsonism. *Ciba Clin Symp* 28(1), 1976.

Nutt JG: Parkinson's disease: Evaluation and therapeutic strategy. *Hosp Pract* 22:107–136, 1987.

Parkes JD: Adverse effects of antiparkinsonian drugs. *Drugs* 21:341–353, 1981.

Pressure Sores

Agency for Health Care Policy and Research, Panel for the Prediction and Prevention of Pressure Ulcers in Adults: *Pressure Ulcers in Adults: Prediction and Prevention.* Clinical Practice Guideline, Number 3, AHCPR Publication No. 92-0047. Rockville, MD, ACPHR, May 1992.

Agris J, Spira M: Pressure ulcers: Prevention and treatment. *Ciba Clin Symp* 31(5), 1979.

Ouslander JG, Osterweil D, Morley J: *Medical Care in the Nursing Home.* McGraw-Hill, New York, 1991, pp 147–164.

Reuler JB, Cooney TG: The pressure sore: Pathophysiology and principles of management. *Ann Intern Med* 94:661–666, 1981.

Rehabilitation

Clark GS, Blue B, Bearer JB: Rehabilitation of the elderly amputee. *J Am Geriatr Soc* 31:439–448, 1983.

Liang MH, Partridge A, Eaton H, et al: Rehabilitation management of homebound elderly with locomotor disability. *Clin Geriatr Med* 4:431–440, 1988.

Sinaki M: Postmenopausal spinal osteoporosis: Physical therapy and rehabilitation principles. *Mayo Clin Proc* 57:699–703, 1982.

Steinberg FU: Rehabilitating the older stroke patient: What's possible? *Geriatrics* 41:85–97, 1986.

Wasson JH, Gall V, McDonald R, Liang MH: The prescription of assistive devices for the elderly: practical considerations. *J Gen Intern Med* 5:46–54, 1990.
Williams TF (ed): *Rehabilitation in the Aging.* New York, Raven Press, 1984.

Stroke

Browne TR, Poskanzer DC: Treatment of strokes. *N Engl J Med* 28:594–602; 650–657, 1969.
Buonanno F, Toole JF: Management of patients with established ("completed") cerebral infarction. *Stroke* 12:7–16, 1981.
Kelly JF, Winograd CH: A functional approach to stroke management in elderly patients. *J Am Geriatr Soc* 33:48–60, 1985.

CHAPTER TEN

CARDIOVASCULAR DISORDERS

In older adults, heart disease is the leading cause of death worldwide and is the most common cause for hospitalization. Physiologic changes of the cardiovascular system in aging may modify the presentation of cardiac disease.

PHYSIOLOGIC CHANGES

In reviewing data on physiologic changes of the cardiovascular system, it is important to recognize the selection criteria of the population studied. Because the prevalence of coronary artery disease may be 50 percent in the eighth and ninth decades, screening for exclusion of occult cardiovascular disease may modify findings.

In a population screened for occult coronary artery disease, there is no change in cardiac output at rest over the third to eighth decades (Gerstenblith et al., 1987) (Table 10-1). There is a slight decrease in heart rate and a compensatory slight increase in stroke volume. This is in contrast to studies in unscreened individuals, where cardiac output has been shown to fall from the second to the ninth decades.

Table 10-1 Resting cardiac function in patients aged 30 to 80 compared with that in 30-year-olds

	Unscreened for occult CAD	Screened for occult CAD
Heart rate	−	−
Stroke volume	− −	+
Stroke volume index	− −	0
Cardiac output	− −	0
Cardiac index	− −	0
Peripheral vascular resistance	+ +	0
Peak systolic blood pressure	+ +	+ +
Diastolic pressure	0	0

Key: CAD, coronary artery disease; +, slight increase; + +, increase; −, slight decrease; − −, decrease; 0, no difference.

During maximal exercise, however, other changes are manifest even in the screened population (Table 10-2). Heart rate response to exercise is decreased in older adults, reflecting a diminished beta-adrenergic responsiveness in aging. Because cardiac output is maintained, the heart affects the Starling curve by increasing cardiac volumes—increasing end-diastolic and end-systolic volumes. With this increase in workload and the work of pumping blood against less

Table 10-2 Performance at maximum exercise in sample screened for coronary artery disease, age 30 to 80

	Compared with 30-year-olds
Heart rate	− −
End-diastolic volume	+ +
Stroke volume	+ +
Cardiac output	0
End-systolic volume	+ +
Ejection fraction	− −
Total peripheral vascular resistance	0
Systolic blood pressure	0

Key: + +, significant increase; − −, significant decrease; 0, no difference.

compliant arteries and a higher blood pressure, cardiac hypertrophy occurs even in the screened elderly population.

Since myocardial reserve mechanisms are utilized to maintain normal function in aging, older persons are more vulnerable to development of dysfunction when disease is superimposed.

Diastolic dysfunction—retarded left ventricular filling and higher left ventricular diastolic pressure—is present both at rest and during exercise in older persons. Older persons are more dependent on atrial contraction, as opposed to ventricular relaxation, for left ventricular filling and thus are more likely to develop heart failure if atrial fibrillation ensues. Heart failure may occur in the absence of systolic dysfunction or valvular disease.

HYPERTENSION

Hypertension is the major risk factor for stroke, heart failure, and coronary artery disease in older adults; all are important contributors to mortality and functional disability. Because hypertension is remediable and its control may reduce the incidence of coronary heart disease and stroke, increased efforts at detection and treatment of high blood pressure are indicated.

Hypertension in older adults is defined as a systolic blood pressure of 160 mmHg or greater and/or a diastolic blood pressure of 95 mmHg or greater. Isolated systolic hypertension is defined as a pressure of 160 mmHg or greater with a diastolic pressure of less than 90 mmHg. With this definition, as many as 40 to 50 percent of individuals over age 65 may be hypertensive.

Diastolic pressure rises with age but stabilizes after age 60, whereas systolic pressure continues to increase, with the incidence rising steeply after age 55 in both sexes, but to a greater degree in women.

Despite the high prevalence of hypertension in older adults, it should not be considered a normal consequence of aging. The Framingham Study has demonstrated that hypertension is the major risk factor for cardiovascular disease in older adults and that the risk increases with each decade (Kannel, 1976). Once coronary artery disease develops, it tends to be more rapidly fatal among patients with hypertension.

Evaluation

The diagnosis should be made on serial blood pressures. In patients with labile hypertension, blood pressure should be averaged to make the diagnosis, because these patients are at no less risk than those with stable hypertension. The history and physical examination should be directed toward assessing the duration, severity, treatment, and complications of the hypertension (Table 10-3). Atherosclerosis may interfere with occlusion of the brachial artery by a blood pressure cuff, leading to erroneously elevated blood pressure determinations, or "pseudohypertension." Such an effect can be determined by the Osler maneuver. The cuff pressure is raised above systolic blood pressure. If the radial artery remains palpable at this pressure, significant atherosclerosis is probably present and may account for a 10- to 15-mmHg pressure error. Initial laboratory evaluation should include complete urinalysis and measurement of serum electrolytes and creatinine levels. A chest film and electrocardiogram should also be included. An intravenous pyelogram is not indicated in the initial evaluation and should be reserved for the patient resistant to therapy.

Table 10-3 Initial evaluation of hypertension in older adults

History
  Duration
  Severity
  Treatment
  Complications
  Other risk factors

Physical examination
  Blood pressure, including Osler maneuver
  Weight
  Funduscopic, vascular, and cardiac examination for end-organ damage
  Abdominal bruit
  Neurologic examination for focal deficits

Laboratory tests
  Urinalysis
  Electrolytes
  Creatinine
  Calcium
  Chest x-ray
  Electrocardiogram

Secondary forms of hypertension are uncommon in older adults but should be considered in treatment-resistant patients and in those with diastolic pressures >115 mmHg (Table 10-4). Primary hyperaldosteronism and pheochromocytoma are uncommon in older adults and are particularly unusual in those past the age of 75. Although also uncommon, renovascular disease should be considered in treatment-resistant patients. It is almost always secondary to atherosclerotic occlusive disease in older adults.

With the use of automated calcium determinations, the frequency of diagnosis of primary hyperparathyroidism is increasing, particularly in postmenopausal women. Because there is a causal link between this disorder and hypertension, the diagnosis and treatment of hyperparathyroidism may ameliorate the elevated blood pressure.

Estrogen therapy in the postmenopausal woman may be associated with hypertension. Such an association can be assessed by withdrawing estrogen therapy for several months and following the blood pressure response.

Treatment

The issue of treatment of systolic/diastolic or isolated systolic hypertension in older individuals has been resolved. The Veterans Administration Cooperative Study (1972), the Hypertension Detection and Follow-Up Program Study (1979), a smaller Australian trial (1980), and more recently the European Working Party on High Blood Pressure in the Elderly (EWPHE) (Amery et al., 1985, 1986), the Systolic Hypertension in the Elderly Program (1991), the Department of Veterans Affairs Cooperative Study of Antihypertensive Agents (Cushman et al., 1991), the Swedish Trial in Old Patients with Hypertension (Dahlof et al., 1991), and the Medical Research Council Trial of Treatment of Hypertension in Older Adults (1992) have all demonstrated that treating hypertension in older adults decreases morbidity

Table 10-4 Secondary hypertension in older persons

Renovascular disease (atherosclerotic)
Hyperparathyroidism (calcium)
Estrogen administration
Renal disease (decreased creatinine clearance)

and mortality from coronary artery disease and stroke. Although there has been concern about the hazard of treating individuals with cerebrovascular disease, the evidence suggests that the presence of cerebrovascular disease is an indication for rather than a contraindication to hypertensive therapy.

Some of the treatment trials that have included individuals to age 84 suggest that there should be no age cutoff above which high blood pressure is not treated (Applegate and Ruttan, 1992). Relatively healthy older persons at any age should be treated unless they have severe comorbid disease that clearly will limit their life expectancy or unless the toxicity of treatment is so great that it outweighs potential benefits.

Several epidemiologic studies and treatment trials have suggested a J-shaped relationship between blood pressure and mortality. Although the J-shaped phenomenon may be related to the higher prevalence of serious cardiovascular or other diseases in the subjects with the lowest blood pressure rather than to the low blood pressure per se, the conservative approach would be to not lower systolic blood pressure below 135 to 140 mmHg or diastolic blood pressure below 80 to 85 mmHg in older adult patients.

Specific Therapy

Although lifestyle changes are not easily accomplished, weight reduction and lowering of dietary sodium intake should be attempted. Each of these measures may lower diastolic pressure by 5 to 10 mmHg. Exercise may also be beneficial in lowering blood pressure. Strenuous exercise is not necessary. A modest walking and running program may have a positive effect on blood pressure reduction (Rippe et al., 1988). Other risk factors—such as smoking, dyslipidemia, and diabetes mellitus—should also be modified.

If dietary measures fail to control blood pressure, drug therapy should be considered. Physiologic and pathologic changes of aging should be considered in individualizing the therapy. Changes in volumes of distribution and hepatic and renal metabolism may alter pharmacokinetics (see Chap. 13). Changes in vessel elasticity and baroreceptor sensitivity may alter responses to posture- and drug-induced falls in blood pressure.

Thiazide diuretics are usually the initial step in therapy (Table 10-5). They are well tolerated, are relatively inexpensive, and can be

Table 10-5 Thiazide diuretics for antihypertensive therapy

Advantages	Adverse effects
Well tolerated	Hypokalemia
No CNS side effects	Volume depletion
Relatively inexpensive	Hyponatremia
Infrequent dosing	Hyperglycemia
Good response rate	Hyperuricemia
Orthostatic hypotension uncommon	
Can be used in conjunction with other agents	

given once a day; results from the European study indicate that 65 percent of older hypertensives can be treated with diuretics as the only medication. The SHEP trial and several other studies have demonstrated that low-dose thiazides (e.g., 12.5 to 25 mg of chlorthalidone) are efficacious in lowering blood pressure while minimizing metabolic side effects (Morledge et al., 1986; Vardan et al., 1987b). Higher doses had a minimal additional effect on blood pressure with a more marked effect on hypokalemia. Postural hypotension is uncommon, but serum potassium should be monitored. Diabetics may have increased requirements for insulin or oral hypoglycemic agents. Although short-term trials of thiazide diuretics have demonstrated increases in serum cholesterol, this effect of the drug does not seem to persist at 1 year (Vardan et al., 1987a). Although beta blockers are also recommended as initial-step therapy, two recent metanalyses have called this into question (Psaty et al., 1997; Messerli et al., 1998). Beta blockers reduced stroke and congestive heart failure but not coronary heart disease, cardiovascular mortality, or all-cause mortality. Beta-blocking agents may be used as the initial drug when another indication for their use exists, such as coronary heart disease, arrhythmias, or essential tremor. All classes of antihypertensive drugs have been shown to be effective in lowering blood pressure in older patients (Joint National Committee, 1992). However, only diuretics and beta blockers have been used in controlled trials of the treatment of uncomplicated hypertension with cardiovascular morbidity and mortality endpoints.

If thiazides alone do not control blood pressure, a second agent is added (Table 10-6) or a thiazide is added if one of the other agents has failed. The choice should be individualized and usually selected from among beta blockers, calcium antagonists, or angiotensin-

Table 10-6 Antihypertensive medications

Agent*	Advantages	Disadvantages
Beta blockers	Useful in associated coronary artery disease or arrhythmias Water-soluble agents have fewer CNS side effects	Contraindicated in cardiac conduction defects, overt heart failure, bradyarrhythmia, reactive airways disease, peripheral vascular disease, and insulin-treated diabetes Propranolol may cause fatigue, somnolence, or depression If cardiac output is decreased, renal blood flow and glomerular filtration rate may fall Must be withdrawn slowly in presence of coronary artery disease
Clonidine	Increased renal perfusion	Somnolence, depression Dry mouth, constipation Rarely, withdrawal hypertensive crisis
Reserpine	Inexpensive	Depression (minimized with low dosage)
Alpha blockers	May be useful in systolic hypertension May be useful in benign prostatic hypertrophy	Orthostatic hypotension with initial dose
Hydralazine	May be useful in systolic hypertension	Reflex tachycardia, aggravation of angina Lupus-like syndrome at high dosage
Calcium channel blockers	Peripheral vasodilator Coronary blood flow maintained Potency increased with age	Headaches Sodium retention Negative inotropic effect Conduction abnormality
Angiotensin-converting enzyme inhibitors	Preload and afterload reduction Use in CHF, diabetes mellitus with proteinuria	Hyperkalemia Hypotension Decreased renal function

* With all these agents, initiation with low dosage and careful titration may minimize side effects.

converting enzyme (ACE) inhibitors. Where beta blockers would be used for treatment of other disorders in association with hypertension, they would be the drug of choice. These agents are contraindicated in patients with cardiac conduction deficits, overt heart failure, brady-arrhythmias, reactive airways disease, peripheral vascular disease, and insulin-dependent diabetes mellitus.

The advantages of beta blockers might make them the general drug of choice in the second step of therapy except that they may not be as effective in older adults as they are in the young. Their mode of action is unknown, but three mechanisms have been proposed: (1) CNS action, (2) decreased cardiac output, and (3) inhibition of renin secretion. Myocardial beta-adrenergic responsiveness decreases with age, and thus the effect of beta blockade on cardiac output may be diminished. Most elderly hypertensives have a low-renin form of hypertension; thus this effect may be less in the aged. However, in those older patients without contraindications who do respond, beta blockers may be the drug of choice.

The more water-soluble beta blockers may be well suited for the geriatric population because they enter the CNS less readily and thus have fewer of the CNS side effects such as somnolence and depression; this would be a particular advantage in the elderly. However, if cardiac output is decreased, renal perfusion and glomerular filtration rate may be affected. One concern with beta blockers is the production of bradycardia with reduced cardiac output. One simple test to moni-tor for this side effect is the patient's response to mild exercise after each dosage increase; a failure to increase pulse by at least 10 beats per minute is an indication to reduce the dosage. If a patient is to be taken off a beta-blocking agent, withdrawal should be done slowly over a period of several days to avoid rebound of original symptoms.

Clonidine may cause somnolence and depression, but it increases renal perfusion. The clonidine transdermal patch may lessen some of these adverse effects. However, local skin reactions may occur in about 15 percent of users. The once-per-week application of the patch may be an asset in improving compliance.

The major disadvantage of reserpine is the high incidence of depression as a side effect. This can be minimized with low dosages.

The major side effect of alpha blockers is orthostatic hypotension: this is especially problematic with initial doses of prazosin. Orthostasis may be induced each time this drug is stopped and restarted when drug dosages are missed. Newer agents with lesser hypotensive effects

are now being used to treat symptomatic benign prostatic hypertrophy.

Although hydralazine is usually a third-step drug, it may occasionally be used as a second-step drug in older adults because reflex tachycardia rarely occurs. If used with diuretics alone, it should be initiated in low dosages, which should be increased slowly. It should not be used in the absence of a beta blocker if coronary artery disease is present.

Calcium antagonists are peripheral vasodilators with the advantage of maintaining coronary blood flow. These agents appear to have increased potency with age, possibly as a result of the decreased reflex tachycardia and myocardial contractility in older adults as compared with younger individuals. Headache, sodium retention, negative inotropic effects—especially in combination with beta blockers—and conduction abnormalities may limit their use

ACE inhibitors are both preload and afterload reducers and thus are particularly useful in the face of congestive heart failure. Long-acting agents may have an advantage in compliance. Renal function, which may deteriorate on administration of these agents, needs to be monitored carefully. These agents may also induce hyperkalemia and should not be used with a potassium-sparing diuretic. Older adults are also more vulnerable to the hypotensive effects of these drugs.

With the newer, more effective agents, drug-resistant hypertension is unusual. In such cases, drug compliance should be monitored and sodium intake assessed. If such factors are not contributing to drug resistance, secondary causes of hypertension should be considered, especially renovascular disease.

STROKE AND TRANSIENT ISCHEMIC ATTACKS

Although the incidence of stroke is declining, it is still a major medical problem affecting approximately 50,000 individuals in the United States every year. Stroke is clearly a disease of older adults; about 75 percent of strokes occur in those over age 65. The incidence of stroke rises steeply with age, being 10 times greater in the 75-to-84 age group than in the 55-to-64 age group.

The causes and outcomes of stroke are listed in Table 10-7. In cerebral infarct, thrombosis, usually arteriosclerotic, is the commonest cause, with embolization from an ulcerated plaque or myocardial

Table 10-7 Stroke

Cause	Relative frequency, percent	Morality rate, percent
Subarachnoid hemorrhage	10	50
Intracerebral hemorrhage	15	80
Cerebral infarction (thrombosis and embolism)	75	40

thrombosis less frequent. Outcomes for survivors are listed in Table 10-8.

Hypertension, diabetes mellitus, and lipid abnormalities are associated with increased risk of cerebrovascular disease; hypertension is the major risk factor. In the Framingham Study (Kannel, 1976), systolic hypertension was associated with a three- to fivefold increased risk for stroke. Hypertension accelerates the formation of atheromatous plaques and damages the integrity of vessel walls, predisposing to thrombotic occlusion and cerebral infarction. Hypertension also promotes growth of microaneurysms in segments of small intracranial arteries. Those lesions are sites of intracranial hemorrhage and lacunar infarcts.

The data associating stroke with transient ischemic attacks are varied. Completed stroke as a sequel of TIA is reported to occur in 12 to 60 percent or more of untreated TIA patients who become asymptomatic; however, some estimates are at 25 percent or less. More TIA patients may die of cardiac disease than of a subsequent stroke (50 percent versus 36 percent, respectively, in a Mayo Clinic 15-year follow-up study) (Robbins, 1978). In retrospective studies of

Table 10-8 Outcome for survivors of stroke

Outcome	Percent
No dysfunction	10
Mild dysfunction	40
Significant dysfunction	40
Institutional care	10

Source: Robbins, 1978.

patients with completed stroke, previous TIA is reported to have occurred in 50 to 75 percent.

The keystone to the diagnosis of stroke is a clear history of sudden, acute neurologic deficit. When the history is not clear, especially if the deficit could have had a gradual onset, consideration should be given to a mass lesion. In such cases, brain scanning with computed tomography is indicated. Electroencephalography is only occasionally helpful in the differential diagnosis. Lumbar puncture is indicated in stroke patients if hemorrhage is suspected but not if there is evidence of increased intracranial pressure. An electrocardiogram should be performed routinely in cases of TIA or stroke because it may relate the episode to myocardial infarction or cardiac arrhythmia. Invasive techniques are not usually necessary in stroke patients.

In older adults, symptoms acceptable as evidence of cerebral ischemia are often misinterpreted. Presenting symptoms for TIA in the carotid and vertebral-basilar systems are given in Table 10-9. When they occur or recur alone without other neurologic symptoms, certain symptoms should not be attributed to vascular causes. These include light-headedness, nonspecific dizziness, vertigo, diplopia, drop attacks, forgetfulness, amnestic attacks, syncope, seizures, episodes of unconsciousness, and drowsy spells (Barnett, 1982).

Treatment

Based heavily on the results of one study (The National Institute of Neurological Disorders and Stroke rt-PA Stroke Study Group, 1995), the FDA approved and committees of the American Heart Association and the American Academy of Neurology published guidelines endorsing the use of t-PA within 3 h of onset of ischemic stroke (Caplan et al., 1997). A metanalysis of thrombolytic therapy revealed an increased risk for early death and intracranial hemorrhage but a decrease in the combined endpoint of death or dependency at 3 to 6 months (Wardlow et al., 1996). Despite the guidelines, thrombolysis has remained controversial and should probably be used only in research settings. Thus, intervention is directed toward prevention of stroke. The primary approach is to manage hypertension appropriately.

Two large, randomized trials including both men and women, one in the United States and the other in Europe, have determined that carotid endarterectomy prevents stroke in patients with neuro-

Table 10-9 TIA: Presenting symptoms

Symptom	Carotid	Vertebrobasilar
Paresis	+++	++
Paresthesia	+++	+++
Binocular vision	0	+++
Vertigo	0	+++
Diplopia	0	++
Ataxia	0	++
Dizziness	0	++
Monocular vision	++	0
Headache	+	+
Dysphasia	+	0
Dysarthria	+	+
Nausea and vomiting	0	+
Loss of consciousness	0	0
Visual hallucinations	0	0
Tinnitus	0	0
Mental change	0	0
Drop attacks	0	0
Drowsiness	0	0
Light-headedness	0	0
Hyperacusia	0	0
Weakness (generalized)	0	0
Convulsion	0	0

Key: +++, most frequent; 0, least frequent.

logic symptoms and severe (70 to 99 percent) stenosis of the internal carotid artery. A third trial, the Veterans Affairs Cooperative Study (Mayberg et al., 1991), which included only men, demonstrated similar results with symptomatic stenosis of >50 percent. The North American Carotid Endarterectomy Trial (1991) found the cumulative risk for stroke ipsilateral to stenosis to be 24 percent in medically treated and 7 percent in surgically treated patients at 18 months after randomization. The European Carotid Surgery Trial (1991) similarly found a lower risk, at 3 percent in its surgical arm than in its medical arm, at 22 percent at 3 years after randomization. Endarterectomy was also found to be beneficial when all strokes and deaths occurring among patients were factored into the analysis. In the VA study, stroke or crescendo TIAs occurred in 7.7 percent of the surgical patients as compared with 19.4 percent in the nonsurgical patients.

The benefit of surgery was more profound in those with stenosis greater than 70 percent.

The efficacy of carotid endarterectomy in preventing stroke in patients with asymptomatic carotid stenosis has not been confirmed in randomized clinical trials, despite the widespread use of operative intervention in such patients. The VA Cooperative Study (Hobson et al., 1993) demonstrated that carotid endarterectomy reduced the overall incidence of ipsilateral neurologic events in a selected group of male patients with asymptomatic carotid stenosis (>50 percent). However, no significant influence of carotid endarterectomy on the combined incidence of stroke and death was found. Identifying carotid artery stenosis in asymptomatic individuals can involve expensive and invasive diagnostic screening procedures. The human and economic costs of screening large numbers of asymptomatic people outweighs the benefits to the number of individuals screening would identify.

The alternative to surgery is drug therapy, although the results have not been dramatic (Rothrock and Hart, 1991). The general trend has been to use aspirin more and anticoagulants less. This is particularly true in older adults, where the complications of anticoagulants are a greater problem. Persantine alone or in combination with aspirin does not appear to be of benefit. Ticlopidine has been used as an antiplatelet agent in stroke prevention, particularly in patients who have failed aspirin. However, bone marrow suppression and monitoring for this complication have limited the usefulness of ticlopidine. Recently clopidogrel, an antiplatelet agent with a lower incidence of bone marrow toxicity, has been approved (Offguson et al., 1998) and will likely replace ticlopidine in stroke prevention therapy.

Both anticoagulants and antiplatelet therapy have been shown to reduce the risk of transient ischemic attacks (TIAs) and stroke in individuals with atrial fibrillation. Combined data from five randomized clinical trials comparing warfarin with control for prevention of ischemic stroke in atrial fibrillation patients demonstrate a 68 percent (95 percent CI, 50 to 79 percent) risk reduction (Prystowsky et al., 1996). Combined data from three randomized clinical trials comparing warfarin with aspirin demonstrate a risk reduction of 47 percent (95 percent CI, 28 to 61 percent) by warfarin relative to aspirin. An International Normalized Ratio (INR) range of 2.0 to 3.0 is safe and effective. For those over 75, close surveillance of INR levels is recommended because of the increased risk of bleeding complications. Those who cannot safely receive anticoagulation should be given aspirin.

Stroke Rehabilitation

Factors in the prognosis for rehabilitation of the older stroke patient are presented in Table 10-10. Although the benefit of stroke rehabilitation is controversial, it should be initiated early in the course if it is to be of benefit. Two studies have suggested that stroke patients fared better in rehabilitative facilities than in skilled nursing facilities (Kane et al., 1996; Schlenker et al., 1997). The Agency for Health Care Policy and Research has published clinical practice guidelines for poststroke rehabilitation (AHCRP, 1995). Generally, most neurologic return occurs during the first month after the stroke. By the end of the third month, little if any further return can be expected. Not all dysfunctions result in the same level of disability. Motor loss is often the least disabling. Perceptual and/or sensory loss, aphasia, loss of balance, hemicorporal neglect, hemianopsia, and/or cognitive damage may cause more severe and often untreatable disabilities.

In the immediate stage, treatment is directed toward avoiding complications such as pressure sores, contractures, phlebitis, pulmonary embolism, aspiration pneumonia, and fecal impaction.

In the next stage of rehabilitation, treatment is directed toward reeducating muscles (affected areas) and enhancing remaining capabilities (unaffected areas). Table 10-11 describes measures to be taken during this phase.

When the patient stops making progress after intensive therapy, the goal of rehabilitation shifts to finding ways for the patient to cope with the dysfunction. At this stage, the patient is assessed for the need for braces and assistive devices for both ambulation and performance of activities of daily living. With a sound program of rehabilitation, the older patient who survives a stroke can return to the community.

Table 10-10 Factors in prognosis for rehabilitation

Prognosis for neurologic return
Mentation
Motivation
Vigor
Availability and implementation of sound program

Table 10-11 Stroke rehabilitation

Acute phase
  Change of patient's position at least every 2 h
  Positioning of patient's joints to prevent contractures
  Positioning of patient to prevent aspiration pneumonia
  Range-of-motion exercises

Later phase
  Perceptual training
  Muscle reeducation exercises
  Functional activities for affected side
  Ambulation training
  ADL training
  Training in transfer technique

CORONARY ARTERY DISEASE

Hypertension is the major risk factor for coronary artery disease in older adults. Hypercholesterolemia and cigarette smoking become less important risk factors in this age group, although they are still significant when associated with other risk factors.

Angina pectoris has a similar presentation in both older adults and in younger patients, with familiar pain characteristics and radiation. Treatment includes reducing factors that precipitated anginal attacks and also pharmacologic intervention. Smokers should be advised to discontinue smoking; physical and emotional stresses that precipitate pain should be modified.

Pharmacologically, episodes of angina pectoris can be treated with sublingual nitroglycerin, which should be taken in the sitting position to avoid severe orthostatic hypotension. Chronic stable angina is treated with nitrates and beta-adrenergic antagonists. These agents have different mechanisms of action and thus may be used in combination with some benefit. Calcium-channel blockers are also of benefit but may be limited by orthostatic hypotension in older patients.

About 20 percent of patients admitted to a coronary care unit with myocardial infarction are over the age of 70. In this age group, incidence among males and females is about equal. The elderly patient with myocardial infarction may present with symptoms other than chest pain (Table 10-12). The mortality rate from acute myocardial infarction increases with age.

**Table 10-12 Presenting symptoms
of myocardial infarction**

Chest pain
Syncope
Confusion
Dyspnea
Worsening congestive heart failure
Rapid deterioration of health

Treatment of the older patient with acute myocardial infarction is similar to that of the young patient. Particular attention should be paid to avoiding drug toxicity and to beginning early mobilization when possible. Early mobilization may decrease deconditioning, orthostatic hypotension, and thrombophlebitis. Despite some conflict, the weight of evidence and opinion is in favor of the usefulness of thrombolysis in patients age 75 years or older with acute myocardial infarction and ST-segment elevation (Ryan et al., 1996a). Although several randomized, controlled trials have shown better outcomes in patients with acute myocardial infarction after primary angioplasty than after thrombolytic therapy, in a community setting there appears to be no benefit in terms of either mortality or the use of resources with one or the other strategy (Every et al., 1996). Primary angioplasty should be an alternative to thrombolytic therapy only if performed in a timely fashion by individuals skilled in the procedure and supported by experienced personnel in high-volume centers (Ryan et al., 1996a).

Indications for coronary artery surgery are controversial, but this surgery can be performed with excellent symptomatic results. Morbidity and mortality, however, are higher than in younger patients. The strongest indication for surgery is angina pectoris refractory to medical management. In patients with left main coronary artery disease, surgery significantly improves survival over medical therapy. Patients with three-vessel disease may also have improved survival. In older adults, however, improved survival must be considered in the light of the patient's projected survival and the higher operative risk.

Long-term administration of beta blockers to patients after myocardial infarction improves survival (Ryan et al., 1996b). Despite these data, physicians are reluctant to administer beta blockers to many

patients, such as older patients (Krumholz et al., 1998) and those with chronic pulmonary disease, left ventricular dysfunction, or non-Q-wave myocardial infarction. However, all these subgroups benefit from beta-blocker therapy after myocardial infarction (Gottlieb et al., 1998). Given the higher mortality rates in these subgroups, the absolute reduction in mortality was similar to or greater than that among patients with no specific risk factors.

VALVULAR HEART DISEASE

Calcific Aortic Stenosis

Pathologically, degenerative calcification of the aortic and mitral valves is common among older adults; it is found at autopsy in about one-third of individuals over age 75. In most cases, aortic valve calcification is of no clinical significance except as a source of aortic systolic murmur. In some patients, however, calcification is extensive enough to result in aortic stenosis. The frequency of aortic stenosis increases with age, appearing at autopsy in about 4 to 6 percent of those over age 65. Isolated aortic stenosis is more common among men than women except over the age of 80, where women predominate. Aortic insufficiency may coexist with calcific aortic stenosis, although regurgitation is usually mild and a regurgitant murmur usually not heard.

The usual clinical presentation of aortic stenosis in older adults consists of fatigue, syncope, angina pectoris, and congestive heart failure. Because systolic murmurs are a frequent finding in older adults, differentiation of mitral regurgitation, aortic sclerosis, or aortic stenosis by auscultation is a challenge. The location of the murmur is usually along the lower left sternal border and apex and often does not radiate to the axilla or carotids. It is characteristically a crescendo-decrescendo systolic murmur ending before the second heart sound. Aspects that may help differentiate mitral regurgitation from aortic murmurs are described in Table 10-13.

Differentiation of aortic stenosis from aortic sclerosis may be difficult in the elderly. The typical murmur and pulse of aortic stenosis may be modified in older adults. Systemic hypertension may shorten the systolic murmur of stenosis, giving it the characteristic of an aortic sclerosis murmur. Loss of vascular elasticity may modify the pulse pressure, so that the typical pulse contour of aortic stenosis is absent.

Table 10-13   Differentiation of systolic murmurs

	Post PCA*	Amyl nitrate	Valsalva	Squatting
Aortic sclerosis	↑ †	↑	↓	↑
Aortic stenosis	↑	↑ ↑	↓	↑
Mitral regurgitation	—	↓	↓	—
IHSS	↑	↑ ↑	↑ ↑	↓ ↓

* Best following a premature ventricular contraction.
† Effect of maneuver on intensity of murmur.

Therefore, the physical examination alone is not reliable in diagnosing aortic stenosis in older adults. Echocardiography may not differentiate aortic stenosis from a nonstenotic calcified valve, and the presence of left ventricular hypertrophy may also not assist in the diagnosis because this may be caused by systemic hypertension. The addition of Doppler flow studies to echocardiography has improved the diagnostic accuracy of noninvasive procedures for aortic stenosis. Left ventricular catheterization remains the most reliable method of assessing aortic stenosis in older adults but should be reserved for patients who are symptomatic and in whom surgery is contemplated.

Surgical mortality for valve replacement is higher in older individuals, but results have recently improved. Significant coexistent coronary artery disease should be treated with bypass surgery at the time of valve replacement. Choice of a valve depends on the size of the patient's aortic valve annulus and ability to tolerate anticoagulation. When anticoagulation is contraindicated, a biological prosthetic valve is preferred. The shorter life span of biological valves should be borne in mind in those between 60 and 70.

Calcified Mitral Annulus

Mitral ring calcification is a disease of older adults and is most frequently found in patients over 70. It is reported in 9 percent of autopsies in individuals over age 50 and has a striking increase with advancing age, particularly in women, in whom it rises from 3.2 percent below age 70 to 44 percent over age 90.

This lesion often results in mitral insufficiency or conduction abnormalities and rarely in stenosis. It is an important contributing

factor to congestive heart failure in older adults and is a site for endocarditis. As many as two-thirds of patients with mitral annulus calcification present with an apical systolic murmur of mitral regurgitation. Echocardiography is the best technique for diagnosing mitral annulus calcification. Regurgitation is usually mild to moderate, and surgery is usually indicated only if endocarditis is superimposed. Prophylaxis for subacute bacterial endocarditis is recommended. There is a higher incidence of cerebral embolism in this disorder, and thus anticoagulation may be indicated.

Mitral Valve Prolapse

Mucoid degeneration affects mainly the mitral valve. This process allows stretching of the mitral valve leaflet under normal intracardiac pressure, with subsequent prolapse into the left atrium during systole. Although the classic murmur is late systolic, the murmur can occur any time in systole. Mucoid degeneration of the mitral valve has been described in about 1 percent of autopsies on patients over 65. It is associated with mitral insufficiency; left atrial dilatation and regurgitant murmurs are common. Mitral insufficiency caused by this disorder is usually well tolerated and rarely requires surgery. Some patients with this syndrome have abnormal electrocardiograms and chest pain suggestive of coronary artery disease; sudden death has been reported. Death directly from the valve disease is usually related to rupture of the chordae tendineae. Mucoid degeneration also predisposes to infective endocarditis. Prophylaxis for subacute bacterial endocarditis is indicated.

Idiopathic Hypertrophic Subaortic Stenosis (IHSS)

In older adults, IHSS may be misdiagnosed as aortic valve stenosis or mitral regurgitation. Presenting symptoms are similar to those of aortic stenosis or coronary artery disease. The presence of a bisferious arterial pulse in the presence of a systolic ejection murmur and in the absence of an aortic regurgitation murmur should suggest IHSS. The IHSS murmur usually does not radiate to the carotids. Squatting, which increases left ventricular filling, usually decreases the murmur of IHSS. Factors that decrease left ventricular volume (Valsalva maneuver, standing) increase the intensity of the murmur.

Documentation of IHSS is accomplished by echocardiography. Therapy usually relies on beta-adrenergic antagonists. Symptoms may be worsened by cardiac glycosides (which increase myocardial contractility) and diuretics (which create volume depletion). Atrial fibrillation is poorly tolerated and may require cardioversion in the rapidly deteriorating patient. In patients refractory to medical therapy, surgery should be considered after cardiac catheterization to assess severity of outflow obstruction and state of coronary artery flow.

ARRHYTHMIAS

Although the prevalence of arrhythmias increases with age, most older patients without clinical heart disease are in normal sinus rhythm. Atrial fibrillation occurs in 5 to 10 percent of asymptomatic ambulatory older adults and more frequently in hospitalized patients. It is usually associated with underlying heart disease; the causes are the same as in younger individuals. Atrial fibrillation does, however, occur more frequently in older patients with thyrotoxicosis. For long-term rate control, verapamil, diltiazem, and beta blockers should be the initial drugs of choice (Prystowsky et al., 1996). Beta-adrenergic blockers are especially effective in the presence of thyrotoxicosis and increased sympathetic tone. Digoxin should be considered as first-line treatment only in patients with congestive heart failure secondary to impaired systolic ventricular function. In some patients, combinations of these drugs may be needed to control ventricular response. The maintenance dose of digoxin is usually lower in older adults because of decreased muscular mass and decreased renal clearance.

The incidence of premature ventricular contractions increases with age and occurs in about 10 percent of electrocardiograms and 30 to 40 percent of Holter monitoring. The decision to treat with antiarrhythmic therapy is difficult except in the immediate post-myocardial infarction period, when it is recommended. Criteria for therapy are the same as in younger patients. The half-life of antiarrhythmic drugs is prolonged in the elderly. Therapy should be initiated at lower doses, and blood levels should be monitored (see Chap. 13).

The sick sinus syndrome is particularly common among older patients. Diagnosis is made by Holter monitor. Symptoms, usually related to decreased organ perfusion, are listed in Table 10-14. There is no satisfactory medical therapy. Symptomatic patients may require

Table 10-14 Manifestations of sick sinus syndrome

Palpitations
Angina pectoris
Congestive heart failure
Dizziness
Syncope
Memory loss
Insomnia

pacemakers, which do not seem to decrease mortality in this syndrome but can alleviate symptoms. A pacemaker may be indicated in patients with cardiac side effects from drugs used to control tachycardias in the bradycardia-tachycardia syndrome.

CONGESTIVE HEART FAILURE

Although congestive heart failure is prevalent in older adults, it is often overdiagnosed. Pedal and pretibial edema is not sufficient to warrant the diagnosis. Venous stasis may produce a similar picture. Care is needed to establish the presence of other signs (e.g., cardiac enlargement, S_3 heart sound, basilar rales, jugular venous distention, enlarged liver). Determination of ejection fraction by two-dimensional echocardiography may assist in diagnosis. The Agency for Health Care Policy and Research has published clinical practice guidelines for the evaluation and care of patients with congestive heart failure (AHCPR, 1994).

Over 75 percent of cases of overt heart failure in older patients are associated with hypertension or coronary heart disease. Diastolic dysfunction, not systolic dysfunction, is the primary cause of heart failure in older patients (Wei, 1992); among those more than 80 years of age who have heart failure, over 50 percent have normal or near-normal systolic function. Patients with preserved systolic function and impaired diastolic function are often treated erroneously with diuretics, vasodilators, and digitalis, which may further reduce ventricular filling or impair relaxation and may actually exacerbate rather than alleviate cardiac decompensation. Calcium-channel blockers may

improve left ventricular diastolic function in older patients with preserved systolic function who have symptoms of heart failure, whether or not they have coronary artery disease. If the calcium-channel blockers lead to hypotension, beta blockers may be initiated with careful monitoring of cardiac function. If patients do not tolerate either one of these agents, ACE-inhibitor therapy may be tried.

The mainstays of therapy for congestive heart failure due to systolic dysfunction in older patients, as in younger patients, are diuretics, vasodilators, dixogin, and inotropic agents. Systolic and diastolic dysfunction often coexist and may need to be treated together. In the acute setting, vasodilation can be accomplished by intravenous infusion of sodium nitroprusside or nitroglycerine or oral administration of either a combination of hydralazine and isosorbide dinitrate or an ACE inhibitor. To improve survival, all patients with chronic symptomatic congestive heart failure that is associated with reduced systolic ejection or left ventricular remodling should be treated with ACE inhibitors (Cohn, 1996). The combination of hydralazine and isosorbide dinitrate has a more favorable effect on left ventricular function and exercise capacity than enalapril but does not have as favorable an effect on survival.

The use of digitalis preparations must be approached with caution. Patients once begun on digoxin tend to remain on it long after the indications have ceased. Subtle signs of toxicity may be missed, as the drug accumulates in the presence of decreased renal function. Because of decreases in lean body mass and glomerular filtration rate, lower doses of digoxin are generally required in the elderly. Initial maintenance doses should be lower; blood levels should be monitored to avoid toxic levels. Because the therapeutic window is narrowed in older adults, patients who have been on digoxin therapy for long periods of time after an acute episode of cardiac decompensation not related to arrhythmias should be considered for discontinuation of digoxin. Weight should be monitored closely so that digoxin can be reinstated before congestive symptoms occur. With such evaluation and monitoring, some older patients on chronic digoxin therapy for other than antiarrhythmic treatment may not require digoxin therapy. Patients with atrial fibrillation should be kept on digoxin.

REFERENCES

Agency for Health Care Policy and Research: *Heart Failure: Evaluation and Care of Patients with Left-Ventricular Systolic Dysfunction.* AHCPR Publication No. 94-0612, 1994.

Agency for Health Care Policy and Research: *Post-Stroke Rehabilitation*. AHCPR Publication No. 95-0662. 1995.

Amery A, Birkenhager W, Brixko P, et al: Efficacy of antihypertensive drug treatment according to age, sex, blood pressure, and previous cardiovascular disease in patients over the age of 60. *Lancet* 2:589–592, 1986.

Amery A, Birkenhager W, Brixko P, et al: Mortality and morbidity results from the European Working Party on High Blood Pressure in the Elderly trial. *Lancet* 1:1349–1354, 1985.

Applegate WB, Rutan GH: Advances in management of hypertension in older persons. *J Am Geriatr Soc* 40:1164–1174, 1992.

Barnett HJM: Thrombotic processes in cerebrovascular disease, in Coleman RW, Hirsh J, Marder VJ, et al (eds): *Hemostasis and Thrombosis*. Toronto, Lippincott, 1982.

Caplan LR, Mohr JP, Kistler JP, et al: Thrombolysis—Not a panacea for ischemic stroke. *N Engl J Med* 337:1309–1310, 1997.

Cohn JN: The management of chronic heart failure. *N Engl J Med* 335:490–498, 1996.

Cushman WC, Khatri I, Materson BJ, et al: Treatment of hypertension in the elderly. *Arch Intern Med* 151:1954–1960, 1991.

Dahlöf B, Lindholm LH, Hansson L, et al: Morbidity and mortality in the Swedish Trial in Old Patients with Hypertension (STOP-Hypertension). *Lancet* 338:1281–1285, 1991.

European Carotid Surgery Trialists' Collaborative Group: MRC European Carotid Surgery Trial: Interim results for symptomatic patients with severe (70%–99%) or with mild (0–29%) carotid stenosis. *Lancet* 337:1235–1240, 1991.

Every NR, Parsons LS, Hlatky M, et al: A comparison of thrombolytic therapy with primary coronary angioplasty for acute myocardial infarction. *N Engl J Med* 335:1253–1260, 1996

Gerstenblith G, Renlund DG, Lakatta EG: Cardiovascular response to exercise in younger and older men. *Fed Proc* 46:1834–1839, 1987.

Gottlieb SS, McCarter RJ, Vogel RA: Effects of beta-blockade on mortality among high-risk and low-risk patients after myocardial infarction. *N Engl J Med* 339:489–497, 1998.

Hobson RW II, Weiss DG, Fields WS, et al: Efficacy of carotid endarterectomy for asymptomatic carotid stenosis. *N Engl J Med* 328:221–227, 1993.

Hypertension Detection and Follow-Up Program Cooperative Group: Five-year findings of the hypertension detection and follow-up program: II. Mortality by race, sex, and age. *JAMA* 242:2572–2577, 1979.

Joint National Committee: The 1992 Report of the Joint National Committee on Detection, Evaluation, and Treatment of High Blood Pressure. Bethesda, MD, National Institutes of Health, 1992.

Kane RL, Chen Q, Blewett LA, et al: Do rehabilitative nursing homes improve the outcomes of care? *J Am Geriatr Soc* 44:545–554, 1996.

Kannel WB: Some lessons in cardiovascular epidemiology from Framingham. *Am J Cardiol* 37:269–282, 1976.

Krumholz HM, Radford MJ, Wang Y, et al: National use and effectiveness of β-blockers for the treatment of elderly patients after acute myocardial infarction. *JAMA* 280:623–629, 1998.

Mayberg M, Wilson E, Yatsu F, et al: Carotid endarterectomy and prevention of cerebral ischemia in symptomatic carotid stenosis. *JAMA* 266:3289–3294, 1991.

Messerli FH, Grossman E, Goldbourt U: Are β-blockers efficacious as first-line therapy for hypertension in the elderly? A systematic review. *JAMA* 279:1903–1907, 1998.

Morledge JH, Ettinger B, Aranda J, et al: Isolated systolic hypertension in the elderly: A placebo-controlled, dose-response evaluation of chlorthalidone. *J Am Geriatr Soc* 34:199–206, 1986.

MRC Working Party: Medical Research Council trial of treatment of hypertension in older adults: principal results. *BMJ* 304:405–412, 1992.

North American Symptomatic Carotid Endarterectomy Trial Collaborators: Beneficial effect of carotid endarterectomy in symptomatic patients with high-grade carotid stenosis. *N Engl J Med* 325:445–453, 1991.

Offguson JJ, Gonzalez ER, Kannel WB, et al: Clinical safety and efficacy of clopidogrel– Implications of the clopidogrel versus aspirin in patients at risk of ischemic events (CAPRIE) study for future management of atherosclerotic disease. *Clin Ther* 20(B):B42–B53, 1998.

Prystowsky EN, Benson DW, Fuster V, et al: Management of patients with atrial fibrillation: a statement for healthcare professionals from the subcommittee on electrocardiography and electrophysiology, American Heart Association. *Circulation* 93:1262–1277, 1996.

Psaty BM, Smith NL, Siscovick DS, et al: Review: Low-dose diuretics, but not high-dose diuretics and β-blockers, reduce coronary heart disease and total mortality. *JAMA* 277:739–745, 1997.

Rippe JM, Ward A, Porcari JP, et al: Walking for health and fitness. *JAMA* 259:2720–2724, 1988.

Robbins S: Stroke in the geriatric patient, in Reichel W (ed): *The Geriatric Patient.* New York, HP Publishing, 1978.

Rothrock JF, Hart RG: Antithrombotic therapy in cerebrovascular disease. *Ann Intern Med* 115:885–895, 1991.

Ryan TJ, Anderson JL, Antman EM, et al: ACC/AHA Guidelines for the management of patients with acute myocardial infarction: executive summary. A report of the American College of Cardiology/American Heart Assoication Task Force on Practice Guidelines (Committee on Management of Acute Myocardial Infarction). *Circulation* 94:2341–2350, 1996a.

Ryan TJ, Anderson JL, Antman EM, et al: ACC/AHA guidelines for the management of patients with acute myocardial infarction: a report of the American College of Cardiology/American Heart Association Task Force on Practice Guidelines (Committee on Management of Acute Myocardial Infarction). *J Am Coll Cardiol* 28:1328–1428, 1996b.

Schlenker RE, Kramer AM, Hrincevich CA, et al: Rehabilitation costs: Implications for prospective payment. *Health Serv Res* 32:651–668, 1997.

SHEP Cooperative Research Group: Prevention of stroke by antihypertensive drug treatment in older persons with isolated systolic hypertension. *JAMA* 265:3255–3264, 1991.

The Australian Therapeutic Trial in Mild Hypertension. *Lancet* 1:1261–1267, 1980.

The National Institute of Neurological Disorders and Stroke rt-PA Stroke Study Group: Tissue plasminogen activator for acute ischemic stroke. *N Engl J Med* 333:1581–1587, 1995.

Vardan S, Dunsky MH, Hill NE, et al: Effect of one year of thiazide therapy on plasma volume, renin, aldosterone, lipids and urinary metanephrines in systolic hypertension of elderly patients. *Am J Cardiol* 60:388–390, 1987a.

Vardan S, Mehrotra KG, Mookherjee S, et al: Efficacy and reduced metabolic side effects of a 15-mg chlorthalidone formulation in the treatment of mild hypertension. A multicenter study. *JAMA* 258:484–488, 1987b.

Veterans Administration Cooperative Study Group on Antihypertensive Agents: Effect of treatment on morbidity in hypertension: III. Influence of age, diastolic pressure, and prior cardiovascular disease. *Circulation* 45:991–1004, 1972.

Wardlow JM, Yamaguchi T, del Zoppo G, et al: Meta-analysis: Thrombolytic therapy increases the risk for early death and intracranial hemorrhage after acute ischemic stroke, in Warlow C, Van Gijn J, Sandercock P (eds): *The Cochrane Database of Systematic Reviews,* 1996.

Wei JY: Age and the cardiovascular system. *N Engl J Med* 327:1735–1739, 1992.

SUGGESTED READINGS

Bloor CM: Valvular disease in the elderly. *J Am Geriatr Soc* 30:466–472, 1982.

Evans JG: "Stroke" predictors, in Sarner M (ed): *Advanced Medicine.* London, Pitman, 1982.

Gersh BJ, Kronmal RA, Schaff HV, et al: Comparison of coronary artery bypass surgery and medical therapy in patients 65 years of age or older. *N Engl J Med* 313:217–224, 1985.

Greenspan AM, Kay HR, Berger BC, et al: Incidence of unwarranted implantation of permanent cardiac pacemakers in a larger medical population. *N Engl J Med* 318:158–163, 1988.

Kannel WB: Hypertension and aging, in Finch CE, Schneider EL (eds): *Handbook of the Biology of Aging.* New York, Van Nostrand Reinhold, 1985.

Lakatta EG: Heart and circulation, in Finch CE, Schneider EL (eds): *Handbook of the Biology of Aging.* New York, Van Nostrand Reinhold, 1985.

Lakatta EG, Yin FCP: Myocardial aging: Functional alterations and related cellular mechanisms. *Am J Physiol* 242:H927–H941, 1982.

Lembo NJ, Dell'Italia LJ, Crawford MH, et al: Bedside diagnosis of systolic murmurs. *N Engl J Med* 318:1572–1578, 1988.

Lindenfeld J, Groves BM: Cardiovascular function and disease in the aged, in Schrier RW (ed): *Clinical Internal Medicine in the Aged.* Philadelphia, Saunders, 1982.

Medical Letter: Drugs for hypertension. *Med Lett* 35:55–58, 1993.

Rich MW: Epidemiology, pathophysiology, and etiology of congestive heart failure in older adults. *J Am Geriatr Soc* 45:968–974, 1997.

Selzer A: Changing aspects of the natural history of valvular aortic stenosis. *N Engl J Med* 317:91–98, 1987.

Stults BM: Digoxin use in the elderly. *J Am Geriatr Soc* 30:158–164, 1982.

Tuck M, Sowers I: Hypertension and aging, in Korenman SG (ed): *Endocrine Aspects of Aging.* New York, Elsevier Biomedical, 1982.

Vallacino R, Sherman FT: Stroke, fractured hip, amputation, pressure sores, and incontinence: Principles of rehabilitation treatment, in Libow LS, Sherman FT (eds): *The Core of Geriatric Medicine.* St Louis, Mosby, 1981.

Winslow CM, Solomon DH, Chassin MR, et al: The appropriateness of carotid endarterectomy. *N Engl J Med* 318:721–727, 1988.

ELEVEN

DECREASED VITALITY

Among older adults, decreased vitality is a common complaint; it has a host of underlying causes. This chapter deals with metabolic factors that may lead to decreased energy in the older adults: endocrine disease, anemia, poor nutrition, lack of exercise, and infection.

ENDOCRINE DISEASE

Carbohydrate Metabolism

Of the elderly population, approximately 50 percent have glucose intolerance with normal fasting blood sugar levels. This abnormality can be demonstrated by oral, intravenous, or either tolbutamide- or glucocorticoid-primed glucose tolerance tests. Although poor diet, obesity, and lack of exercise may account for some of these findings (Hollenbeck et al., 1984), aging itself is associated with deteriorating glucose tolerance. Most data now suggest a change in peripheral glucose utilization as the major factor in this phenomenon (Fink et al., 1984), although abnormal insulin secretion is also a contributing factor.

Glucose intolerance, however, should not be diagnosed as diabetes mellitus. The diagnosis of diabetes should be made on the basis of a fasting plasma glucose of 126 mg/dL or greater on at least two occasions. This is particularly important in older adults because the prevalence of glucose intolerance is so high. It follows, therefore, that for older patients, glucose tolerance testing is not indicated in the diagnosis of diabetes mellitus; the fasting plasma glucose is the diagnostic criterion.

The therapeutic goal for most older diabetic patients is the same as that in younger patients: normal fasting plasma glucose without hypoglycemia. However, in those with short life expectancies, the therapeutic goal may be modified to eliminate symptoms associated with hyperglycemia. This can be accomplished by lowering the blood sugar to levels that avoid glycosuria. The use of oral hypoglycemic agents has remained controversial and has become an individual physician-patient choice. In older patients with visual problems, arthritis, or memory deficits, where insulin administration by injection may be complicated, oral agents may be the therapy of choice.

Chlorpropamide should be avoided in older adults because of the known side effect of the syndrome of inappropriate antidiuretic hormone (SIADH) and associated hyponatremia as well as its prolonged time of action. Shorter-acting sulfonylureas—such as acetohexamide, tolazamide, glyburide, or glipizide—are more appropriate agents for the older patient. In some patients, once-a-day dosing with these agents may be adequate, and these agents do not produce SIADH. Although tolbutamide also does not produce this syndrome, it is short-acting and necessitates multiple daily doses, thereby increasing problems in compliance.

Sulfonylureas act primarily by increasing beta-cell insulin secretion. Recently three new agents for the treatment of type 2 diabetes mellitus have become available in the United States, each with a different mechanism of action. Acarbose reduces postprandial plasma glucose by inhibiting small intestine brush border alpha glucosidases. It has a small effect on metabolic control and causes frequent gastrointestinal distress with bloating and flatulence. Metformin, a biguanide, exerts its major metabolic effect by inhibiting hepatic glucose production. It leads to significant improvement in glucose control when used alone or in combination with a sulfonylurea (Inzucchi et al., 1998). As opposed to sulfonylureas, which often lead to weight gain, metformin therapy is associated with weight loss, a benefit to most type 2 diabetic

patients. Weight should be monitored closely in thin diabetic patients. A serious side effect of metformin is lactic acidosis. It should not be used in patients with renal insufficiency or congestive heart failure. In patients 80 years old or older, creatinine clearance should be measured before therapy is initiated. Metformin should be discontinued during illnesses associated with volume depletion and prior to surgery. Initial excitement for troglitazone has waned because of its potential for liver toxicity. Troglitazone, a thiazolidinedione, lowers blood sugar by improving target-cell insulin sensitivity. Besides the potential for hepatic toxicity, which requires frequent liver function testing, troglitazone therapy may be associated with marked weight gain. Therapy with these agents might best await the next generation of thiazolidinediones without hepatic toxicity. A step-care approach to the treatment of type 2 diabetes is presented in Table 11-1.

With the results of the Diabetes Control and Complications Trial (DCCT) in type 1 diabetes mellitus, close control of plasma glucose is now in vogue, although its efficacy or feasibility has not been assessed in the older adult (Colwell, 1996). Because atherosclerosis is the major complication of diabetes in this age group and because close control has not been shown to affect this complication, the risk of hypoglycemia with close control must be weighed carefully in designing a treatment plan. Counterregulatory hormones, especially catecholamines and glucagon, are important reactants to hypoglycemia, and catecholamine responsiveness is diminished in older adults. It is important to observe patients closely for hypoglycemic reactions and their ability to respond to this stress as a management regimen is prescribed.

Because most patients with adult-onset diabetes are obese, weight reduction should be attempted, although only about 10 percent will maintain a prolonged weight loss. Dietary fats should be reduced. Aerobic exercise is of benefit in both delaying the onset of non-insulin-dependent diabetes mellitus and in improving insulin resistance in individuals with established disease. Other atherosclerotic risk factors such as smoking, dyslipidemia, and hypertension should be eliminated or treated.

Angiotensin-converting enzyme (ACE) inhibitors have been found to attenuate progression of nephropathy in both type 1 and type 2 diabetic patients with hypertension and in normotensives with microalbuminuria. They also attenuate decline in renal function in normotensive, normoalbuminuric type 2 diabetic patients (Ravid et

Table 11-1 Step-care approach to the treatment of type 2 diabetes

Step	Criteria and recommendation	Monitoring
Step 1: Evaluation and nonpharmacologic approaches	Newly diagnosed or current therapy ineffective: initiate or reinforce diet, exercise, home blood glucose monitoring, formal diabetes education. Current therapy effective: continue therapy.	Success: continue step 1. Failure for 2–3 months: go to step 2. Severe hyperglycemia (fasting blood glucose >300): go to step 5.
Step 2: Oral monotherapy	Obese or dyslipidemic: first line—metformin; second line—(troglitazone) or acarbose. Nonobese: first line—sulfonylurea or metformin; second line—acarbose.	Success: continue step 2. Failure: go to step 3.
Step 3: Oral combination therapy	Previously on metformin: add sulfonylurea. Previously on sulfonylurea: add metformin or (troglitazone). Previously on (troglitazone): add sulfonylurea. Previously on acarbose, obese: add metformin. Previously on acarbose, nonobese: add sulfonylurea.	Success: continue step 3. Failure: go to step 4.
Step 4: Insulin initiation	FBG <200–240: eliminate one drug, start bedtime NPH. FBG >200–240: eliminate one drug, start bid NPH/regular.	Success: continue step 4. Failure (HbA1c >8.5% and insulin >30 U/day): go to step 5.
Step 5: Insulin + oral therapy	On insulin monotherapy: add (troglitazone) or metformin. Or insulin + sulfonylurea or insulin + metformin: discontinue first oral agent and add (troglitazone).	Success: continue step 5. Failure: consult specialist.

Source: Modified from White, 1996. (The author's bias is not to use troglitazone.)

al., 1998), but further research is needed to determine if this therapy forestalls overt nephropathy. The antihypertensive regimen of diabetics should include an ACE inhibitor, and such therapy should be initiated in normotensive albuminuric patients. Earlier use of ACE inhibitors in type 2 diabetics awaits further data.

Older adults have an increased incidence of hyperosmolar nonketotic (HNK) coma. Characteristic symptoms and signs help the physician distinguish this syndrome from diabetic ketoacidotic (DKA) coma. Table 11-2 contrasts HNK and DKA. Whereas DKA frequently develops over hours, HNK typically develops over days to weeks. Focal or generalized seizures are common in HNK and unusual in uncomplicated DKA. The fluid deficit is greater in HNK, thus leading to a higher serum sodium and more marked rise in blood urea nitrogen. Therapy in HNK must therefore address the volume and hyperosmolar state of the patient. Because these patients may be quite sensitive to insulin, lowering of glucose should be done cautiously. Volume replacement should be initiated with normal saline. This therapy alone may reduce blood glucose levels, as renal perfusion is enhanced and glucose is lost in the urine. If, after 1 h of volume repletion, blood glucose levels are not reduced, a bolus of 20 U of regular insulin should be administered intravenously. If glucose levels do not respond, an insulin drip may be started. Such an approach should allow repletion of volume without lowering serum osmolarity too rapidly.

Thyroid

Although thyroid function is generally normal in aging, the physician should be aware of the norms for thyroid function tests for this age

Table 11-2 Hyperosmolar nonketotic (HNK) coma and diabetic ketoacidosis (DKA)

	HNK[a]	DKA
Time of development	Days to weeks	Hours
Seizures	Common	Uncommon
Fluid deficit	Marked	Present
Serum sodium	↑ ↑	↑
Blood urea nitrogen	↑ ↑	↑

[a] Double arrow signifies a higher increase than for a single arrow. Correction factor for sodium: 100 mg/dL of glucose = 1.6 meq/L of sodium.

group (Table 11-3) (Kabadi and Rosman, 1988; Hershman et al., 1993). The majority of data indicate that T_4 levels are normal while T_3 levels may be low in healthy older people. Some older adults have normal T_3 levels; it has been suggested that the low T_3 levels reported in several studies are caused by undiagnosed illness and the low-T_3 syndrome described below. Thyroid-stimulating hormone (TSH) levels are also normal, while the TSH response to thyroid-releasing hormone (TRH) is decreased in males (Harman et al., 1984) and normal in females. Thus, the TRH test is less valuable in older males. Metabolic clearance of thyroid hormones is decreased in aging. With intact feedback loops, normal thyroid function is maintained despite this change. However, with exogenous replacement of thyroid hormone, such regulatory mechanisms are not maintained; thyroid replacement doses in older adults should be lower to take into account the lower metabolic clearance (Rosenbaum and Barzel, 1982). Laboratory evaluation tests most useful in thyroid disease are summarized in Table 11-4.

Hypothyroidism Hypothyroidism is primarily a disease of those aged 50 to 70. Goiter is rarely seen with hypothyroidism in the elderly except when it is iodide-induced. Diagnosis is usually made by a low free T_4 and an elevated TSH. Because total T_4 levels may be depressed in seriously ill patients, diagnosis of hypothyroidism should not be made on the basis of low T_4 levels alone. In seriously ill patients, a circulatory plasma factor interferes with T_4 and T_3 binding to thyroid hormone–binding proteins; this results in a low total T_4 level but maintenance of normal free T_4 and TSH. This factor also interferes with T_3 binding and resin uptake in vitro and thus leads to a low free T_4 index determination. Laboratory characteristics of the low-T_4

Table 11-3 Thyroid function in the normal elderly

Normal	Decreased
T_4	TSH response to TRH in males
Free T_4	Thyroid hormone production rate
Free T_4 index	Metabolic clearance rate of thyroid hormone
T_3	
TSH	

Table 11-4 Laboratory evaluation of thyroid disease in the elderly*

	Hypothyroidism	Hyperthyroidism
T_4	E	E
Free T_4 index	E	E
TSH	E	E
Free T_4	E	E
T_3	O	D
Radioactive iodine uptake	O	D
TRH test	D (Females)	D (Females)
	O (Males)	O (Males)
Reverse T_3	D	D
TSH stimulation	D	O
T_3 suppression	O	O

 * E, test for initial evaluation; D, helpful in confirming diagnosis or in differentiation of difficult cases; O, not helpful in diagnosis or not indicated. Where a free T_4 is available, the T_4 and free T_4 index need not be performed.

syndrome associated with nonthyroidal illness are listed in Table 11-5. Not all free-T_4 methods distinguish the low-T_4 syndrome from hypothyroidism; physicians should be aware of the type of determination and interpretation used in their laboratory. The T_3 level may be in the normal range in hypothyroidism and thus is not a helpful test. The low T_3 level associated with a host of acute and chronic nonthyroidal illnesses also contributes to the poor specificity of this test in hypothyroidism. About 75 percent of circulating T_3 is derived from peripheral conversion from T_4. The enzymes that convert T_4 to T_3 or reverse T_3 are under metabolic control. During illness, more T_4

Table 11-5 Thyroid-function tests in nonthyroidal illness

	Low-T_4 syndrome	Low-T_3 syndrome
T_4	Decreased	Normal
T_4 index	Decreased	Normal
Free T_4	Normal or increased	Normal
T_3	Decreased	Decreased
Reverse T_3	Normal or increased	Normal or increased
TSH	Normal	Normal

is converted to reverse T_3, leading to the characteristic laboratory findings of the low-T_3 syndrome.

The radioactive iodine uptake is also not helpful because normal values are so low that they overlap with hypothyroidism. The TRH stimulation test can be used in females, but decreased responsiveness to TRH in older males does not allow this test to distinguish normal from pathologic states. In males, a TSH stimulation test may help confirm the presence of hypothyroidism.

Hypothyroidism may be accompanied by other laboratory abnormalities. Creatine phosphokinase (CPK) levels, including the MB fraction, may be elevated. A normocytic, normochromic anemia, which responds to thyroid hormone replacement, may be present. There is an increased incidence of pernicious anemia in hypothyroidism, but the microcytic anemia of iron deficiency remains the commonest anemia associated with hypothyroidism.

The symptoms and signs of hypothyroidism may be overlooked when such complaints as fatigue, memory loss, and decreased hearing are ascribed to aging without further investigation. The prevalence of undiagnosed hypothyroidism in healthy older people has varied from 0.5 to 2 percent in multiple studies; a general screening program is thus not cost-effective. The prevalence among older adults who are ill, however, is sufficient to support screening for hypothyroidism in this population, comprising individuals who have already presented themselves for care.

Therapy for hypothyroidism should be started at 0.025 to 0.05 mg of sodium levothyroxine (Synthroid) per day and increased by the same dose at 1- to 3-week intervals. The decreased metabolic clearance rate of thyroid hormone in aging may lead to a lower maintenance dose of T_4. The physician should monitor heart rate response and symptoms of angina and, in the laboratory, the TSH level. When indicated for symptomatic cardiovascular disease, a beta blocker may be added to the T_4 regimen. In patients with coronary artery disease, therapy can be initiated with triiodothyronine 5 μg/day and increased by 5 μg at weekly intervals to a level of 25 μg/day, at which time the patient can be converted to T_4 therapy. Because T_3 has a shorter half-life than T_4, symptoms will remit more rapidly after discontinuance of therapy if the patient develops cardiovascular complications. A beta blocker can also be added to the T_3 regimen.

Myxedema Coma   Most patients with myxedema coma are over age 60 (Table 11-6). In about 50 percent of the cases, the coma is induced

Table 11-6 Myxedema coma

Usually over 60 years old
50 percent induced by hypnotics
Neck scar
Hypothermia
Delayed relaxation of tendon reflex
Respiratory failure and apnea

in the hospital by treating hypothyroid patients with hypnotics. A neck scar, from previous thyroid surgery, is a clue to the cause of coma. Because patients with this disorder die of respiratory failure, hypercapnia requires prompt attention. These patients should be treated in an intensive care setting, with intubation and respiratory assistance instituted at the first sign of respiratory failure. The CSF protein level is often over 100 mg/dL and should not in itself be used as an indicator of other CNS pathology. Therapy includes a large initial dose (500 mg) of T_4 intravenously. Although studies have not been done to demonstrate the efficacy of glucocorticoids in this syndrome, it is generally recommended that these patients receive 200 mg of hydrocortisone per day in divided doses for the first 1 or 2 days. Patients with concomitant adrenal insufficiency will require continued steroid therapy.

Hyperthyroidism About 20 percent of hyperthyroid patients are older adults; 75 percent have classic signs and symptoms. Ophthalmopathy is infrequent. Although about one-third have no goiter, toxic multinodular goiter is more frequent than in the young. Severe nonthyroidal disease may disguise thyrotoxicosis (apathetic hyperthyroidism). Congestive heart failure, stroke, and infection are common disorders associated with masked hyperthyroidism. There should be a high threshold of suspicion for hyperthyroidism in older adults. Unexplained heart failure or tachyarrhythmia, recent onset of a psychiatric disorder, or profound myopathy should raise questions about masked hyperthyroidism. The triad of weight loss, anorexia, and constipation, which may raise the possibility of neoplastic disease, occurs in 15 percent of older thyrotoxic patients. Diagnosis is made by T_4, T_3, and/or radioactive iodine uptake (Table 11-4). The new ultrasensitive TSH assays can differentiate hyperthyroidism from normal. In the absence

of acute nonthyroidal disease, this test alone may confirm the clinical diagnosis of hyperthyroidism. In the presence of acute illness, concomitant determination of TSH and free T_4 may be more appropriate (Sawin et al., 1991). A T_3 suppression test should not be done in older adults because of the risk of angina or myocardial infarction.

Therapy is usually by radioactive iodine ablation. Often patients are first treated with antithyroid medications to control hyperthyroidism and deplete the thyroid gland of hormone prior to the radioactive iodine treatment. Surgery is reserved for patients with thyroid glands that are causing local obstructive symptoms.

Severe thyrotoxicosis is treated with antithyroid drugs (preferably propylthiouracil because it blocks conversion of T_4 to T_3) to inhibit new hormone synthesis, iodides to block thyroid hormone secretion, and beta blockers to decrease the peripheral manifestations of thyroid hormone action. In older adults with underlying cardiac disease, beta blocker therapy may be a problem; thus the cardiovascular response must be closely monitored. In patients allergic to antithyroid medications or where beta blockers are contraindicated, calcium ipodate (Oragrafin), 3 g every 3 days, can be used because it inhibits peripheral conversion of T_4 to T_3.

Goiter and Thyroid Cancer   The prevalence of multinodular goiter increases with age. At autopsy, multinodular goiter is found in 70 percent of females over age 60.

In the evaluation of a thyroid nodule for possible malignancy, several tests are available to assist in the decision for surgery (Table 11-7). Hyperfunctioning nodules on scan are less likely to be malignant than normo- or hypofunctioning nodules and necessitate therapy only on the basis of overall thyroid function. Fine-needle aspiration biopsy

Table 11-7 Tests for thyroid nodule

Thyroid scan
Ultrasound
Needle aspiration
Soft tissue films for psammoma bodies of papillary carcinoma
Thyroid function tests
Serum calcitonin for medullary carcinoma
Antithyroid antibodies for chronic thyroiditis

is the diagnostic procedure of choice. Cystic lesions should be aspirated. If cytology of the aspirate is not malignant, the nodule need not be resected unless it recurs or enlarges.

Soft tissue x-rays of the neck may assist in the diagnosis of papillary carcinoma of the thyroid if psammoma bodies are demonstrated. Elevated serum calcitonin levels may indicate medullary carcinoma of the thyroid. Anaplastic carcinoma of the thyroid, a rapidly progressive and fatal neoplasm, occurs mostly in females over age 60.

Hyperparathyroidism

One-third of patients with hyperparathyroidism are over age 60. Symptoms are the same in older adults as in those who are younger but may be overlooked. Bone demineralization, weakness, and joint complaints may be ascribed to aging when they may actually indicate parathyroid disease. In patients with mild elevation of calcium and no symptoms, the surgical risks must be carefully weighed.

Table 11-8 contrasts some of the basic patterns of the common laboratory tests in hyperparathyroidism with those of other metabolic bone diseases common in older adults.

Vasopressin Secretion

Basal vasopressin levels are unaltered in normal older individuals. Infusion of hypertonic saline, however, leads to a greater increase in plasma vasopressin in older as compared with younger persons (Helderman et al., 1978). In contrast to the response to the hyperosmo-

Table 11-8 Laboratory findings in metabolic bone disease

Disease	Ca	P	Alk	PTH
Hyperparathyroidism	High	Low/normal	High/normal	High
Osteomalacia	Low/normal	Low	High/normal	High
Hyperthyroidism	High	High	High/normal	Low
Osteoporosis	Normal	Normal	Normal	Normal/high
Paget's disease	Normal/high	Normal/high	High	Normal

Key: Ca, calcium; P, phosphorus; Alk, alkaline phosphatase; PTH, parathyroid hormone.

lar challenge, volume changes related to the assumption of upright posture are associated with less of a vasopressin response in older subjects as compared with the young (Rowe et al., 1982). Both these findings might be explained by impaired baroreceptor input to the supraoptic nucleus. Volume expansion decreases osmoreceptor sensitivity. Hypertonic saline infusion results in volume expansion and thus decreases osmoreceptor sensitivity. If baroreceptor input is impaired in older adults, volume expansion would lead to a lesser dampening effect, and thus the vasopressin response to hyperosmolar stimuli would be increased.

Hyponatremia is a serious and often overlooked problem of the older patient. This syndrome is often associated with one of three general causes: (1) decreased renal blood flow with a decreased ability to excrete a water load, (2) diuretic administration leading to water intoxication (this condition is rapidly corrected by discontinuing diuretics), and (3) excess vasopressin secretion. Although a host of pulmonary disorders (e.g., pneumonia, tuberculosis, tumor) and central nervous system disorders (e.g., stroke, meningitis, subdural hematoma) are associated with SIADH in any age group, older adults seem more prone to develop this complication. Certain drugs such as chlorpropamide and barbiturates may cause this syndrome more frequently in older individuals.

In addition to treatment directed at correcting the underlying cause, water restriction and hypertonic saline are indicated when the patient is symptomatic or the sodium level is below 120 meq/L. Dimethylchlorotetracycline therapy may be needed in resistant patients with SIADH. This agent induces a partial nephrogenic diabetes insipidus and thus corrects the hyponatremia. Serum creatinine and blood urea nitrogen should be closely monitored.

Ectopic Hormonal Syndromes

Because the incidence of malignancy increases with age, ectopic hormone syndromes are seen more often in older adults. The ectopic adrenocorticotropic hormone (ACTH) syndrome, seen with small cell carcinoma of the lung, often presents with hypokalemia. The hyponatremia of the ectopic antidiuretic hormone syndrome is also associated with small cell carcinoma of the lung. Ectopic parathyroid hormone (PTH) secretion and its associated hypercalcemia has been described with renal cell carcinoma and hepatomas. The hypercalce-

mia associated with squamous cell carcinoma of the lung appears not to be an ectopic PTH syndrome but hypercalcemia due to a related protein.

Iatrogenic Endocrine Disease

Endocrine disease can also be induced iatrogenically. Two endocrine syndromes related to drug therapy in older patients are hyperglycemia induced by diuretics (thiazides, furosemide) and hyponatremia induced by chlorpropamide.

Anabolic Hormones

Aging is associated with a decline in anabolic hormones (Lamberts et al., 1997). The declining activity of the growth hormone insulin-like growth factor I (IGF-I) axis with advancing age may contribute to the decrease in lean body mass and the increase in mass of adipose tissue that occur with aging. One study demonstrated improvement of these deficits in older men deficient in IGF-I who were treated with growth hormone (Rudman et al., 1990), but other studies have not found such benefits. A multiple site trial for benefits and side effects of such treatment in older adults is presently under way.

Normal male aging is accompanied by a decline in testicular function, including a fall in serum levels of total testosterone (T) and bioavailable T. Only some men become hypogonadal. Androgens have many important physiologic actions, including effects on muscle, bone, and bone marrow. However, little is known about the effects of the age-related decline in testicular function on androgen target organs. Studies in small numbers of older hypogonadal males have demonstrated significant increases in lean body mass and significant decreases in biochemical parameters of bone resorption with testosterone treatment. However, there was also a significant increase in hematocrit and a sustained stimulation of prostate-specific antigen (Tenover, 1992). Again, further trials are under way.

ANEMIA

Anemia is common in older adults but should not be attributed simply to old age. Increased weakness, fatigue, and a mild anemia should not be dismissed as a manifestation of aging. In healthy older individu-

als, there is generally no change in normal levels of hemoglobin from younger adult values.

Signs and symptoms of anemia may be subtle. Some of these manifestations are listed in Table 11-9. Anemia should be considered in these circumstances. If anemia is present, a diagnostic evaluation is indicated to define the cause. The appearance of the peripheral blood smear along with the history and physical examination should direct the diagnostic evaluation as described below.

Iron Deficiency

Iron deficiency is the most common cause of anemia in older adults. Laboratory findings include hypochromia, microcytosis, low reticulocyte count, decreased serum iron, increased total iron-binding capacity (TIBC), low transferrin saturation, and absent bone marrow iron stores. A low serum iron and elevated TIBC indicate iron deficiency even in the absence of changes in red cell morphology. Because transferrin is reduced in many diseases, the TIBC may be normal or low in older patients with iron deficiency. However, a transferrin saturation of <10 percent would suggest iron deficiency even in the presence of a low TIBC. A low serum ferritin level is valuable in confirming the diagnosis because serum ferritin levels are below 12 mg/L in iron-deficiency anemia. Because inflammatory disease can elevate ferritin levels and liver disease can influence ferritin levels in either direction, the diagnosis of iron deficiency on the basis of a ferritin level must be made with a knowledge of the clinical situation.

Once iron deficiency is identified, it should be treated, and the cause of the anemia must be identified and corrected. Poor dietary intake of iron may contribute to iron deficiency in older adults. A dietary evaluation is important, both for foods that contain iron and

Table 11-9 Signs and symptoms of anemia

Weakness	Ischemic chest pain
Postural hypotension	Congestive heart failure
Syncope	Exertional dyspnea
Falls	Pallor
Confusion	Tachycardia
Worsened dementia	

for substances such as tea, which inhibit iron absorption. However, even in the presence of poor nutrition, evaluation for a bleeding lesion must be completed.

The stool should be examined for occult blood. Evaluation for a gastrointestinal lesion should be carried out in a patient with unexplained iron deficiency even if the stool is negative for occult blood. Although gastrointestinal bleeding may be caused by drugs (especially certain analgesics, steroids, and alcohol), a gastrointestinal lesion must be excluded. Diverticulosis is a common cause of bleeding. Vascular ectasia of the cecum and ascending colon is increasingly a recognized cause of bleeding in older adults.

Replacement of iron should usually be by daily oral administration. The hemoglobin should improve in 10 days and be normal in about 6 weeks. Normal bone marrow iron stores should occur in an additional 4 months. If the anemia does not improve, one should consider noncompliance, continued bleeding, or an incorrect diagnosis. In unreliable patients or when oral iron is not tolerated, parenteral iron replacement with iron dextran is indicated. Tolerance should be monitored with a test dose, and the patient should be closely observed for an acute reaction. Parenteral iron should not be used routinely but it is an important therapeutic modality in the appropriate patient.

Chronic Disease

The anemia of chronic disease may display many similarities with iron deficiency. In older adults, this anemia is frequently associated with chronic inflammatory diseases or neoplasia. There is a defect in bone marrow red cell production and a shortening of erythrocyte life span. The finding of hypochromia, low reticulocyte count, and low serum iron may lead to confusion with iron deficiency. When a high TIBC does not confirm the presence of iron deficiency, a ferritin level can differentiate the two anemias. It is low in iron deficiency and high-normal or elevated in the anemia of chronic disease. Treatment is addressed to the underlying chronic illness, because there is no specific therapy for this type of anemia.

Sideroblastic Anemia

Sideroblastic anemia should be considered in an older patient with hypochromic anemia who does not have iron deficiency or a chronic

disease. Serum iron and transferrin saturation are increased. Hence, synthesis is defective, leading to increased iron stores and the diagnostic finding of ringed sideroblasts in the marrow.

In older adults, sideroblastic anemia is commonly of the acquired type. The idiopathic group is usually refractory; only a few patients have a partial response to pyridoxine, but all should have a trial of pyridoxine. Although the prognosis is fairly good, about 10 percent of patients develop acute myeloblastic leukemia. Secondary sideroblastic anemia may be associated with underlying diseases such as malignancies and chronic inflammatory diseases. Certain drugs and toxins can induce sideroblastic anemia (e.g., ethanol, lead, isoniazid, chloramphenicol). The drug-induced syndromes are corrected by administering pyridoxine. Tests that will assist in the differential diagnosis of hypochromic anemias are listed in Table 11-10.

Vitamin B$_{12}$ and Folate Deficiency

Both vitamin B$_{12}$ and folate deficiency may occur on a nutritional basis, although folate deficiency is the more common. Older people who live alone or are alcoholics are most likely to have poor nutrition. Poor dietary intake of fresh fruits and vegetables may lead to folate deficiency; lack of meat, poultry, fish, eggs, and dairy products may lead to vitamin B$_{12}$ deficiency. Vitamin B$_{12}$ deficiency also occurs with the loss of intrinsic factor (pernicious anemia) and in gastrointestinal disorders associated with malabsorption of vitamin B$_{12}$.

Table 11-10 Differential tests in hypochromic anemia

Item	Iron deficiency	Chronic disease	Sideroblastic anemia
Serum iron	Low	Low	High
Total iron-binding capacity	Usually increased*	Low	Normal
Transferrin saturation	Low	Low	High
Ferritin	Low	High	Normal
Bone marrow iron	Absent	Adequate	Increased ringed sideroblasts

* May be normal or even low in older adults.

The laboratory findings are similar in the two deficiencies and include macrocytosis, hyperchromasia, hypersegmented neutrophils, and megaloblasts in the marrow. Leukopenia and thrombocytopenia may be present, and serum lactic dehydrogenase (LDH) and bilirubin may be increased. The two are differentiated by measuring serum vitamin B_{12} and folate levels.

Treatment is with vitamin B_{12} or folic acid, as appropriate. However, because folate will correct the hematologic disorder but not the neurologic abnormalities of vitamin B_{12} deficiency, a correct diagnosis is essential before treatment.

NUTRITION

Recently there has been emphasis on perinatal nutrition; in the past, nutrition during growth has been extensively examined, but little has been done in nutrition of adulthood and senescence. A discussion of nutrition and aging is therefore limited by the lack of adequate studies, defined methods, and standards. Although it is generally accepted that intake moderately above recommended allowances is optimal, animal studies demonstrate increased longevity with lower caloric levels than recommended. In establishing nutritional requirements in humans, we must contend with the multiple factors that confound interpretation of available data, e.g., genetic factors, social environment, economic status, selection of food, and weak methods of assessing nutritional status.

Several national surveys have been performed to assess nutrition in older adults. Taken as a whole, these surveys do not indicate poor nutritional status or marked deficiency among older individuals in the United States and suggest that intake relates more to health and poverty than to age. However, obesity is a significant problem. In a study of 500 older individuals admitted to a hospital with long-term illness, 35 percent were found to have significant primary nutritional problems, 15 percent were undernourished, and 20 percent were obese. Of 107 older patients admitted to a county hospital, 5 to 10 percent were found to have low vitamin A and vitamin C levels. Of 234 ambulant, well subjects, 5 percent of males and 13 percent of females had a low hematocrit, 8 percent had low vitamin C levels, and 18 to 21 percent had a low thiamine level (6 percent by transketolase assay). Again, these data suggest a low prevalence of nutri-

tional deficiency in older adults and provide no basis for recommending massive vitamin replacement.

Vitamins, Protein, and Calcium

Table 11-11 summarizes nutritional requirements in older adults and demonstrates that there is no general increase in vitamin requirements with age. Studies on vitamin metabolism and requirements reveal no correlation between age and the requirement for vitamins A, B_1, B_2, or C. Vitamin B_6 and vitamin B_{12} requirements also do not increase with age.

Studies on protein requirements are not in agreement. Based on nitrogen balance studies, estimates of protein requirement varied from 0.5 to more than 1.0 g/kg daily. Data on amino acid requirements are also conflicting: some data show increased requirements with age, and other data show no change.

For calcium, estimated requirements vary from 850 to 1020 mg/day. All these studies exceed the required dietary allowance for calcium of 800 mg/day. Data on the correlation of calcium intake and osteoporosis are conflicting. Although calcium supplementation alone does not seem to reverse postmenopausal osteoporosis, it is an important adjunct to estrogen replacement therapy. It may be necessary to use a calcium supplement to ensure adequate intake.

Nutritional Deficiency and Physiologic Impairments

There is little evidence to correlate age-associated nutritional deficiency with clinical findings. In a study on the consequences of vitamin A levels, there was no significant correlation with dark adaptation, epithelial cells excreted, or percent keratinization. In other studies, there was no correlation between vitamin C levels and gingivitis or

Table 11-11 Nutritional requirements in older persons

Vitamins	Unchanged in older persons
Protein	0.5 to >1.0 g/kg/day
Amino acids	Unchanged to increased
Calcium	850–1020 mg/day
Calories	Declines by 12.4 cal/day per year (maturity to senescence)

vitamin B_{12} and lactic acid, lactic dehydrogenase, or hematocrit. Older people with limited sun exposure may be at risk of vitamin D deficiency.

The highest prevalence of osteoporosis is among postmenopausal women. In a study using radiographs of the dorsal and lumbar spine, osteoporosis was present in 50 percent of women aged 65 to 70 and increased to 90 percent in women over age 90. In males, the numbers were 15 and 30 percent in the same age groups. Data are conflicting on correlation of dietary calcium intake and osteoporosis. Problems in assessing this correlation include reduced calcium intake in older adults, altered calcium and phosphorus ratio, decreased protein intake, and acid-base balance.

Reversal of Deficiency by Supplementation

There is no impairment of vitamin or protein absorption in older adults. Data have demonstrated conclusively that low vitamin levels in older adults can be reversed by administration of oral supplementation. Because these deficiencies can be corrected by dietary supplementation, they are most likely related to decreased intake.

Caloric Needs

A study of 250 individuals aged 23 to 99 demonstrated an age-associated decline in total caloric intake at the rate of 12.4 cal/day for a year. A yearly decline in basal metabolic rate accounted for 5.23 cal/day, while 7.6 cal/day related to reduction in other requirements, including physical exercise.

Dietary Restriction and Food Additives

Rats, mice, *Drosophila,* and other lower organisms have demonstrated that caloric restriction delays maturation and increases life span. The mechanism, however, is not understood. Animals fed isocaloric diets but decreased protein have increased life span. Based on the free radical theory of aging, it has been proposed that reducing agents would prolong life. Although the data are conflicting, some studies have supported this hypothesis.

In certain animal models, caloric restriction has also been shown to decrease incidence and delay onset of disease, including chronic

glomerulonephritis, muscular dystrophy, and carcinogenesis. In humans, however, body weight below ideal is not associated with increased life span (discussed below). In animal experiments, nutrition is maintained during caloric variation. This may not be true in humans, and thus may lead to the differing results.

NUTRITIONAL ASSESSMENT

Because people age at different rates, there is a need for age- and sex-specific normative data as indicators of nutritional status. Unfortunately, adequate data are not available. Such data also need to distinguish among community-dwelling, institutionalized, and hospitalized older adults.

Certain parameters are, however, used in assessing nutritional status in older adults. Some anthropometric variables are probably effective estimators of major aspects of body composition (Table 11-12). They cannot provide a complete description of the nutritional status of an individual and are not highly correlated with biochemical or hematologic indicators of nutritional status.

Although weight is a global measure, it can be obtained easily from adults and is useful in the absence of edema. Weight/stature ratio is best correlated with total body fat. Triceps and subscapular skin folds are highly correlated with the percentage of body fat in older adults. Upper arm circumference is correlated with lean body mass and may be particularly helpful in edematous patients in whom weight is misleading. The effect of the aging process on lean body mass is so great that it remains a poor reflection of nutritional status in older adults.

Table 11-12 Assessment of body composition

Assessment	Component
Weight	Global
Weight/stature	Total fat
Skin fold	Percent fat
Upper arm circumference	Lean body mass

Serum albumin is a practical indicator of malnutrition in older adults. However, liver disease, proteinuria, and protein-losing enteropathies must be excluded. A low serum albumin may be indicative of malnutrition, but a normal or increased serum albumin concentration does not necessarily indicate normality. Thyroxine-binding prealbumin and/or retinol-binding protein are more sensitive indices than are albumin and transferrin. However, the effect of age on these proteins has not been defined.

In animals, dietary deprivation of protein results in anemia. Because anemia is one of the earliest manifestations of protein-calorie malnutrition, its presence should alert the physician to the possibility of malnutrition. Total lymphocyte count may be a very good marker for nutritional problems. An initial evaluation of the immune system may be obtained with a skin test. *Candida* antigen can be utilized because virtually all people over age 11 have a delayed-type sensitivity.

Although there are presently no clear-cut criteria for the diagnosis of malnutrition in older adults, some important factors need to be considered in evaluating a given patient, as shown in Table 11-13. Table 11-14 presents some factors that put older patients at risk for malnutrition. Individuals with such problems should be considered for evaluation of nutritional status.

Special Considerations

As discussed in Chap. 12, sensory loss, especially in taste and smell, may lead to decreased appetite in the elderly and thus predispose to malnutrition. Dentures may cover the roof of the mouth and secondary taste areas, adding to the sensory loss. Poor dentition may also put the patient at risk for malnutrition because the patient will select soft foods often high in sugars or carbohydrates and low in nutrients.

Table 11-13 Critical questions in assessing a patient for malnutrition

Is there any reason to suspect malnutrition?
If so, of which nutrient(s) and to what extent?
What are the pathophysiologic mechanisms (e.g., alteration in nutrient intake, digestion and absorption, metabolism, excretion, or requirements)?
What etiology underlies the pathophysiologic mechanism(s)?

Table 11-14   Factors that place older adults at risk for malnutrition

Drugs (e.g., reserpine, digoxin, antitumor agents)
Chronic disease (e.g., congestive heart failure, renal insufficiency, chronic
    gastrointestinal disease)
Depression
Dental and periodontal disease
Decreased taste and smell
Low socioeconomic level
Physical weakness
Isolation
Food fads

Good dental care and especially prevention are thus important factors in nutrition of the older patient.

Although the influence of dietary fiber on colonic carcinoma and diverticular disease is controversial, the use of dietary fiber to maintain bowel regularity has significant support, especially in older adults, where constipation may present a difficult clinical problem. When dietary intake of fiber is low, bran can be used as a supplement, particularly in cereals, breads, or as bran powder. Intake of bran can be adjusted to maintain normal bowel movements.

Although the food industry is slowly responding, most canned foods still contain large amounts of added sodium and sugar. Because some of these are less expensive than fresh or frozen foods, older adults with limited incomes may use such prepared foods exclusively. When refined carbohydrates or sodium need to be restricted, these patients should be educated about the use of canned products.

Until recently, actuarial tables have been used to support the position that obesity is associated with excess mortality. Data from the Framingham Study (Andres, 1981), however, indicate that modest increases in adiposity may even prolong life. However, in older adults, the Framingham Study demonstrated increasing mortality with increasing relative body weight above ideal weight. Thus, minimally excessive weight may not be as beneficial to older adults as it is in younger individuals.

INFECTIONS

Although it is proposed that alterations in host defense mechanisms predispose older adults to certain infections, there is little evidence

to support this hypothesis. It may well be that environmental factors, physiologic changes in other than the immune system, and specific diseases are the major elements in the increased frequency of certain infections in older adults (Table 11-15).

Because the elderly more often have acute and chronic illnesses necessitating hospitalization and have longer hospital stays, they are at greater risk for nosocomial infections. Such hospitalizations put older patients at greater risk for gram-negative and *Staphylococcus aureus* infections. Physiologic alterations (Chap. 1)—such as occur in the lungs, bladder function, and the skin—and glucose homeostasis may also predispose older adults to infections.

The incidence of malignancies is increased in older adults. Many of these neoplastic disorders, especially those of the hematologic sys-

**Table 11-15 Factors predisposing
to infection in older adults**

More frequent and longer hospital stays:
   Nosocomial infections
      Gram-negative bacilli
      Staphylococcus aureus

Physiologic changes:
   Lung
   Bladder
   Skin
   Glucose homeostasis

Chronic disease:
   Malignancy
      Multiple myeloma and leukemia
      Immunosuppression from therapy

Diabetes mellitus
   Urinary tract infection
   Soft tissue infections
   Osteomyelitis

Prostatic hypertrophy
   Urinary tract infection

Host defenses:
   Phagocytosis unaltered
   Complement unaltered
   Cellular and humoral immunity diminished

tem, are associated with a higher frequency of infection. Immunosuppression during therapy is also a predisposing factor. The prevalence of diabetes mellitus is higher in older adults, thus predisposing them to more frequent urinary tract, soft tissue, and bone infections. Prostatic hypertrophy with obstruction predisposes the older male to urinary tract infections.

Phagocytic function appears to be unaltered in aging, as is the complement system. Cell-mediated immunity and, to a lesser extent, humoral immunity, is diminished in aging. The role that these changes play in predisposing older individuals to infection has not been well defined.

With the predisposing factors described above, the spectrum of pathogens causing common infections in the elderly is often different than that in younger adults (Table 11-16). The frequency of gram-negative bacilli increases in each category.

Many infections occur more frequently in older adults and are often associated with a higher morbidity and mortality (Yoshikawa and Norman, 1987). Atypical presentation of infection in some older patients may delay diagnosis and treatment. Underreporting of symptoms, impaired communication, coexisting diseases, and altered physiologic responses to infection may contribute to altered presentations.

Table 11-16 Pathogens of common infections in older adults

Infection	Common pathogens in adults	Common pathogens in older adults
Pneumonia	*S. pneumoniae* Anaerobic bacteria	*S. pneumoniae* Anaerobic bacteria *H. influenzae* Gram-negative bacilli
Urinary tract	*E. coli*	*E. coli* *Proteus* sp. *Klebsiella* sp. *Enterobacter* sp. Enterococcus
Meningitis	*S. pneumoniae* N. meningitidis	*S. pneumoniae* *Listeria monocytogenes* Gram-negative bacilli
Septic arthritis	*N. gonorrhoeae* *S. aureus*	*S. aureus* Gram-negative bacilli

As an example, failure of patients to seek medical evaluation is one factor in the higher morbidity and mortality of appendicitis in the elderly. Difficulties in communication may also alter presentation. Infections not directly involving the central nervous system may cause confusion in the elderly, particularly in individuals with preexisting dementia. The mechanism by which this occurs has not been defined. Acute unexplained functional deterioration should also alert the physician to a potential acute infectious process.

Existing chronic disease may mask an acute infection. Septic arthritis usually occurs in a previously abnormal joint. It may be difficult to distinguish clinically between exacerbation of the underlying arthritis and acute infection. Therefore, the physician should not be hesitant to examine synovial fluid in elderly patients with acute exacerbation of joint disease.

Febrile response may be blunted or absent in some older individuals with bacterial infections. This may obscure diagnosis and delay therapy. A poor febrile response may also be a negative prognostic factor. Conversely, a febrile response is more likely to indicate a bacterial rather than viral illness in older patients, particularly in the very old.

Antibiotic therapy in older adults, as in the young, is directed to the specific organism isolated. However, when empiric antimicrobial therapy is initiated, consideration should be given to including a third-generation cephalosporin and/or aminoglycoside because gram-negative infections are more common regardless of the site. With all antibiotics, but particularly with the aminoglycosides, renal function must be considered and monitored for toxicity. Monitoring of drug blood level and renal function is mandatory with the aminoglycosides.

Since 1984, the incidence of tuberculosis is on the rise again. Older persons of both sexes among all racial and ethnic groups are especially at risk for tuberculosis. This cohort has lived through a period of higher incidence of tuberculosis, has probably not been treated with isonicotinic acid hydralazide (INH) prophylaxis, and may have predisposing factors such as physiologic changes, malnutrition, and underlying disease that may lead to reactivation. Older patients are also at increased risk for primary infection. This is particularly the case for older patients in long-term-care institutions (Stead, 1981). Tuberculosis screening programs should be implemented in long-term-care facilities because of this increased risk and because of the potential to prevent active disease among patients whose skin test

converts to a strongly positive reaction (Stead and To, 1987; Stead et al., 1987) (see Chap. 15). The American Thoracic Society now recommends preventive therapy for certain types of patients regardless of age, including insulin-dependent diabetic patients, those on steroids and other immunosuppressive treatment, patients with end-stage renal disease, and patients who have lost a large amount of weight rapidly (American Thoracic Society, 1986). A useful rule in geriatric care is to suspect tuberculosis when a patient is inexplicably failing.

Several studies have suggested an association of bacteriuria with increased mortality in the elderly (Dontas et al., 1981; Evans et al., 1982; Platt et al., 1982; Sourander and Kasanen, 1972). However, others have not confirmed this finding (Heinamaki et al., 1986; Nicolle et al., 1987a; Nordenstam et al., 1986). Most of these studies did not differentiate between the effect of bacteriuria and age and/or concomitant disease on mortality. When Nordenstam et al. adjusted for age, they concluded that fatal diseases associated with bacteriuria may account for the increase in mortality among older patients with bacteriuria.

Several previous studies in elderly hospitalized or institutionalized patients have not revealed antimicrobial therapy for bacteriuria to be effective because of the high rate of recurring infection (Alling et al., 1975; Brocklehurst et al., 1977; Nicolle et al., 1983, 1987b). One study in older ambulatory nonhospitalized women with asymptomatic bacteriuria demonstrated that short-course antimicrobial therapy is effective in eliminating bacteriuria in most of the women for at least a 6-month period (Boscia et al., 1987b). Survival was not an outcome measure.

Bacteriuria in older persons is common and usually asymptomatic. At present, in the absence of obstructive uropathy, no evidence exists to support the routine use of antimicrobial therapy for asymptomatic bacteriuria in older persons (Boscia et al., 1987a). Among bacteriuric patients with urinary incontinence and no other symptoms of urinary tract infection, the bacteriuria should be eradicated as part of the initial assessment of the incontinence (see Chap. 7).

DISORDERS OF TEMPERATURE REGULATION

Temperature dysregulation in the elderly demonstrates the narrowing of homeostatic mechanisms that occurs with advancing age.

Older persons are less able to adjust to extremes of environmental temperatures. Hypo- and hyperthermic states are predominantly disorders of older adults. Despite underreporting of these disorders, there is evidence that morbidity and mortality increase during particularly hot or cold periods, especially among ill elderly (Hope et al., 1984; Collins et al., 1977; Rango, 1984). Much of this illness is caused by an increased incidence of cardiovascular disorders (myocardial infarct and stroke) or infectious diseases (pneumonia) during these periods.

Studies in the United Kingdom reveal that hypothermia is a common finding among older adults during the winter, when homes are heated below 70°F. As might be expected, there are similar seasonal occurrences in the United States and Canada.

Pathophysiology

The basic pathophysiology of hypo- and hyperthermic states in older adults is represented in Table 11-17. The thermoregulatory center maintains body temperature through control of sweating, vasoconstriction and vasodilation, chemical thermogenesis, and shivering. Impaired temperature perception, diminished sweating (Foster et al., 1976) in hyperthermia, and abnormal vasoconstrictor response in hypothermia are major pathophysiologic mechanisms in these disorders.

Table 11-17 Pathophysiology of temperature dysregulation

Hyperthermia	Hypothermia
Higher threshold of central temperature to sweating	Diminished sensation to cold
Diminished or absent sweating	Impaired sensation to change in temperature
Impaired warmth perception	Abnormal autonomic vasoconstrictor response to cold
Abnormal peripheral blood flow response to warming	Impaired shiver response
Compromised cardiovascular reserve	Diminished thermogenesis

Hypothermia

Hypothermia is defined as a core temperature (rectal, esophageal, tympanic) below 35°C. Essential to the diagnosis is early recognition with a low-recording thermometer. Ordinary thermometers will not serve. The factors predisposing to hypothermia are listed in Table 11-18. Underlying infections are common (Kramer et al., 1989; Darowski et al., 1991).

Table 11-19 illustrates the clinical spectrum of hypothermia. Because early signs are nonspecific and subtle, a high index of suspicion

Table 11-18 Factors predisposing to hypothermia

Decreased heat production
  Hypothyroidism
  Hypoglycemia
  Starvation and malnutrition
  Immobility and decreased activity
    (e.g., stroke, arthritis, parkinsonism)

Increased heat loss
  Decreased subcutaneous fat
  Exposure to cold (immersion)

Thermoregulatory impairment

Hypothalamic and CNS dysfunction
  Heat trauma
  Hypoxia
  Tumor
  Cerebrovascular disease

Drug-induced impairment
  Alcohol
  Barbiturates
  Major and minor tranquilizers
  Glutethimide
  Reserpine
  Tricyclic antidepressants
  Salicylates, acetaminophen
  General anesthetics

Old age

Miscellaneous
  Sepsis
  Cardiovascular disease
  Bronchopneumonia

Table 11-19   Clinical presentation of hypothermia

Early signs (32–35°C)	Later signs (28–30°C)	Late signs (<28°C)
Fatigue	Cold skin	Very cold skin
Weakness	Hypopnea	Rigidity
Slowness of gait	Cyanosis	Apnea
Apathy	Bradycardia	No pulse—ventricular fibrillation
Slurred speech	Atrial and ventricular arrhythmias	Areflexia
Confusion		
Shivering (±)	Hypotension	Unresponsiveness
Cool skin	Semicoma and coma	Fixed pupils
Sensation of cold (±)	Muscular rigidity	
	Generalized edema	
	Slowed reflexes	
	Poorly reactive pupils	
	Polyuria or oliguria	

must exist to allow an early diagnosis. A history of known or potential exposure is helpful, but older patients can become hypothermic at modest temperatures. Frequently the most difficult differential diagnosis in more severe hypothermia is hypothyroidism. A previous history of thyroid disease, a neck scar from previous thyroid surgery, and a delay in the relaxation phase of the deep tendon reflexes may assist in diagnosing hypothyroidism. Patients may sometimes be mistaken for dead. Case reports reveal patients who have survived after being discovered without respiration and pulse.

Complications of severe hypothermia are listed in Table 11-20. The most significant early ones are arrhythmias and cardiorespiratory arrests. Later complications involve the pulmonary, gastrointestinal, and renal systems. ECG abnormalities are frequent (Table 11-21). The most specific ECG finding is the J wave (Osborn wave) following the QRS complex. This abnormality disappears as temperature returns to normal.

General supportive therapy for severe hypothermia consists of intensive care management of complicated multisystem dysfunctions (Table 11-22). Every attempt should be made to assess and treat any contributing medical disorder (e.g., infection, hypothyroidism,

Table 11-20 Complications of severe hypothermia

Arrhythmias
Cardiorespiratory arrest
Bronchopneumonia
Aspiration pneumonia
Pulmonary edema
Pancreatitis
Gastrointestinal bleeding
Acute tubular necrosis
Intravascular thrombosis

Table 11-21 ECG abnormalities in hypothermia

Bradycardia
Prolonged PR interval, QRS complex, and QT segment
J wave (Osborn wave)
Atrial fibrillation
PVCs
Ventricular fibrillation
Muscle tremor artifact

Table 11-22 Supportive therapy for hypothermia

Use intensive care unit (for temperature below 30°C).
Maintain continuous ECG monitoring.
Treat sepsis (unless proven otherwise).
Use intravenous fluid replacement (assess individually).
Arrhythmias are resistant to cardioversion and drug therapy (drugs given during hypothermia may cause problems when patient is rewarmed).
Treat only severe hyperglycemia.
Use caution when correcting severe acidosis with HCO_3.
If central venous pressure necessary, avoid entrance into the heart.
Follow blood gases to assess respiratory function.
O_2 therapy, suctioning and endotracheal intubation may be required.
Monitor chest films—pneumonia is common.
In myxedema, treat with levothyroxine 500 μg IV and corticosteroids

hypoglycemia). Hypothermia in older patients should promptly be treated as sepsis unless proven otherwise. While patients should have continuous ECG monitoring, central lines should be avoided if possible because of myocardial irritability. Because there is delayed metabolism, most drugs have little effect on a severely hypothermic patient, but they may cause problems once the patient is rewarmed. It is preferable to stabilize the patient and immediately undertake specific rewarming techniques (Table 11-23). Serious arrhythmias, acidosis, and fluid and electrolyte disorders will usually respond to therapy only after rewarming has been accomplished.

Passive rewarming is generally adequate for those with mild hypothermia (>32°C). Active external rewarming has been associated with increased morbidity and mortality because cold blood may suddenly be shunted to the core, further decreasing core temperature; peripheral vasodilatation can precipitate hypovolemic shock by decreasing circulatory blood volume. For more severe hypothermia (<32°C), core rewarming is necessary. Several techniques for core rewarming have been used (Table 11-23), but positive results have been reported only from small, uncontrolled studies. Peritoneal dialysis and inhalation rewarming may be the most practical techniques in the

Table 11-23 Specific rewarming techniques

Passive rewarming
    Removal from environmental exposure
    Insulating material
    Placement in warm environment (>70°F)

Active external rewarming
    Immersion in heated water (42°C or 107.6°F)
    Electric blankets
    Heated objects (water bottle)

Active core rewarming
    Intragastric balloon
    Colonic irrigation
    Mediastinal irrigation via thoracotomy
    Hemodialysis
    Peritoneal dialysis
    Extracorporeal blood rewarming
    Inhalation rewarming
    Cardiopulmonary bypass

majority of institutions. For reviews of treatment in the field and in the hospital, see Danzl and Pozos (1994) and The Medical Letter (1994).

Mortality is usually greater than 50 percent for severe hypothermia. It increases with age and is particularly related to underlying disease.

Hyperthermia

Heat stroke is defined as a failure to maintain body temperature and is characterized by a core temperature of >40.6°C (105°F), severe central nervous system dysfunction (psychosis, delirium, coma), and anhidrosis (hot, dry skin). The two groups primarily affected are older adults who are chronically ill and the young undergoing strenuous exercise. Mortality is as high as 80 percent once this syndrome is manifest.

Table 11-24 illustrates predisposing factors relevant to older adults. Usually there are multiple factors, but most often there is a prolonged heat wave. Again, the diagnosis requires a high level of suspicion. In view of the poor survival, efforts must be directed toward prevention. Older patients should be cautioned about the dangers of hot weather. For those at particularly high risk, temporary relocation to more protected environments should be considered.

Early manifestations of heat exhaustion are nonspecific (Table 11-25). Later, severe central nervous system dysfunction and anhidrosis develop.

Table 11-26 lists some of the more serious complications resulting from heat damage to organ systems. Once the full syndrome has developed for any length of time, the prognosis is very poor. While management at this stage requires intense multisystem care, the key is rapid specific therapy consisting of cooling to 102°F within the first hour. Ice packs and ice-water immersion are superior to convection cooling with alcohol sponge baths or electric fans.

Prevention appears to be the most appropriate approach to management of temperature dysregulation in older adults. Education of older adults to their susceptibility to hypo- and hyperthermia in extremes of environmental temperature, education as to appropriate behavior in such conditions, and close monitoring of the most vulnerable older adults should help reduce the morbidity and mortality from these disorders.

Table 11-24 Factors predisposing to heat stroke

Exogenous heat gain
  High ambient temperature
  Increased risk in:
    Extremes of age
    Debilitating illness
    Alcohol ingestion

Increased heat production
  Exercise and exertion
  Infection (febrile state)
  Agitated and tremulous states
  Drugs (amphetamines)
  Hyperthyroidism

Impaired heat dissipation
  Lack of acclimatization
  High ambient temperature
  High humidity
  Obesity
  Heavy clothing
  Cardiovascular disease
  Dehydration
  Extremes of age
  Central nervous system lesions
  Drugs
    Phenothiazines
    Anticholinergics
    Diuretics
    Propranolol
  Sweat gland dysfunction
  Potassium depletion

Table 11-25 Clinical presentation of hyperthermia

Early signs	Later signs
Dizziness	CNS dysfunction
Weakness	Psychosis
Sensation of warmth	Delirium
Anorexia	Coma
Nausea	Anhidrosis
Vomiting	Hot, dry skin
Headache	
Dyspnea	

Table 11-26 Complications of heat stroke

Myocardial damage
  Congestive heart failure
  Arrhythmias

Renal failure (20–25%)

Cerebral edema
  Seizures
  Diffuse and focal findings

Hepatocellular necrosis
  Jaundice
  Liver failure

Rhabdomyolysis
  Myoglobinuria

Bleeding diathesis
  Disseminated intravascular coagulation

Electrolyte disturbances

Acid-base disturbances
  Metabolic acidosis
  Respiratory alkalosis

Infection
  Aspiration pneumonia
  Sepsis

Dehydration and shock

ACKNOWLEDGMENT

The authors wish to thank Dr. T. T. Yoshikawa for his assistance in preparing material for an earlier version of the section on infections in this chapter.

The authors wish to acknowledge the assistance of Dr. Alan Robbins in preparing an earlier version of the material on temperature regulation in this chapter.

REFERENCES

Alling B, Brandberg A, Seeberg S, et al: Effect of consecutive antibacterial therapy on bacteriuria in hospitalized geriatric patients. *Scand J Infect Dis* 7:201–207, 1975.

American Thoracic Society: Treatment of tuberculosis and tuberculosis infection in adults and children. *Am Rev Respir Dis* 134:355–363, 1986.

Andres R: Aging, diabetes and obesity: Standards of normality. *Mt Sinai J Med* 48:489–495, 1981.

Boscia JA, Abrutyn E, Kaye D: Asymptomatic bacteriuria in elderly persons: treat or do not treat? *Ann Intern Med* 106:764–766, 1987a.

Boscia JA, Kobasa WD, Knight RA, et al: Therapy vs no therapy for bacteriuria in elderly ambulatory nonhospitalized women. *JAMA* 257:1067–1071, 1987b.

Brocklehurst JC, Bee P, Jones D, et al: Bacteriuria in geriatric hospital patients, its correlates and management. *Age Ageing* 6:240–245, 1977.

Collins KJ, Dore C, Exton-Smith AN, et al: Accidental hypothermia and impaired temperature homeostasis in the elderly. *BMJ* 1:353–356, 1977.

Colwell JA. Intensive insulin therapy in type II diabetes: rationale and collaborative clinical trial results. *Diabetes* 45(3):S87–S90, 1996.

Danzl DF, Pozos RS: Accidental hypothermia. *N Engl J Med* 331:1756–1760, 1994.

Darowski A, Najim Z, Weinberg JR, et al: Hypothermia and infection in elderly patients admitted to hospital. *Age Ageing* 20:100–106, 1991.

Dontas AS, Kasviki-Charvati P, Papanayiotou PC, et al: Bacteriuria and survival in old age. *N Engl J Med* 304:939–943, 1981.

Edward K, Larson EB: Benefits of exercise for older adults. *Clin Geriatr Med* 8:35–50, 1992.

Evans DA, Kass EH, Hennekens CH, et al: Bacteriuria and subsequent mortality in women. *Lancet* 1:156–158, 1982.

Fink RI, Kolterman OG, Koa M, et al: The role of the glucose transport system in the post receptor defect in insulin action associated with human aging. *J Clin Endocrinol Metab* 58:721–725, 1984.

Foster KG, Ellis FT, Dore C, et al: Sweat responses in the aged. *Age Ageing* 5:91–101, 1976.

Harman SM, Wehmann RE, Blackman MR: Pituitary-thyroid hormone economy in healthy aging men: basal indices of thyroid function and thyrotropin responses to constant infusions of thyrotropin releasing hormone. *J Clin Endocrinol Metab* 58:320–326, 1984.

Heinamaki P, Haavisto M, Hakulinen T, et al: Mortality in relation to urinary characteristics in the very aged. *Gerontology* 32:167–171, 1986.

Helderman JH, Vestal RE, Rowe JW, et al: The response of arginine vasopressin to intravenous ethanol and hypertonic saline in man: the impact of aging. *J Gerontol* 33:39–47, 1978.

Hershman JM, Pekary AE, Berg L, et al: Serum thyrotropin and thyroid hormone levels in elderly and middle-aged euthyroid persons. *J Am Geriatr Soc* 41:823–828, 1993.

Hollenbeck CB, Haskell W, Rosenthal M, et al: Effect of habitual physical activity on regulation of insulin-stimulated glucose disposal in older males. *J Am Geriatr Soc* 33:273–277, 1984.

Hope W, Donnel HD Jr, McKinley TW, et al: Illness and death due to environmental heat: Georgia and St Louis, 1983. Leads from the MMWR. *JAMA* 252:20–23, 1984.

Inzucchi SE, Maggs DG, Spollett GR, et al: GI Efficacy and metabolic effects of metrormin and troglitazone in type II diabetes mellitus. *N Engl J Med* 338:867–872, 1998.

Kabadi MM, Rosman PM: Thyroid hormone indices in adult healthy subjects: no influence of aging. *J Am Geriatr Soc* 36:312–316, 1988.

Kramer MR, Vandijk J, Rosin AJ: Mortality in elderly patients with thermo-regulatory failure. *Arch Intern Med* 149:1521–1523, 1989.

Lamberts SWJ, van den Beld AW, van der Lely A-J: The endocrinology of aging. *Science* 278:419–424, 1997.

Nicolle LE, Bjornson J, Harding GKM, et al: Bacteriuria in elderly institutionalized men. *N Engl J Med* 309:1420–1425, 1983.

Nicolle LE, Henderson E, Bjornson J, et al: The association of bacteriuria with resident characteristics and survival in elderly institutionalized men. *Ann Intern Med* 106:682–686, 1987a.

Nicolle LE, Mayhew WJ, Bryan L: Prospective randomized comparison of therapy and no therapy for asymptomatic bacteriuria in institutionalized elderly women. *Am J Med* 83:27–33, 1987b.

Nordenstam GR, Brandberg CA, Oden AS, et al: Bacteriuria and mortality in an elderly population. *N Engl J Med* 314:1152–1156, 1986.

Platt R, Polk BF, Murdock B, et al: Mortality associated with nosocomial urinary tract infection. *N Engl J Med* 307:637–642, 1982.

Rango N: Exposure related hypothermia mortality in the United States, 1970–79. *Am J Public Health* 74:1159–1160, 1984.

Ravid M, Brosh D, Levi Z, et al: Use of enalapril to attenuate decline in renal function in normotensive, normoalbuminuric patients with type 2 diabetes mellitus. *Ann Intern Med* 128:982–988, 1998.

Rosenbaum RL, Barzel US: Levothyroxine replacement dose for primary hypothyroidism decreases with age. *Ann Intern Med* 96:53–55, 1982.

Rowe JW, Minaker KC, Sparrow D, et al: Age-related failure of volume-pressure-mediated vasopressin release. *J Clin Endocrinol Metab* 56:661–664, 1982.

Rudman D, Feller AG, Nagroj HS, et al: Effects of human growth hormone in men over 60 years old. *N Engl J Med* 323:1–6, 1990.

Sawin CT, Geller A, Kaplan MM, et al: Low serum thyrotropin (thyroid-stimulating hormone) in older persons without hyperthyroidism. *Arch Intern Med* 151:165–168, 1991.

Sourander LB, Kasanen A: A 5-year follow-up of bacteriuria in the aged. *Gerontol Clin* 14:274–281, 1972.

Stead W: Tuberculosis among elderly persons: An outbreak in a nursing home. *Ann Intern Med* 94:606–610, 1981.

Stead WW, To T: The significance of the tuberculin skin test in elderly persons. *Ann Intern Med* 107:837–842, 1987.

Tenover JS: Effects of testosterone supplementation in the aging male. *J Clin Endocrinol Metab* 75:1092–1098, 1992.

The Medical Letter: Treatment of hypothermia. *Med Lett* 36:116–117, 1994.

White JR. The pharmacologic management of patients with type 2 diabetes mellitus in the era of new oral agents and insulin analogs. *Diabetes Spectrum* 9:227–232, 1996.

Yoshikawa TT, Norman DC: *Aging and Clinical Practice: Infectious Diseases. Diagnosis and Management.* New York, Igaku-Shoin, 1987.

SUGGESTED READINGS

Avery CE, Pestle RE: Hypothermia and the elderly: perceptions and behavior. *Gerontologist* 27:523–526, 1987.

Collins KJ, Exton-Smith AN, James MH, et al: Functional changes in autonomic nervous responses with ageing. *Age Ageing* 9:17–24, 1980.

Collins KJ, Exton-Smith AN: Thermal homeostasis in old age. *J Am Geriatr Soc* 31:519–524, 1983.

Davis PJ, Davis FB: Hyperthyroidism in patients over the age of 60 years. *Medicine* 53:161–181, 1974.

Doucet J, Trivalle C, Chassagne P, et al: Does age play a role in clinical presentation of hypothyroidism? *J Am Geriatr Soc* 42:984–986, 1994.

Elahi D, Muller DC, Tzarkoff SP, et al: Effect of age and obesity on fasting levels of glucose, insulin, glucagon, and growth hormone. *J Gerontol* 37:385–391, 1982.

Federman DD: Hyperthyroidism in the geriatric population. *Hosp Pract* 61–76, 1991.

Foley CJ, Libow LS, Sherman FT: Clinical aspects of nutrition, in Libow LS, Sherman FT (eds): *The Core of Geriatric Medicine.* St Louis, Mosby, 1981.

Gambert SR: Effect of age on thyroid hormone physiology and function. *J Am Geriatr Soc* 33:360–365, 1985.

Gardner ID: The effect of aging on susceptibility to infection. *Rev Infect Dis* 2:801–810, 1980.

Grieco MH: Use of antibiotics in the elderly. *Bull NY Acad Med* 56:197–208, 1980.

Hudson LD, Conn RD: Accidental hypothermia: associated diagnoses and prognosis in a common problem. *JAMA* 227:37–40, 1974.

Jackson RA, Blix PM, Matthews JA, et al: Influence of aging on glucose homeostasis. *J Clin Endocrinol Metab* 55:840–848, 1982.

Khogali M, Weiner JS: Heat stroke: report on 18 cases. *Lancet* 2:276–278, 1980.

Knochel JP, Dallas MD: Environmental heat illness: an eclectic review. *Arch Intern Med* 133:841–864, 1974.

Korenman SG (ed): *Endocrine Aspects of Aging.* New York, Elsevier, 1982.

Lipschitz DA: An overview of anemia in older patients. *Older Patient* 2:5–11, 1988.

MacMillan AL, Corbett JL, Johnson RH, et al: Temperature regulation in survivors of accidental hypothermia of the elderly. *Lancet* 2:165–169, 1967.

Moolten SE: Nutrition in the elderly, in Somers AR, Fabian DR (eds): *The Geriatric Imperative: An Introduction to Gerontological and Clinical Geriatrics.* New York, Appleton-Century-Crofts, 1981.

Morley JE, Mooradian AD, Silver AJ, et al: Nutrition in the elderly. *Ann Intern Med* 109:890–904, 1988.

Morley JE, Silver AJ, Fiatarone M, et al: Geriatric grand rounds: nutrition and the elderly. *J Am Geriatr Soc* 34:823–832, 1986.

Nielsen, HK, Toft P, Koch J, et al: Hypothermic patients admitted to an intensive care unit: a fifteen year survey. *Dan Med Bull* 39:190–193, 1992.

O'Keeffe K: Accidental hypothermia: A review of 63 cases. *J Am Coll Emerg Phys* 6:491–496, 1977.

Phais JP, Kauffman CA, Bjornson A, et al: Host defenses in the aged: evaluation of components of the inflammatory and immune responses. *J Infect Dis* 138:67–73, 1978.

Poehlman ET, Horton ES: Regulation of energy expenditure in aging humans. *Annu Rev Nutr* 10:255–275, 1990.

Reaven GM, Reaven EP: Age, glucose intolerance, and non-insulin-dependent diabetes mellitus. *J Am Geriatr Soc* 33:286–290, 1985.

Report of the Third Ross Roundtable on Medical Issues: *Assessing the Nutritional Status of the Elderly: State of the Art.* Columbus, Ohio, Ross Laboratories, 1982.

Reuler J: Hypothermia: pathophysiology, clinical settings, and management. *Ann Intern Med* 89:519–527, 1978.

Rockstein M, Sussman ML (eds): *Nutrition, Longevity, and Aging.* New York, Academic Press, 1976.

Rosenthal MJ, Hartnell JM, Morley JE, et al: UCLA geriatric grand rounds: diabetes in the elderly. *J Am Geriatr Soc* 35:435–447, 1987.

Rosin AJ, Exton-Smith AN: Clinical features of accidental hypothermia with some observations on thyroid function. *BMJ* 1:16–19, 1964.

Sawin CT, Castelli WP, Hershman JM, et al: The aging thyroid: thyroid deficiency in the Framingham Study. *Arch Intern Med* 145:1386–1388, 1985.

Semenza JC, Rubin CH, Falter KH, et al: Heat-related deaths during the July 1995 heat wave in Chicago. *N Engl J Med* 335:84–90, 1996.

Simon HB: Hyperthermia (review article). *N Engl J Med* 329:483–487, 1993.

Stead WW, To T, Harrison RW, et al: Benefit-risk considerations in preventive treatment for tuberculosis in elderly persons. *Ann Intern Med* 107:843–845, 1987.

Thomas FB, Mazzaferi EL, Skillman TB: Apathetic thyrotoxicosis: a distinctive clinical and laboratory entity. *Ann Intern Med* 72:679–685, 1970.

Treatment of hypothermia. *Med Lett Drugs Ther* 28:123–124, 1986.

Trevino A, Bazi B, Beller BM, et al: The characteristic electrocardiogram of accidental hypothermia. *Arch Intern Med* 127:470–473, 1971.

Trivalle C, Doucet J, Chassagne P, et al: Differences in the signs and symptoms of hyperthyroidism in older and younger patients. *J Am Geriatr Soc* 44:50–53, 1996.

Vogel JM: Hematologic problems of the aged. *Mt Sinai J Med* 47:150–165, 1980.

Walsh JR, Cassel CK, Madler JJ: Iron deficiency in the elderly: it's often nondietary. *Geriatrics* 36:121–132, 1981.

Walsh JR: Hematologic disorders in the elderly. *West J Med* 135:445–446, 1981.

Wheeler M: Heat stroke in the elderly: Symposium on geriatric medicine. *Med Clin North Am* 60:1289–1296, 1976.

Wong KC: Physiology and pharmacology of hypothermia. *West J Med* 138:227–232, 1983.

Wongsurawat N, Davis BB, Morley JE: Thermoregulatory failure in the elderly. *J Am Geriatr Soc* 38:899–906, 1990.

Yoshikawa TT: Antimicrobial therapy for the elderly patient. *J Am Geriatr Soc* 38:1353–1372, 1990.

Yoshikawa TT: Geriatric infectious diseases: An emerging problem. *J Am Geriatr Soc* 31:34–39, 1983.

Yoshikawa TT: Important infections in elderly persons. *West J Med* 135:441–445, 1981.

Yoshikawa TT: Infectious diseases. *Clin Geriatr Med* 8:701–945, 1992.

Yoshikawa TT: Tuberculosis in aging adults. *J Am Geriatr Soc* 40:178–187, 1992.

CHAPTER TWELVE

SENSORY IMPAIRMENT

Because as many as 75 percent of older adults have significant visual and auditory dysfunction not reported to their physicians, adequate screening for these problems is important. These disorders may limit functional activity and lead to social isolation and depression. Correction of remediable conditions may improve ability to perform daily activities.

VISION

Physiologic and Functional Changes

The visual system undergoes many changes with age (Table 12-1). Decreases in visual acuity in old age may be caused by morphological changes in the choroid, pigment epithelium, and retina, or by decreased function of the rods, cones, and other neural elements. Older patients frequently have difficulties turning their eyes upward or sustaining convergence. Intraocular pressure slowly increases with age.

The refractive error may become either more hyperopic or more myopic. In the young, hyperopia may be overcome by the accommoda-

Table 12-1 Physiologic and functional changes of the eye

Functional change	Physiologic change
Visual acuity	Morphologic change in choroid, pigment epithelium, or retina Decreased function of rods, cones, or other neural elements
Extraocular motion	Difficulty in gazing upward and maintaining covergence
Intraocular pressure	Increased pressure
Refractive power	Increased hyperopia and myopia Presbyopia Increased lens size Nuclear sclerosis (lens) Ciliary muscle atrophy
Tear secretion	Decreased tearing Decreased lacrimal gland function Decreased goblet cell secretion
Corneal function	Loss of endothelial integrity Posterior surface pigmentation

tive power of the ciliary muscle on the young lens. However, with age, this latent hyperopia becomes manifest because of loss of accommodative reserve.

Other older patients may show an increase in myopia with age, caused by changes within the lens. The crystalline lens increases in size with age as old lens fibers accumulate in the lens nucleus. The nucleus becomes more compact and harder (nuclear sclerosis), increasing the refractive power of the lens and worsening the myopia.

Another definitive refractive change of aging is the development of presbyopia from nuclear sclerosis of the lens and atrophy of the ciliary muscle. As a result, the closest distance at which one can see clearly slowly recedes with age. At approximately age 45, the near point of accommodation is so far that comfortable reading and near work become cumbersome and difficult. Corrective lenses are then needed to enable the patient to move that point closer to the eyes.

Diminished tear secretion in many older patients, especially post-menopausal women, may lead to dryness of the eyes, which can cause irritation and discomfort. This condition may endanger the intactness

of the corneal surface. The treatment consists mainly in substitution therapy, with artificial tears instilled at frequent intervals.

The corneal endothelium often undergoes degenerative changes with aging. Because these cells seldom proliferate during adult life, the cell population is decreased. This may leave an irregular surface on the anterior chamber side, where pigments may accumulate. This type of endothelial dystrophy is frequently seen in older patients, and dense pigment accumulation may slightly decrease visual acuity. In some patients, the endothelial dystrophy will spontaneously progress and lead to corneal edema. Such cases require corneal transplants.

Blindness

The prevalence of visual problems and blindness increases with age (Fig. 12-1). The most common causes of blindness are cataracts, glaucoma, macular degeneration, and diabetic retinopathy. Screening for these disorders should include testing visual acuity, performing an

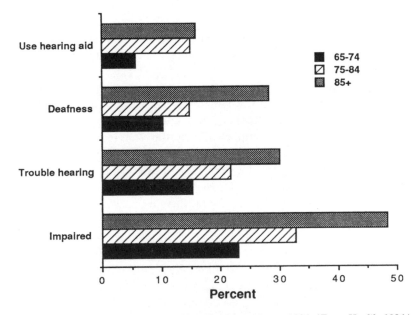

Figure 12-1 Prevalence of vision problems in older persons, 1984, *(From Havlik, 1986.)*

ophthalmoscopic evaluation, and checking intraocular pressure (Table 12-2).

Senile Cataract Opacification of the crystalline lens is a frequent complication of aging. In the Framingham Study, the prevalence of cataracts was associated with age and reached 46 percent at ages 75 to 85 (Kini et al., 1978).

The cause of age-related cataracts is unknown, but the opacifications in the lens are associated with the breakdown of the g-crystalline proteins. Epidemiologic data and basic research suggest that ultraviolet light may be a contributing factor in cataract development (Straatsma et al., 1985). The pathologic process may occur in either the cortex or the nucleus of the lens. Cortical cataracts have various stages of development. Early in the process, opacities are in the periphery and do not decrease visual acuity. At the mature stage, opacifications are more widespread and involve the pupillary area, leading to a slow decrease in visual acuity. In the mature stage, the entire lens becomes opaque. The nuclear cataract does not have these stages of development but is a slowly progressing central opacity, which frequently shows a yellowish discoloration, therefore preventing certain colors from reaching the retina.

Cataracts of mild degree may be managed by periodic examination and optimum eyeglasses for an extended period. Ultraviolet lenses may be of benefit. When a cataract progresses to the point where it interferes with activities, cataract surgery is generally indicated. The surgeon may use several methods to remove it, and the decision regarding the best method for each patient should be made by the ophthalmologist.

In intracapsular cataract extractions, the entire cataract and surrounding capsule are removed in a single piece. This removes the entire opacity. In extracapsular cataract extractions, the cataractous

Table 12-2 Ophthalmologic screening

Visual acuity	Ability to read newspaper-sized print
Lens, fundus	Ophthalmoscopic examination
Intraocular pressure	Tonometry
	Visual fields

lens material and a portion of the capsule are removed. The posterior capsule is left in place to hold an intraocular lens implant.

After cataract removal, the eye has decreased refractive power. Three methods of restoring useful vision are available: eyeglasses, contact lenses, and intraocular lenses (Table 12-3). Approximately 95 percent of those who undergo cataract surgery now receive intraocular lens implants.

Eyeglasses required after surgery are usually thick and heavy. These correct the focus of the eye and permit excellent vision through the central portion. However, they increase the apparent size of the object by about 25 percent, introduce optical distortion, and interfere with peripheral vision. Patients must learn to turn the head instead

Table 12-3 Methods of restoring vision after cataract surgery

Eyeglasses
Are thick and heavy
Provide good central vision
Interfere with peripheral vision
Introduce optical distortion
Increase image size by 25%
Cannot be used after surgery on one eye if other eye is normal

Contact lenses
Correct central and peripheral vision
Increase image size by 6%
Are difficult for some patients to handle
Most require daily insertion and removal
About 50–70% can use extended-wear lenses
Can be used after surgery on one or both eyes
Require reading glasses

Intraocular lenses
Correct central and peripheral vision
Increase image size by 1%
Can be used after surgery on one or both eyes
Are useful for older adults unable to wear contact lenses
Require bifocal eyeglasses
Introduce added surgical and postsurgical complications

of the eyes to see clearly to the side. Eyeglasses can be used for patients who have had surgery on both eyes or surgery on one eye and decreased vision in the other. However, eyeglasses cannot usually be used for patients who have had surgery in one eye and have normal vision in the other eye because of the difference in image size.

Contact lenses correct the focus of the eye, permit both central and peripheral vision, and increase apparent object size by 6 percent. However, handling contact lenses is difficult for some individuals, and most lenses must be removed and inserted daily. Extended-wear contact lenses are available, and about 50 to 70 percent of elderly patients are able to wear them after surgery. Contacts are useful in patients who have had cataract surgery in one or both eyes. The lenses correct for distant vision, but eyeglasses are required for reading.

The intraocular lens is surgically placed inside the iris and is expected to remain permanently in place. This lens corrects the focus of the eyes and permits central and peripheral vision; object size is increased by only 1 percent. It is appropriate for patients with cataracts in one or both eyes and is particularly useful for patients unable to wear a contact lens. Bifocal eyeglasses are usually required to aid distant or near vision.

Glaucoma   The glaucomas are a group of eye disorders characterized by increased intraocular pressure, progressive excavation of the optic nerve head with damage to the nerve fibers, and a specific loss in the visual field. Most cases of primary glaucoma occur in older patients. In the Framingham Study, prevalence of open-angle glaucoma increased with age to 7.2 percent at ages 75 to 85, with men having much higher rates than women (Kini et al., 1978).

Angle-closure glaucoma is an acute and relatively infrequent type of glaucoma, characterized by a sudden painful attack of increased intraocular pressure accompanied by a marked loss in vision. The treatment consists of normalizing the intraocular pressure by the application of miotic eye drops or other medication (such as carbonic anhydrase inhibitors or osmotic agents). The definitive treatment, however, is surgical excision of a peripheral piece of iris or, more frequently now, by laser iridectomy, ensuring free flow of aqueous humor. Because the disease is usually bilateral, some physicians propose prophylactic iridectomy on the second eye.

Chronic open-angle glaucoma is the more frequent variety of primary glaucoma. It is characterized by an insidious onset, slow

progression, and the appearance of typical defects of the visual fields. Early in the disease, intraocular pressure is only moderately elevated, and optic nerve head excavation progresses slowly and sometimes asymmetrically.

While central visual acuity may remain normal for a long time, the defects in the peripheral visual field are characteristic and gradually progressive. Initially there is a paracentral scotoma, which may coalesce. A nasal step of the visual field is another important sign. Finally, the entire field will constrict and eventually involve the visual centers.

The treatment is usually medical, with miotics of various kinds used first. Beta-blocking agents may also be used and have the advantage of not changing the diameter of the pupil. However, care should be taken because these agents may be systemically absorbed. In severe cases, combination drops may be used with systemic medications such as carbonic anhydrase inhibitors. Surgery or laser therapy is indicated only if disease progresses on maximal medical therapy.

Age-Related Macular Degeneration The macular area of the retina lying at the posterior pole of the globe is the site of highest visual acuity. This area depends entirely on choriocapillaries for nutrition. Any disturbance in the vessel wall of the choroidal capillaries, in the permeability or thickness of Bruch's membrane, or in the retinal pigment epithelium may interfere with exchange of nutrients and oxygen from the choroidal blood to the central retina. Such disturbances occur frequently in older patients. Senile degeneration of the macula is one of the most frequent causes of visual loss in older adults and is the commonest cause of legal blindness (20/200 or worse). In the Framingham Study, the prevalence was 28 percent at ages 75 to 85, with a higher rate in women than in men (Kini et al., 1978).

Ophthalmoscopic findings vary and do not always parallel loss of vision. In the "dry" form of degeneration, there are areas of depigmentation alternating with zones of hyperpigmentation caused mainly by changes in the retinal pigment epithelium. In another form, the degeneration involves Bruch's membrane, leading to the pigmentation of well-circumscribed, roundish yellow areas.

The second type of degeneration is an exudative or "wet" type. Here there is an elevated focus in the macular area, which at first

contains serous fluid but later contains blood derived from blood vessels sprouting from the choroid to the subretinal space. The blood may become organized and form a plaque.

In all these cases, central visual acuity will be markedly affected. These patients will gradually lose the ability to read or see any other details. Most macular degeneration is not treatable; however, laser treatment applied at a specific stage of exudative macular degeneration has been effective in preventing central visual loss in some patients (Folk, 1985). Total blindness does not occur, as patients retain peripheral vision and therefore are able to perform activities that do not necessitate acute central vision.

Diabetic Retinopathy In the geriatric population, a significant amount of visual loss is attributed to diabetic retinopathy. The Framingham Study showed an age-associated increase in prevalence up to 7 percent at ages 75 to 85 years (Kini et al., 1978). In the adult-onset diabetic with background changes, the visual loss is usually related to vascular changes in and around the macula. Leakage of serous fluid from vessels surrounding the macula leads to macular edema and deterioration of visual acuity. This may respond to laser photocoagulation. Hemorrhages within the macula may lead to more permanent visual loss. A loss of retinal capillaries may lead to macular ischemia and poor prognosis of visual recovery.

General Factors

Table 12-4 summarizes the general patterns of signs and symptoms associated with common visual problems of older adults. In addition to the specific treatment discussed above, some simple techniques such as use of a magnifying glass, large-print reading material, and reduction of glare can help maximize visual function (see Table 12-5).

Health care providers should also be aware of the significant systemic absorption of ophthalmic medications (Anand and Eschmann, 1988). These agents may lead to other organ-systems dysfunction and interact with other medications (Table 12-6). The patient's other medical problems and medications should be assessed and the minimum dose to achieve the desired effect should be used. Patients should also be monitored for systemic toxicity.

Table 12-4 Signs and symptoms associated with common visual problems in older adults

Signs and symptoms	Cataract	Open-angle glaucoma	Angle-closure glaucoma	Macular degeneration	Temporal arteritis	Diabetic retinopathy
Pain			x		x	
Red eye			x			
Fixed pupil			x			
Retinal vessel changes					x	x
Retinal exudates				x		x
Optic disk changes		x			x	
Sudden visual loss			x		x	
Loss of peripheral vision		x				
Glare intolerance	x					
Elevated intraocular pressure		x	x			
Loss of visual acuity	x	x		x		x

Table 12-5 Aids to maximize visual function

Magnifying glass
Soft light, flat paint to avoid glare
Tinted glasses to reduce glare
Night light to assist in adaptation
Large-print newpapers, books, and magazines

Table 12-6 Potential adverse effects of ophthalmic solutions

Drug	Organ system	Responses
Beta blockers (e.g., timolol)	Cardiovascular	Bradycardia, hypotension, syncope, palpitation, congestive heart failure
	Respiratory	Bronchospasm
	Neurologic	Mental confusion, depression, fatigue, lightheadedness, hallucinations, memory impairment, sexual dysfunction
	Miscellaneous	Hyperkalemia
Adrenergics (e.g., epinephrine, phenylephrine)	Cardiovascular	Extrasystoles, palpitation, hypertension, myocardial infarction
	Miscellaneous	Trembling, paleness, sweating
Cholinergic/ anticholinesterases (e.g., pilocarpine, echothiophate)	Respiratory	Bronchospasm
	Gastrointestinal	Salivation, nausea, vomiting, diarrhea, abdominal pain, tenesmus
	Miscellaneous	Lacrimation, sweating
Anticholinergic (e.g., atropine)	Neurologic	Ataxia, nystagmus, restlessness, mental confusion, hallucination, violent and aggressive behavior
	Miscellaneous	Insomnia, photophobia, urinary retention

Source: Anand and Eschmann, 1988.

HEARING

This section covers four areas related to hearing problems in older adults: a review of the major parts of the auditory system, tests used to evaluate the hearing system, effects of aging on hearing performance, and specific pathologic disorders affecting the auditory system.

Hearing problems are common in the elderly, especially in a highly industrialized society where noise and age interact to cause hearing loss (Fig. 12-2). This loss is usually of the sensorineural type due to damage of the hearing organ, the peripheral nervous system, and/or the central nervous system. These hearing problems are not usually amenable to medical or surgical intervention and thus require hearing aids, aural rehabilitation, and understanding as the major avenues of remediation.

The Auditory System

On a functional basis, the auditory system can be divided into three major parts: peripheral, brainstem, and cortical areas (Table 12-7).

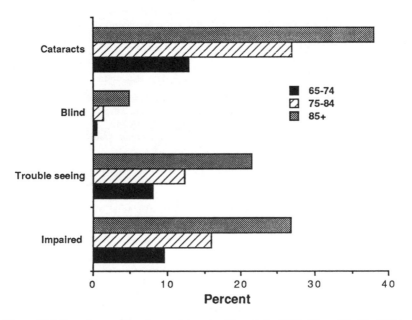

Figure 12-2 Prevalence of hearing problems in older adults, 1984. *(From Havlik, 1986.)*

Table 12-7   Peripheral and central auditory nervous system

A. External ear and peripheral hearing mechanism
   1. Auricle
   2. Tympanic membrane
   3. Ossicular chain
   4. Eustachian tube
   5. Cochlea
      a. Bony labyrinth
      a. Membranous labyrinth
   6. Cochlear nerve
B. Auditory areas in the brainstem
   1. Entrance of the VIIIth cranial nerve
   2. Cochlear nucleus
   3. Superior olivary complex
   4. Lateral lemniscus
   5. Inferior colliculus
   6. Medial geniculate
   7. Auditory radiations (brainstem-to-cortex tract)
C. Auditory areas in the cortex
   1. Temporal lobe
   2. Parietal lobe
   3. Corpus callosum

Each part of the hearing system has unique functions, which combine to allow hearing and understanding of speech. These functions are listed in Table 12-8.

The main functions of the peripheral auditory system are to change sound into a series of electrical impulses and to transmit those to the brainstem. The major brainstem function is binaural interaction. Binaural interaction allows localization of sound and extraction of a signal from a noisy environment. The cortex brings sound to consciousness and allows interpretation of speech and initiation of appropriate reactions to sound signals.

Assessment

Assessment of hearing function can be divided into three kinds of hearing tests: standard, binaural, and difficult speech. The standard tests are useful for evaluating the peripheral system, binaural tests for evaluating the brainstem, and difficult speech tests for evaluating

Table 12-8 Functional components of the auditory system

A. Transmission of signals in the periphery
   1. Molecular motion (ear canal)
   2. Mechanical vibration (eardrum and ossicles)
   3. Hydromechanical motion (inner ear)
   4. Electrical impulse (eighth nerve)
B. Binaural interaction in the brainstrem
   1. Localization and lateralization of sound
   2. Extraction of signals from environmental noise
C. Speech processing in the cortex
   1. Conscious sensation of hearing
   2. Interpretation of speech
   3. Initiation of response to sound

cortical problems (Table 12-9). Standard tests are performed by presenting pure tones or single words at varying intensity. An audioscope (Welch-Allyn, Inc.) that will deliver pure tones is now available for the office screening of hearing deficits (Lichtenstein et al., 1988). Tympanic membrane movement is assessed with a probe. Loudness comparison assesses the individual's ability to balance intensity of sound coming from both ears; lateralization tests the individual's ability to fuse sounds from both ears; and masking level differences assesses the ability to pick out specific sounds from a background of noise. Monotic degraded tasks present difficult sounds such as noise

Table 12-9 Assessment of hearing function

A. Standard test measures
   1. Sensitivity for tones and speech
   2. Speech discrimination/understanding
   3. Movement of tympanic membrane
B. Binaural tests
   1. Loudness comparison
   2. Lateralization
   3. Masking level differences
C. Difficult speech tests
   1. Monotic degraded tasks
   2. Dichotic tasks

Table 12-10   Effects of aging on the hearing mechanism

Atrophy and disappearance of cells in the inner ear
Angiosclerosis in the inner ear
Calcification of membranes in the inner ear
Bioelectric and biomechanical imbalances in the inner ear
Degeneration and loss of ganglion cells and their fibers in the eighth cranial nerve
Eighth nerve canal closure, with destruction of nerve fibers
Atrophy and cell loss at all auditory centers in the brainstem
Reduction of cells in auditory areas of the cortex

background, filtered sound, and time-compressed speech; dichotic tasks simultaneously present sense and nonsense speech, which the individual is asked to repeat.

Aging Changes

Many changes in the peripheral and central auditory system during aging have effects on the hearing mechanism (Table 12-10). These changes lead to diminished performance by older subjects (Table 12-11), including the loss of sensitivity and distortion of signals that succeed in passing to higher levels, difficulty in localizing signals and in taking advantage of two-ear listening, difficulty understanding speech under unfavorable listening conditions, and problems with language, especially when aging is compounded by stroke.

Three major factors enhance the progression of hearing loss with

Table 12-11   Hearing performance in older adults

A. Peripheral pathology
   1. Hearing loss for pure tones
   2. Hearing loss for speech
   3. Problems understanding speech
B. Brainstem pathology
   1. Problems localizing sounds
   2. Problems in binaural listening
C. Cortical pathology
   1. Problems with difficult speech
   2. Language problems

advancing age: previous middle-ear disease, vascular disease, and exposure to noise. These factors alone do not, however, account for the hearing loss of old age, called *presbycusis*. Although clinically and pathologically complex, this is a distinct progressive sensorineural hearing loss associated with aging. The deterioration is not limited to the peripheral sensory receptor. Presbycusis affects 60 percent of individuals over age 65 in the United States. However, only a fraction of these have a functional deficit necessitating aural rehabilitation.

Sensitivity

Beginning with the third decade of life, there is a deterioration in the hearing threshold. At first, sensitivity at the high frequencies declines gradually. This age-associated loss has been confirmed in populations not exposed to high levels of noise. This gradual impairment is sensorineural and can be tested by pure-tone audiometry, which reveals useful information about the physiologic condition of hearing but does not disclose some important aspects of deterioration.

Speech

Although there is a close relationship between pure tone loss and ability to hear speech, the audiogram does not precisely measure hearing for speech. To assess this auditory function, speech audiometry can be performed by presenting the undistorted test words above threshold intensities in the absence of background noise.

Older people with hearing impairment may have difficulty understanding speech under less favorable conditions, as with background noise, under poor acoustic conditions, or when speech is rapid. This difficulty may be caused in part by the longer time required by higher auditory centers to identify the message. Such hearing loss may necessitate testing of desired signals with the presentation of a competing signal. This will more accurately reflect hearing of speech in social circumstances.

Speech occurring in rooms that cause long reverberations is also much less intelligible to the elderly. Auditory temporal discrimination and auditory reaction time and frequency discrimination also decline with age. Because consonant sounds are of higher frequency and shorter duration, the loss of high-frequency hearing in the elderly may affect these sounds, which encode much of speech information. Lipreading may compensate to some extent for this effect on understanding speech, but other factors of processing information still remain.

Loudness

A common auditory problem of the elderly is abnormal loudness perception. This can occur as hypersensitivity to sounds of high intensity and appears as increased "loudness recruitment," in which gradually increasing loudness such as amplified sound is unpleasantly harsh and difficult to tolerate. In older adults with hearing impairment, this abnormality is manifest when a speaker is asked to speak louder or the output of a hearing aid is increased. It may result from a sensorineural loss attributable to changes in the hair cells of the inner ear.

Localization

Sound localization contributes to effectiveness of signal detection and helps with discrimination. Loss of directional hearing results in greater hearing difficulty in a noisy environment. Localization is disturbed in older adults with hearing loss and may be partly caused by the aging brain's deranged processing of interaural intensity differences and time delays. A strongly asymmetrical hearing loss also disturbs localization.

Tinnitus

Tinnitus, an internal noise generated within the hearing system, occurs in many types of hearing disorders at all ages but is much more frequent in older adults. Tinnitus, however, is not necessarily associated with hearing loss and may occur in older adults without hearing impairment. Estimates of prevalence in those aged 65 to 74 are about 11 percent (Fisch, 1978). Treatment is generally unsatisfactory.

Other Hearing Disorders

One of the most easily treatable but too easily overlooked causes of hearing loss is cerumen that occludes the external auditory canal (see Table 12-12). Cerumen usually affects low-frequency sounds and complicates existing hearing impairments.

Hearing loss in the geriatric patient may be caused by scarring of the tympanic membrane. In tympanosclerosis, there is calcification of the tympanic membrane that results in stiffening of the drumhead.

Otosclerosis may cause fixation of the ossicular chain and lead to a conduction hearing loss. The bony capsule may also be affected,

**Table 12-12 Disorders of
hearing in older adults**

Cerumen plug
Tympanosclerosis
Otosclerosis
Paget's disease
Ototoxic medications
Sound trauma
CNS lesions
Pseudo-deafness (depression)

leading to sensorineural loss. Paget's disease may also lead to both kinds of hearing loss and should be evaluated radiologically and by an alkaline phosphatase determination.

Ototoxic medication is an acquired cause of hearing loss producing cochlear damage. The aminoglycoside antibiotics require special caution. At high doses, ethacrynic acid and furosemide may be ototoxic. High doses of aspirin may cause a reversible hearing impairment. Unfortunately, except for aspirin, removal of the offending drug usually does not reverse the sensorineural loss.

Sound trauma is an environmental factor with neurosensory consequences. Superimposed on the changes of aging, sound trauma can have a severe impact on a patient's communicative ability.

Vascular or mass lesions may affect hearing at one of several levels, including the middle and inner ear, auditory nerve, brainstem, and cortex.

Aural Rehabilitation

Every individual who has communication difficulties caused by a permanent hearing loss should have an ear, nose, and throat evaluation to rule out remediable disease and then an audiological evaluation to assess the roles of amplification and aural rehabilitation. Factors that should be considered during the evaluation for a hearing aid are listed in Table 12-13. In the severely impaired, aural rehabilitation with speech reading may be necessary in addition to a hearing aid. Family counseling may also improve utilization and satisfaction with an aid.

Table 12-13   Factors in evaluation for a hearing aid

Exclude contraindicating medical or other correctable problem
Greatest satisfaction is achieved with aid if loss is 55–80 dB; there is only partial
help if loss is greater than 80 dB
Less satisfaction is achieved when poor discrimination is present
Aid is specifically designed for face-to-face conversation; patient's expectations
should be realistic
Aid may need to be combined with lipreading
Loudness perception abnormalities may make aid unacceptable
More severe hearing loss requires aid worn on the body rather than behind-the-ear
device
Assess for monaural or binaural aids
Assess for patient's ability to handle aid independently
Assess patient's motivation for using an aid

Improvements and modifications in design and construction of hearing aids have enabled a greater proportion of the hearing-impaired population to profit from amplification. The old adage that hearing aids will not help people with sensorineural loss is simply not true. The aid can be adjusted to a specific frequency rather than all frequencies, thus decreasing loudness problems, improving discrimination, and making the aid more acceptable. Binaural aids improve sound localization and discrimination.

The hearing aid that is worn on the body provides the greatest amplification but is necessary only for patients with the most severe hearing loss. The controls are large and therefore more easily managed by some elderly persons. However, many elderly people prefer behind-the-ear or in-the-ear devices. The in-the-ear devices are small, cosmetically more acceptable, but more difficult to manipulate.

Although expensive, cochlear implants can restore hearing in individuals with severe hearing loss not corrected by hearing aids.

TASTE

During aging there is a significant loss of lingual papillae and an associated diminution of ability to taste. Salivary secretion also diminishes, thus decreasing solubilization of flavoring agents. Upper dentures may cover secondary taste sites and decrease taste acuity.

Olfactory bulbs also show significant atrophy with old age. Taste and olfactory changes together may account for the lessened interest in food shown by older adults.

ACKNOWLEDGMENT

The authors wish to thank Dr. Douglas Noffsinger for his assistance in preparing material for an earlier version of the section on hearing in this chapter.

REFERENCES

Anand KB, Eschmann E: Systemic effects of ophthalmic medication in the elderly. *NY State J Med* 88:134–136, 1988.

Fisch L: Special senses: the aging auditory system, in Brocklehurst JC (ed): *Textbook of Geriatric Medicine and Gerontology.* New York, Churchill Livingstone, 1978.

Folk JC: Aging macular degeneration. Clinical features of treatable disease. *Ophthalmology* 92:594–602, 1985.

Havlik RJ: Aging in the eighties: impaired senses for sound and light in persons age 65 years and over. *NCHS Advance data,* No. 125, 1986.

Kini MM, Liebowitz HM, Colton T, et al: Prevalence of senile cataract, diabetic retinopathy, senile macular degeneration, and open-angle glaucoma in the Framingham Eye Study. *Am J Ophthalmol* 85:28–34, 1978.

Lichtenstein MJ, Bess FH, Logan SA: Validation of screening tools for identifying hearing-impaired elderly in primary care. *JAMA* 259:2875–2878, 1988.

Straatsma BR, Foos RY, Horowitz J, et al: Aging related cataract: Laboratory investigation and clinical management. *Ann Intern Med* 102:82–92, 1985.

SUGGESTED READINGS

Blodi FC: Eye problems of the elderly. *Ophthalmologica* 181:121–128, 1980.

Capino DG, Liebowitz HM: Age-related macular degeneration. *Hosp Pract* 23:23–25, 29–30, 36–38, 1988.

Koopmann CF Jr: Symposium of Geriatric Otolaryngology. *Otolaryngol Clin North Am* 15(2):293–312, 1982.

Kornzweig AL: Visual loss in the elderly, in Reichel W (ed): *The Geriatric Patient.* New York, HP Publishing, 1978.

Lavizzo-Mourey RJ, Siegler EL: Hearing impairment in the elderly. *J Gen Intern Med* 7:191–198, 1992.

Liesegang TJ: Cataracts and cataract operations. *Mayo Clin Proc* 59:622–632, 1984.

Mader S: Hearing impairment in elderly persons. *J Am Geriatr Soc* 32:548–553, 1984.

Margolis M, Levy B, Sherman FT: Hearing disorders, in Libow LS, Sherman FT (eds): *The Core of Geriatric Medicine.* St Louis, Mosby, 1981.

Marmor MF: Age-related eye diseases and their effects on visual function, in Faye EE, Stuen CS (eds): *The Aging Eye and Low Vision.* New York, The Lighthouse, 1992.

Marmor MF: Normal age-related vision changes and their effects on vision, in Faye EE, Stuen CS (eds): *The Aging Eye and Low Vision.* New York, The Lighthouse, 1992.

Mulrow CD, Lichtenstein MJ: Screening for hearing impairment in the elderly: rationale and strategy. *J Gen Intern Med* 6:249–258, 1991.

Roush J (ed): Aging and hearing impairment. *Semin Hearing* 6:99–219, 1985.

Ruben RJ: Otolaryngologic problems, in Reichel W (ed): *The Geriatric Patient.* New York, HP Publishing, 1978.

Uhlmann RF, Rees TS, Psatz BM, et al: Validity and reliability of auditory screening tests in demented and non-demented older adults. *J Gen Intern Med* 4:90–96, 1989.

PART
THREE

GENERAL MANAGEMENT
STRATEGIES

THIRTEEN

DRUG THERAPY

Geriatric patients are frequently prescribed multiple drugs in complex dosage schedules. In some instances this is justified because of the presence of multiple chronic medical conditions on which acute illnesses are superimposed. In most instances, however, complex drug regimens are unnecessary; they are excessively costly and predispose to noncompliance and adverse drug reactions. Many older patients are prescribed multiple drugs, take over-the-counter drugs, and are then prescribed additional drugs to treat the side effects of medications they are already taking. This scenario can result in an upward spiral in the number of drugs being taken and commonly leads to polypharmacy.

Several important considerations, some pharmacologic and others nonpharmacologic, influence the safety and effectiveness of drug therapy in the geriatric population. This chapter focuses on these considerations and attempts to give practical suggestions for prescribing drugs for this population. Drug therapy for specific geriatric conditions is discussed in several other chapters throughout this text.

NONPHARMACOLOGIC FACTORS INFLUENCING DRUG THERAPY

Discussions of geriatric pharmacology frequently center around age-related changes in drug pharmacokinetics and pharmacodynamics. Although these changes are sometimes of clinical importance, non-pharmacologic factors can play an even greater role in the safety and effectiveness of drug therapy in the geriatric population. Several steps make drug therapy safe and effective (Fig. 13-1). Many factors can interfere with this scheme in the geriatric population, and, as can be seen, most of them come into play before pharmacologic considerations arise.

Effective drug therapy can be hampered by inaccurate diagnoses. Many older patients tend to underreport symptoms; complaints of others may be vague and multiple. Symptoms of physical diseases frequently overlap with symptoms of psychological illness. To add to this complexity, many diseases present with atypical symptoms. Thus, making the correct diagnoses and prescribing the appropriate drugs are often difficult tasks in the geriatric population.

There is a tendency among health care professionals to treat symptoms with drugs rather than to evaluate the symptoms thoroughly. Because older patients tend to have multiple problems and complaints and may consult several health care professionals, they often end up with prescriptions for several drugs. Moreover, older patients or their family members sometimes exert pressure on health care professionals to prescribe medication, thus adding to the tendency for polypharmacy.

All too frequently, neither the patients nor the health care professionals have a clear picture of the total drug regimen. New patients undergoing initial geriatric assessment should be asked to empty their medicine cabinets and bring all bottles to their first appointments. Medication records, such as the one shown in Fig. 13-2, carried by the patient and maintained as an integral part of the overall medical record may help to eliminate some of the polypharmacy and noncompliance common in the geriatric population. Such records should be updated at each patient visit. Drug regimens should be simplified whenever possible and patients instructed to discard old medications.

Compliance plays a central role in the success of drug therapy in all age groups (Fig. 13-1). In addition to the tendency for polyphar-

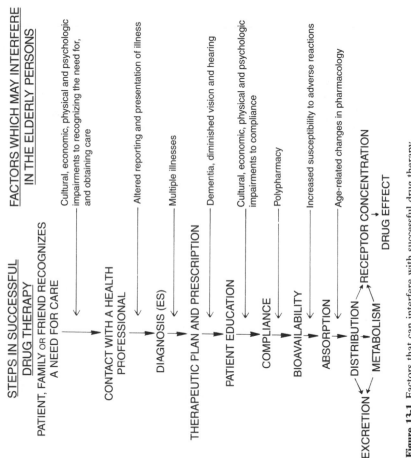

Figure 13-1 Factors that can interfere with successful drug therapy.

NAME _____ DOCTOR _____ PHONE: ( ) _____

MEDICATION NAME	REASON FOR USE	DESCRIBE OR TAPE MEDICINE HERE	WHEN TO TAKE MEDICINE				SPECIAL NOTES

REMEMBER

BRING THIS CHART TO ALL DOCTOR APPOINTMENTS
INCLUDE ALL THE MEDICATIONS YOU ARE TAKING
DO NOT CHANGE THE WAY YOU TAKE THE MEDICATIONS WITHOUT CALLING THE DOCTOR
DO NOT SHARE MEDICATIONS
IF YOU HAVE ANY QUESTIONS, CALL THE DOCTOR

Figure 13-2 Example of a medication record.

macy and complex dosage schedules, older patients face other potential barriers to compliance. The chronic nature of illness in the geriatric population can play a role in noncompliance. The consequences of these illnesses are often delayed (as opposed to the more dramatic effects of acute illnesses), and chronic illnesses necessitate ongoing prophylactic or suppressive rather than relatively short and time-limited courses of therapy. Compliance tends to be poor for these types of drug regimens. Diminished hearing, impaired vision, and poor short-term memory are relatively common in the geriatric population, and all can interfere with patient education and compliance. Problems with transportation can make getting to a pharmacy difficult. Outpatient prescriptions are not covered by Medicare, thus forcing older persons to pay for their drugs from a limited income. Some older people have "Medigap" insurance, which covers some medication costs, and capitated programs commonly offer drug benefits (often limited to a formulary). Even if the older person gets to the pharmacy, can afford the prescription, understands the instructions, and remembers when to take it, the use of childproof bottles and tamper-resistant packaging may hinder compliance in those with arthritic or weak hands.

Several strategies might improve compliance in the geriatric population (Table 13-1). As few drugs as possible should be prescribed, and the dosage schedule should be as simple as possible. Drugs should be given on the same dosage schedules whenever possible (e.g., twice daily, three times daily), and the administration should correspond

Table 13-1 Strategies to improve compliance in the geriatric population

1. Making drug regimens and instructions as simple as possible.
   a. Use the same dosage schedule whenever feasible (e.g., once or twice per day)
   b. Time the doses in conjunction with a daily routine.
2. Instruct relatives and caregivers on the drug regimen.
3. Enlist others (e.g., home health aides, pharmacists) to help ensure compliance.
4. Make sure the older patient can get to a pharmacist (or vice versa), can afford the prescriptions, and can open the container.
5. Use aids (such as special pillboxes and drug calendars) whenever appropriate.
6. Keep updated medication records (Fig. 13-2).
7. Review knowledge of and compliance with drug regimens regularly.

to a daily routine in order to enhance the consistency of taking the drugs and compliance. For many drugs, once-daily dosing is available and should be prescribed when clinically appropriate. Relatives or other caregivers should be instructed in the drug regimen, and they as well as others (e.g., home health aides and pharmacists) should be enlisted to help the older patients comply. Specially designed pill dispensers, dosage calendars, and other innovative techniques can be useful. (At a minimum, prescriptions should instruct the pharmacist not to use the childproof container whenever appropriate.) Geriatric patients (as well as their health care professionals) should keep an updated record of the drug regimen (Fig. 13-2). Medications should be brought to appointments, and patients and families should show all medications to their physicians, particularly on initial visits to new primary care physicians or at a consultation with a specialist. Health care professionals should regularly inquire about other medications being taken (prescribed by other physicians or purchased over the counter) and review their patients' knowledge of and compliance with the drug regimen.

ADVERSE DRUG REACTIONS AND INTERACTIONS

Primum nonnocere ("first, do no harm"), a watchword phrase in the practice of medicine, is nowhere more applicable than when drugs are being prescribed for the geriatric population. Adverse drug reactions are the most common forms of iatrogenic illness (see Chap. 4). The incidence of adverse drug reactions in hospitalized patients increases from about 10 percent in those between 40 to 50 years of age to 25 percent in those above age 80 (Seidel et al., 1966; Steel et al., 1981; Lazarou et al., 1998). They account for between 3 and 10 percent of hospital admissions (Caranasos et al., 1974; Williamson and Chopin, 1980) and result in several billion dollars in yearly health care expenditures. Many drugs commonly prescribed for geriatric patients produce distressing and sometimes potentially disabling or life-threatening adverse reactions (Table 13-2). Psychotropic drugs and cardiovascular agents are common causes of serious adverse reactions in the geriatric population. In part, this is because of the narrow therapeutic-toxic ratio of many of these drugs. In some instances, age-related changes in pharmacology, such as diminished renal excretion

Table 13-2 Examples of common and potentially serious adverse drug reactions in the geriatric population

Drug	Common adverse reactions
Analgesics	
Anti-inflammatory agents	Gastric irritation and ulcers Chronic blood loss
Narcotic	Constipation
Antimicrobials	
Aminoglycosides	Renal failure Hearing loss
Antiparkinsonian drugs	
Dopaminergic agents	Nausea Delirium Hallucinations Postural hypotension
Anticholinergics	Dry mouth Constipation Urinary retention Delirium
Cardiovascular drugs	
Angiotensin converting enzyme (ACE) inhibitors	Cough Impaired renal function
Antiarrhythmics	Diarrhea (quinidine) Urinary retention (disopyramide)
Anticoagulants	Bleeding complications
Antihypertensives	Hypotension Sedation and/or other changes in mental function
Calcium channel blockers	Decreased myocardial contractility Edema Constipation
Diuretics	Dehydration Hyponatremia Hypokalemia Incontinence

(continued)

Table 13-2 Examples of common and potentially serious adverse drug reactions in the geriatric population *(Continued)*

Drug	Common adverse reactions
Cardiovascular drugs	
Digoxin	Arrhythmias Nausea Anorexia
Nitrates	Hypotension
Hypoglycemic agents	
Insulin Oral agents	Hypoglycemia
Psychotropic drugs	
Antidepressants	(see Chap. 6)
Antipsychotics	Sedation Hypotension Extrapyramidal movement disorders
Lithium	Weakness Tremor Nausea Delirium
Sedative and hypnotic agents	Excessive sedation Delirium Gait disturbances
Others	
Alendronate	Esophageal ulceration
Aminophylline	Gastric irritation Tachyarrhythmias
Carbamazepine	Anemia Hyponatremia Neutropenia
Cimetidine	Mental status changes
Terbutaline	Tremor

and prolonged duration of action, predispose to adverse reactions. Some side effects can have a therapeutic benefit and may be key factors in drug selection (see below).

Because symptoms can be nonspecific or may mimic other illnesses, adverse drug reactions may be ignored or unrecognized. In some instances, another drug is prescribed to treat these symptoms, thus contributing to polypharmacy and increasing the likelihood of an adverse drug interaction. The problem of polypharmacy is exacerbated by visits to multiple physicians who may prescribe still more drugs. Medication records kept by the patient (Fig. 13-2) as well as the physician's medical record should help to prevent unnecessary polypharmacy when many physicians are involved. Several drugs commonly prescribed for the geriatric population can interact, with adverse consequences (Table 13-3). The more common types of potential adverse drug interactions are drug displacement from protein-binding sites by other highly protein-bound drugs, induction or suppression of the metabolism of other drugs, and additive effects of different drugs on blood pressure and mental function (mood, level of consciousness, etc.). In addition to the potential to interact with other drugs, several drugs can interact adversely with underlying medical conditions in the geriatric population, creating "drug-patient" interactions (Table 13-4). A good example of this problem is the increased risk of hospitalization for congestive heart failure among older patients taking diuretics who are told to take a nonsteroidal anti-inflammatory drug (Heerdink et al., 1998).

Health care professionals should have a thorough knowledge of the more common drug side effects, adverse reactions to drugs, and potential drug interactions in the geriatric population. Careful questioning about side effects should be an important part of reviewing the drug regimen at each visit. Many institutions use computers to detect potential adverse drug interactions and prevent their occurrence. Several software programs are now available that can assist in identifying potential adverse drug interactions. With or without this computer capability, special attention should be given to the potential for a newly prescribed drug to interact with drugs already being taken or with underlying medical or psychological conditions.

Table 13-3 Examples of potentially clinically important drug-drug interactions

Interaction	Examples	Potential effects
Interference with drug absorption	Antacids interacting with digoxin, INH, antipsychotics Enteral tube feedings and liquid phenytoin Iron and ciprofloxacin	Diminished drug effectiveness
Displacement from binding proteins	Warfarin, oral hypoglycemics, aspirin, chloral hydrate, other highly protein-bound drugs (see Table 13-6)	Enhanced effects and increased risk of toxicity
Altered distribution	Digoxin and quinidine	Increased risk of toxicity
Altered metabolism	Ketoconazole, erythromycin, SSRIs, with antihistamines, calcium channel blockers, others*	Decreased metabolism, increased levels of toxicity
Altered excretion	Lithium and diuretics	Increased risk of toxicity and electrolyte imbalance
Pharmacologic antagonism	Levodopa and clonidine	Decreased antiparkinsonian effects
Pharmacologic synergism	Tricyclic antidepressants and antihypertensives	Increased risk of hypotension

Key: INH, isonicotine hydrazine; SSRI, selective serotonin inhibitor.
* See text.

Table 13-4 Examples of potential clinically important drug-patient interactions

Drug	Patient factors	Clinical implications
Diuretics	Diabetes	Decreased glucose tolerance
	Poor nutritional status	Increased risk of dehydration and electrolyte imbalance
	Urinary frequency, urgency	Incontinence may result
Angiotensin converting enzyme (ACE) inhibitors	Renovascular disease	Worsening renal function
	Stress incontinence	Precipitate incontinence
Beta blockers	Diabetes	Sympathetic response to hypoglycemia may be masked
	Chronic obstructive lung disease	Increased bronchospasm
	CHF	Decreased myocardial contractility
	Peripheral vascular disease	Increased claudication
Narcotic analgesics	Chronic constipation	Worsening symptoms, fecal impaction
Tricyclic antidepressants	CHF, angina	Tachycardia, decreased myocardial contractility, postural hypotension exacerbating cardiovascular conditions
Tricyclic antidepressants, antihistamines, and other drugs with anticholinergic effects	Constipation, glaucoma and other visual impairments, prostatic hyperplasia, reflux esophagitis	Worsening of symptoms
Antipsychotics	Parkinsonism	Worsening of immobility
Psychotropics	Dementia	Further impairment of cognitive function
Nonsteroidal anti-inflammatory drugs	CHF, on diuretics	Increased risk of exacerbation of CHF

AGING AND PHARMACOLOGY

Several age-related biological and physiologic changes are relevant to drug pharmacology (Table 13-5). With the exception of changes in renal function, however, the effects of these age-related changes on dosages of specific drugs for individual patients are variable and difficult to predict. In general, an understanding of the physiologic status of each patient (taking into account factors such as state of hydration, nutrition, and cardiac output) and how that status affects the pharmacology of a particular drug is more important to clinical efficacy than are age-related changes. New technology in drug delivery

Table 13-5 Age-related changes relevant to drug pharmacology

Pharmacologic parameter	Age-related changes

Absorption	Decreases in
	    Absorptive surface
	    Splanchnic blood flow
	Increased gastric pH
	Altered gastrointestinal motility

Distribution	Decreases in
	    Total body water
	    Lean body mass
	    Serum albumin
	Increased fat
	Altered protein binding

Metabolism	Decreases in
	    Liver blood flow
	    Enzyme activity
	    Enzyme inducibility

Excretion	Decreases in
	    Renal blood flow
	    Glomerular filtration rate
	    Tubular secretory function

Tissue sensitivity	Alterations in
	    Receptor number
	    Receptor affinity
	    Second-messenger function
	    Cellular and nuclear responses

systems, such as oral sustained-release preparations and skin patches, have been developed for many medications. Such technology may be useful in designing strategies to account for the effect of aging changes on pharmacology and to make many drugs safer in the geriatric population. Given these caveats, the effects of aging on each pharmacologic process are briefly discussed below.

Absorption

Several aging changes occur that can affect drug absorption (Table 13-5). Studies of several drugs, however, have failed to document any clinically meaningful alterations in drug absorption with increasing age. Absorption, therefore, appears to be the pharmacologic parameter least affected by increasing age.

Distribution

In contrast to absorption, clinically meaningful changes in drug distribution can occur with increasing age. Serum albumin, the major drug-binding protein, tends to decline, especially in hospitalized patients. Although the decline is numerically small, it can substantially increase the amount of free drug available for action. This effect is of particular relevance for highly protein-bound drugs, especially when they are used simultaneously and compete for protein-binding sites (see Table 13-3).

Age-related changes in body composition can prominently affect pharmacology by altering the volume of distribution (Vd). The elimination half-life of a drug varies with the ratio Vd/drug clearance. Thus, even if the rate of clearance of a drug is unchanged with age, changes in Vd can affect a drug's half-life and duration of action.

Because total body water and lean body mass decline with increasing age, drugs that distribute in these body compartments (such as most antimicrobial agents, digoxin, lithium, and alcohol) may have a lower Vd and can, therefore, achieve higher concentrations from given amounts of drugs. On the other hand, drugs that distribute in body fat (such as many of the psychotropic agents) have a large Vd in the geriatric patients. The larger Vd will thus cause a prolongation of

the half-life unless the clearance increases proportionately (which is unlikely to happen with increasing age).

Metabolism

The effects of aging on drug metabolism are complex and difficult to predict. They depend on the precise pathway of drug metabolism in the liver and on several other factors (such as gender and amount of smoking). There is evidence that the first, or preparative, phase of drug metabolism (including oxidations, reductions, and hydrolyses) declines with increasing age, and that the decline is more prominent in men than in women. In contrast, the second phase of drug metabolism (biotransformation, including acetylation and glucuronidation) appears to be less affected by age (Greenblatt et al., 1982). There is also evidence that the ability of environmental factors (most importantly smoking) to induce drug-metabolizing enzymes declines with age. Even when liver function is obviously impaired (by intrinsic liver disease, right-sided congestive heart failure, etc.), the effects of aging on the metabolism of specific drugs cannot be precisely predicted. It is *not* safe to assume, however, that geriatric patients with normal liver function tests can metabolize drugs as efficiently as can younger individuals.

The cytochrome P450 system in the liver has been extensively studied. Over thirty isoenzymes have been identified and classified into families and subfamilies. Genetic mutations in some of these enzymes, while relatively uncommon, can impair metabolism of specific drugs. Although aging may affect this system, the effects of commonly used drugs are probably more important. Ketoconazole, erythromycin, and the selective serotonin reuptake inhibitors (SSRIs, especially fluoxetine) can inhibit the metabolism of several drugs (see Chap. 6). Potentially fatal ventricular arrhythmias can be caused by high levels of the antihistamines terfenadine and astemizole, resulting from inhibition of these enzymes.

Excretion

Unlike those of metabolism, the effects of aging on renal functions are somewhat more predictable. The tendency for renal function to decline with increasing age can affect the pharmacokinetics of several

drugs (and their active metabolites) that are eliminated predominantly by the kidney (Table 13-6). These drugs will be cleared from the body more slowly, their half-lives (and duration of action) will be prolonged, and there will be a tendency to accumulate to higher (and potentially toxic) drug concentrations in the steady state.

Several considerations are important in determining the effects of age on renal function and drug elimination:

1. There is wide interindividual variation in the rate of decline of renal function with increasing age. Thus, although renal function is said to decline by 50 percent between the ages of 20 and 90, this is an *average* decline. A 90-year-old individual may not have a creatinine clearance of only 50 percent of normal. Applying average declines to individual elderly patients can result in over- or under-dosing.
2. Muscle mass declines with age; therefore, daily endogenous creatinine production declines. Because of this decline in creatinine production, serum creatinine may be normal at a time when renal function is substantially reduced. Serum creatinine, therefore, does not reflect renal function as accurately in the elderly as it does in younger persons.
3. A number of factors can affect renal clearance of drugs and are often at least as important as age-related changes. State of hydration, cardiac output, and intrinsic renal disease, among other factors, should be considered in addition to age-related changes in renal function.

Several formulas and nomograms have been used to estimate renal function in relation to age. The most widely used and accepted formula is shown in Table 13-7. This formula is useful in *initial estimations* of creatinine clearance for the purpose of drug dosing in the geriatric population. Clinical factors (such as state of hydration and cardiac output), which vary over time, should be considered in determining drug dosages.

When drugs with narrow therapeutic-toxic ratios are being used, actual measurements of creatinine clearance and drug blood levels (when available) should be utilized.

Tissue Sensitivity

A proportion of the drug (or its active metabolite) will eventually reach its site of action. Age-related changes at this point—that is,

Table 13-6 Important considerations in geriatric prescribing

Drug	Major route of elimination	Other pharmacologic considerations	Other considerations
		Analgesics	
Nonnarcotic			
Acetaminophen	Hepatic	No substantial age-related change in kinetics Liver toxicity may occur in high doses	Analgesic effects of noninflammatory condition similar to aspirin and other anti-inflammatory agents
Aspirin	Renal	Highly protein-bound Half-life may be prolonged at higher dosages	Enteric-coated preparations useful
Nonsteroidal anti-inflammatory agents	Renal (naproxen, ibuprofen) Hepatic (indomethacin)	Highly protein-bound	(see Chap. 9)
Narcotic	Hepatic	Blood levels may be higher, pain relief longer	Lower doses generally effective for analgesia Constipation a major problem
		Antimicrobials	
Antibacterial			
Aminoglycosides (gentamicin, tobramycin, amikacin)	Renal	Half-life prolonged	Nephrotoxicity and ototoxicity are major problems Blood levels important
Aztreonam	Renal	Half-life prolonged	

Drug	Elimination	Pharmacokinetics	Comments
Cephalosporins	Renal	Half-life prolonged	
Clindamycin	Hepatic		
Erythromycin	Hepatic		
Quinolones	Renal, hepatic	Relatively long half-life allows twice a day dosage	Can increase warfarin effects
Penicillins	Renal	Half-life prolonged	Carbenicillin and ticarcillin—high parenteral doses give a large sodium load
	Hepatic (nafcillin, cloxacillin)	Highly protein-bound (nafcillin, cloxacillin, oxacillin)	
Sulfonamides	Renal	Highly protein-bound	Increased effects of warfarin
Tetracyclines	Renal; Hepatic (doxycycline)	Half-life prolonged	
Vancomycin	Renal	Half-life prolonged	Ototoxicity, nephrotoxicity; Blood levels important; Poor oral absorption makes oral preparation useful for *Clostridium difficile*–associated diarrhea
Antitubercular			
Ethambutol	Renal		
Isoniazid	Hepatic	Genetic variation in rate of metabolism; no substantial age-related change	Hepatotoxicity increases with age
Rifampin	Hepatic		
Antifungal			
Amphotericin	Nonrenal		Nephrotoxicity a major problem

(continued)

Table 13-6 Important considerations in geriatric prescribing (Continued)

Drug	Major route of elimination	Other pharmacologic considerations	Other considerations
		Antiparkinsonian agents	
Amantadine	Renal		
Bromocriptine	Hepatic		
Carbidopa-levodopa	Hepatic		Cardiovascular toxicity increased
Pergolide	Hepatic		Postural hypotension may occur
Pramipexole	Renal		
Ropinirole	Hepatic		Syncope and hallucinations relatively common
Trihexyphenidyl	Nonrenal		
		Cardiovascular drugs	
Antiarrhythmic			
Disopyramide	Renal, hepatic		Can cause urinary retention
Encainide	Hepatic		
Lidocaine	Hepatic	Volume of distribution increased Half-life prolonged Clearance unchanged	Blood levels helpful
Procainamide	Renal	Clearance decreased Steady-state levels higher	Blood levels helpful
Quinidine	Nonrenal	Highly protein-bound Clearance decreased Half-life prolonged	Blood levels helpful

Drug	Route	Effect	Comments
Tocainide	Renal, hepatic		
Verapamil	Hepatic	Clearance decreased; Pharmacologic effects more pronounced and prolonged	Interacts with and raises digoxin blood levels
Anticoagulant			
Heparin	Nonrenal		
Sulfinpyrazone	Renal		
Warfarin	Hepatic	Highly protein-bound; Sensitivity to effects increased	Multiple drug interactions
Antihypertensives			
Atenolol	Renal		See Chap. 10 for more detailed discussion of antihypertensive therapy
Captopril	Renal		
Clonidine	Renal		
Diltiazem	Hepatic	Clearance decreased	Use carefully with sinus node dysfunction
Enalapril/lisinopril	Renal	Pharmacologic effects more pronounced and prolonged	
Hydralazine	Hepatic	Highly protein-bound; Blood levels higher	
Metoprolol	Hepatic		
Methyldopa	Renal		
Nadolol	Renal		
Nifedipine	Hepatic		
Propranolol	Hepatic	Highly protein-bound; Blood levels higher; Clearance decreased; Half-life prolonged; Sensitivity to effects decreased	

(continued)

Table 13-6 Important considerations in geriatric prescribing (*Continued*)

Drug	Major route of elimination	Other pharmacologic considerations	Other considerations
		Cardiovascular drugs	
Prazosin	Hepatic	Highly protein-bound	
Reserpine	Renal		
Terazosin	Renal, hepatic	Highly protein-bound	
Diuretics			
Furosemide	Renal	Highly protein-bound	Older patients predisposed to dehydration and electrolyte imbalance
Thiazides	Renal		Potassium supplementation not always necessary
Triamterene	Hepatic		Glucose intolerance or diabetes may worsen
Digoxin	Renal (15–40% nonrenal)	Decreased clearance Half-life prolonged	Many with heart failure and sinus rhythm may not need digoxin (see Chap. 10)
		Hypoglycemic agents	
Oral			
Acetohexamide	Renal, hepatic	Highly protein-bound (all oral hypoglycemics)	See Chap. 11 for more detailed discussion of hypoglycemic therapy in the elderly
Chlorpropamide	Renal	Long half-life	May cause hyponatremia

Drug	Route	Comments
Glipizide	Hepatic	
Glyburide	Hepatic	
Metformin	Renal	May cause lactic acidosis
		Must be withheld 48 h before and after iodinated contrast media
Tolazamide	Hepatic	
Tolbutamide	Hepatic	
Troglitazone	Hepatic	Serum transaminase monitoring required
Insulin	Renal, hepatic	Renal metabolism may be decreased
		Sensitivity to effects may be decreased

Psychotropic drugs		
Antidepressants (tricyclic, tetracyclic)	Hepatic	Highly protein-bound
		Blood levels may be higher
		See Chap. 6 for more detailed discussion on antidepressant drugs
Selective serotonin reuptake inhibitors (SSRIs)	Hepatic	Can inhibit cytochrome p450 isoenzymes
		May cause inappropriate antidiuretic hormone secretion and hyponatremia
Lithium	Renal	Clearance decreased
		Blood levels important
Antipsychotics	Hepatic	Highly protein-bound
		See Tables 13-9 and 13-11
Sedatives and hypnotics		
Benzodiazepines	Hepatic	Highly protein-bound
	Renal (oxazepam)	Diazepam half-life prolonged
		See Tables 13-10 and 13-11
Chloral hydrate	Hepatic	Highly protein-bound
Diphenhydramine	Hepatic	
		Anticholinergic side effects may be a problem
Zolpidem	Hepatic	Highly protein-bound

(continued)

Table 13-6 Important considerations in geriatric prescribing (*Continued*)

Drug	Major route of elimination	Other pharmacologic considerations	Other considerations
		Other drugs	
Aminophylline	Hepatic	Half-life prolonged	Lower doses may give therapeutic blood levels Blood levels helpful
Carbamazepine	Hepatic	Highly-protein bound	Several drugs can affect metabolism Blood levels helpful
Cimetidine	Renal	Half-life prolonged Steady-state blood levels higher	Can cause mental changes at high doses
Famotidine	Renal, hepatic		
Gabapentin	Renal	Clearance decreased	
Nizatidine	Renal		
Oxybutynin	Hepatic		Prominent anticholinergic effects Blood levels helpful
Phenytoin	Hepatic		Low albumin results in higher free drug than levels indicate
Prophylthiouracil	Hepatic, renal		
Raloxifene	Hepatic		Increased risk of thromboembolism
Ranitidine	Renal		
Sildenafil	Hepatic	Half-life prolonged	
Terbutaline	Hepatic		
Thyroxine	Hepatic	Clearance decreased	Maintenance dose lower Effects can be monitored by TSH blood levels (see Chap. 11)
Tolterodine	Hepatic	Blood levels higher	Can have anticholinergic effects

Table 13-7   Renal function in relation to age*

Creatinine clearance $= \dfrac{(140 - \text{age}) \times \text{body weight (kg)}}{72 \times \text{serum creatinine level}}$ ($\times$ 0.85 for women)

* Several other factors can influence creatinine clearance (see text).
Source: From Cockcroft and Gault, 1976, with permission.

responsiveness to given drug concentrations (without regard to pharmacokinetic changes)— are termed *pharmacodynamic changes.* Older persons are often said to be more sensitive to the effects of drugs. For some drugs, this appears to be true. For others, however, sensitivity to drug effects may decrease rather than increase with age. For example, older persons seem to be more sensitive to the sedative effects of given blood levels of benzodiazepines (e.g., diazepam) but less sensitive to the effects of drugs mediated by beta-adrenergic receptors (e.g., isoproterenol, propranolol). There are several possible explanations for these changes (see Table 13-5). The effects of age-related pharmacodynamic changes on dosages of specific drugs for individual geriatric patients remain largely unknown.

GERIATRIC PRESCRIBING

General Principles

There is no simple rule for prescribing drugs for the geriatric population. Certain factors that influence drug pharmacology, such as changes in renal function, are readily quantifiable; thus specific recommendations for prescribing drugs in patients with renal failure can be made (Bennett et al., 1994).

Several considerations make the development of specific recommendations for geriatric drug prescribing very difficult. These include the following:

1. Multiple interacting factors influence age-related changes in drug pharmacology.
2. There is wide interindividual variation in the rate of age-related changes in physiologic parameters that affect drug pharmacology. Thus, precise predictions for individual older persons are difficult to make.

Table 13-8 General recommendations for geriatric prescribing

Evaluate geriatric patients thoroughly in order to identify all conditions that could
 (1) benefit from drug treatment; (2) be adversely affected by drug treatment;
 (3) influence the efficacy of drug treatment.
Manage medical conditions without drugs as often as possible.
Know the pharmacology of the drug(s) being prescribed.
Consider how the clinical status of each patient could influence the pharmacology
 of the drug(s).
Avoid potential adverse drug interactions.
For drugs or their active metabolites eliminated predominantly by the kidney, use a
 formula or nomogram to approximate age-related changes in renal function and
 adjust dosages accordingly.
If there is a question about drug dosage, start with smaller doses and increase
 gradually.
Drug blood concentrations can be helpful in monitoring several potentially toxic
 drugs used frequently in the geriatric population.
Help to ensure compliance by paying attention to impaired intellectual function,
 diminished hearing, and poor vision when instructing patients and labeling
 prescriptions (and by using other techniques listed in Table 13-1).
Monitor older patients frequently for compliance, drug effects, and toxicity.

---

3. The clinical status of each patient (including such factors as state
 of nutrition and hydration, cardiac output, intrinsic renal and liver
 disease) must be considered in addition to the effects of aging.
4. As more research studies with newer drugs are carried out in well-
 defined groups of older subjects, more specific recommendations
 will be possible.

Adherence to several general principles can make drug therapy
in the geriatric population safer and more effective (Table 13-8).
Cardiovascular drugs, which account for a substantial proportion of
adverse drug reactions, are also discussed in Chap. 10. Because psychotropic drugs are so commonly used and potentially toxic, they are
discussed in greater detail below.

GERIATRIC PSYCHOPHARMACOLOGY

Psychotropic drugs can be broadly categorized as antidepressants
(discussed in detail in Chap. 6), antipsychotics (Table 13-9), and seda-

Table 13-9 Examples of antipsychotic drugs*

Drug	Approximate equivalent dose, mg	Geriatric daily dose range, mg	Relative sedation	Potential for side effects	
				Hypotension	Extrapyramidal effects[†]
Chlorpromazine (Thorazine, others)	100	10–300	Very high	High	Moderate
Haloperidol (Haldol)	2	0.25–6	Low	Low	Very high
Loxapine (Loxitane)	10	10–100		Moderate	High
Olanzapine (Zyprexa)	—[‡]	2.5–10§	Low	Low	Low
Quetiapine (Seroquel)	—[‡]	12.5–100§	Low	Low	Low
Risperidone (Risperdal)	—[‡]	0.25–8	Low	Low	Low
Thioridazine (Mellaril)	100	10–300	High	Moderate	Low
Thiothixene (Navane)	5	1–5	Low	Low	Very high

* Other agents are also available.
† Rigidity, bradykinesia, tremor, akathisia.
‡ Not available.
§ Geriatric dosage ranges not well studied.

tives and hypnotics (Table 13-10). These drugs are probably the most misused and overused class of drugs in the geriatric population. Several studies have shown that over half of nursing home residents are prescribed at least one psychotropic drug (Buck, 1988; Harrington et al., 1992), and that these prescriptions are changed commonly (Garrard et al., 1992). Ironically, there is also evidence that antidepressants may be underused in nursing homes, where there is a high prevalence of depression (Heston et al., 1992). Other studies suggest that psychotropic drugs are commonly prescribed inappropriately in the nursing home setting (Beers et al., 1988, 1992). This is of special concern because of the frequency of adverse reactions to these drugs. Federal rules and regulations contained in the Omnibus Budget Reconciliation Act (OBRA) of 1987 were implemented in 1990 and contained specific guidelines on the use of psychotropic drugs in nursing homes. The OBRA guidelines are discussed in detail elsewhere (Ouslander et al., 1997). These guidelines emphasize avoiding the use of frequent "as needed" dosing for nonspecific symptoms (e.g., agitation, wandering) and the inappropriate use of these drugs as chemical restraints.

Several considerations can be helpful in preventing the misuse of psychotropic drugs in the geriatric population:

1. Psychological symptoms (depression, anxiety, agitation, insomnia, paranoia, disruptive behavior) are often caused or exacerbated by medical conditions in geriatric patients. A thorough medical evaluation should therefore be done before symptoms are attributed to psychiatric conditions alone and psychotropic drugs are prescribed.

2. Reports of psychiatric symptomatology such as agitation are often presented to physicians by family caregivers and nursing home personnel who are inexperienced in the description, interpretation, and differential diagnosis of these symptoms. "Agitation" or "disruptive behavior" may, in fact, have been a reasonable response to an inappropriate interaction or situation created by the caregiver. Psychotropic drugs should, therefore, be prescribed only after the physician has clarified what the symptoms are and what correctable factors might have precipitated them.

3. Psychological symptoms and signs, like physical symptoms and signs, can be nonspecific in the geriatric patient. Paranoid psychosis, for example, can be the manifestation of an underlying depression. Therefore, appropriate drug treatment often depends on an

Table 13-10 Examples of sedatives and hypnotic agents*

Drug (brand name)	Geriatric daily dose range, mg	Relative rapidity of effect after oral administration	Half-life, h	Active metabolites
		Benzodiazepines		
Longer-acting[†]				
Clonazepam (Klonopin)	0.5–5	Intermediate	20–100	No
Clorazepate (Tranxene)	7.5–15	Fast	50–100	Yes
Diazepam (Valium)	1–5	Fast	40–200	Yes
Flurazepam (Dalmane)	15	Fast	18–50	Yes
Shorter-acting				
Alprazolam (Xanax)	0.25–0.75	Fast	2–5	No
Estrazolam (ProSom)	0.5–2	Intermediate	10–24	No
Lorazepam (Ativan)	10–30	Slow	5–15	No
Oxazepam (Serax)	7.5–15	Fast	5–15	No
Temazepam (Restoril)	0.0625–0.125	Intermediate	2–5	No
Triazolam (Halcion)				
		Others		
Chloral hydrate (Noctec, etc.)	500–1500	Fast	7–10	Yes
Buspirone (BuSpar)[‡]	10–30	Fast	2–3	Yes
Zolpidem (Ambien)	5	Very fast	2–3	No

* Several other agents are also available.
† Longer-acting benzodiapines should be avoided in geriatric patients.
‡ Must be used chronically to be an effective antianxiety agent.

405

accurate psychiatric diagnosis. Psychiatrists and psychologists experienced with geriatric patients should be consulted, when available, in order to identify and help target psychotropic drug treatment to the major psychiatric problem(s).

4. Many nonpharmacologic treatment modalities can either replace or be used in conjunction with psychotropic drugs in managing psychological symptoms. Behavioral modification, environmental manipulation, supportive psychotherapy, group therapy, recreational activities, and other, related techniques can be useful in eliminating or diminishing the need for drug treatment. (See Suggested Readings and Chap. 5).

5. Within each broad category of psychotropic drug, there are considerable differences among individual agents with regard to effects, side effects, and potential interactions with other drugs and medical conditions. Rational prescription of these drugs necessitates careful consideration of the characteristics of each drug in relation to the individual patient.

6. Because geriatric patients are, in general, more sensitive to the effects and side effects of psychotropic drugs, initial doses should be lower, increases should be gradual, and monitoring should be frequent.

7. Careful, ongoing assessment of the response of target symptoms and behaviors to psychotropic drugs is essential. In addition to reports from patients themselves, objective observations by trained and experienced professionals should be continuously evaluated in order to adjust psychotropic drug therapy. Several scales are available that may be helpful in monitoring response (Teri et al., 1997).

All psychotropic drugs must be used judiciously in geriatric patients because of their potential side effects. The most common and potentially disabling side effects of psychotropic drugs fall into four general categories: changes in cognitive status (e.g., sedation, delirium, dementia) and extrapyramidal, anticholinergic, and cardiovascular effects. Research has documented that psychotropic drugs can contribute to cognitive impairment (Larson et al., 1987) and are associated with hip fractures in the geriatric population (Ray et al., 1987).

Anticholinergic and cardiovascular side effects are most prominent with the tricyclic antidepressants. Antipsychotic drugs with alpha-adrenergic blocking properties, including chlorpromazine and thiorid-

azine, also have cardiovascular side effects, most notably hypotension. Extrapyramidal side effects are most common with several antipsychotic drugs (Table 13-9). These effects—which include pseudoparkinsonism (rigidity, bradykinesia, tremor), akathisia (restlessness), and involuntary dystonic movements (such as tardive dyskinesia)— can be severe and may cause substantial disability. Rigidity and bradykinesia can lead to immobility and the complications discussed in Chap. 9. Akathisia (a feeling of restlessness) can make the patient appear more anxious and agitated and lead to the inappropriate prescription of more medication. Tardive dyskinesia can cause permanent disability because of continuous orolingual movements and difficulty with eating. In addition to side effects, many psychotropic drugs interact with each other and with other drug classes. Some of these interactions may be clinically important and can enhance the risk of toxicity (Steffens and Krishnan, 1998).

Optimal efficacy of psychotropic drugs necessitates consideration of characteristics of the drugs in relation to several clinical factors in each patient (Table 13-11). In general, the antipsychotic agents should be reserved for treatment of psychoses (i.e., paranoid states, delusions, and hallucinations), which are common in dementia patients. These drugs may also be useful for severe physical and/or verbal agitation that does not respond to nonpharmacologic interventions. OBRA regulations and good clinical practice dictate that environmental and behavioral interventions should be attempted before psychotropic drugs are prescribed. There is no clear choice of one antipsychotic agent over another based on controlled clinical trials. Some of the newer agents, such as risperidone, olanzapine, and quetiapine, have less extrapyramidal side effects than older drugs. They are clearly the drugs of choice for psychosis and agitation that occurs in dementia of Parkinson's disease and dementia associated with Lewy bodies (see Chap. 5). In some situations, intermittent agitation, especially at night, is best treated by a short-acting benzodiazepine (Table 13-10). When antipsychotics fail or cause side effects and sedation is not desired, carbamazepine and valproic acid may be useful alternatives in some patients. Both of these drugs, however, have the potential for hematologic and hepatic toxicity and must be used cautiously in the geriatric population.

A variety of nonpharmacologic measures can be effective in geriatric patients with agitation or excessive anxiety. Specific behavioral and other nonpharmacologic therapeutic approaches are described in

Table 13-11 Clinical considerations in prescribing psychotropic drugs

Clinical indicator	Most useful types	Comments
Depression with psychomotor retardation	Less sedating antidepressant (e.g., paroxetine, sertraline)	See Chap. 6
Depression with prominent anxiety	Antidepressant with antianxiety effects (e.g., nefazadone)	
Agitation without psychosis that occurs at night	Short-acting sedative (e.g., lorazepam) or a hypnotic (e.g., chloral hydrate, temazepam)	Should generally be used on an "as needed" basis Nonpharmacologic intervention may be more appropriate
Psychoses without prominent agitation (e.g., delusions and hallucinations in patients with depression or dementia)	Less sedating antipsychotic (e.g., risperidone, olanzapine)	Extrapyramidal effects may occur Risperidone may cause postural hypotension if not titrated slowly
Severe physical or verbal agitation poorly controlled by nonpharmacologic intervention	More sedating antipsychotic (e.g., thioridazine, loxapine)	More potent antipsychotics Extrapyramidal effects may be prominent Akathisia can make patient appear more agitated
Insomnia	Chloral hydrate Temazepam Zolpidem	Underlying cause(s) should be sought; nonpharmacologic interventions often helpful

detail in some of the Suggested Readings at the end of this chapter (see also Chap. 5). These measures, however, are often unavailable, impractical, inappropriate, or unsuccessful. Patients with severe impairment of cognitive function can be especially difficult to manage with nonpharmacologic measures alone, particularly when their physical and/or verbal agitation is interfering with their care (or the care of others around them). Thus, drug treatment of agitation is necessary in these patients.

Insomnia, like agitation, can be the manifestation of depression or physical illness. It is a very common complaint in geriatric patients, and causes of sleep disorders should be sought (see Chap. 6). Nonpharmacologic measures (such as increasing activity during the day, diminishing nighttime noise, and ensuring cooler nighttime temperatures) are sometimes helpful. When a drug is needed, chloral hydrate or small doses of a benzodiazepine (e.g., temazepam) are often effective (Table 13-10). Low doses of trazadone (e.g., 50 mg) are also safe and effective. Melatonin, a naturally occurring hormone available over the counter, has gained increasing popularity as a hypnotic. Geriatric sleep disturbances are associated with changes in the melatonin cycle. Doses of 1 to 3 mg have been reported to improve the initiation and maintenance of sleep. The long-term effects of chronic hypnotic use in the geriatric population are unknown, but rebound insomnia can become a problem in patients who use hypnotics (especially benzodiazepine hypnotics and melatonin) regularly and then discontinue them. Whatever the indication, it is extremely important that after a psychotropic drug is prescribed, the patient be closely monitored for the effects of the drug on the target symptoms and side effects and that the drug regimen be adjusted accordingly.

REFERENCES

Beers M, Avorn J, Soumerai SB, et al: Psychoactive medication use in intermediate-care facility residents. *JAMA* 260:3016–3020, 1988.

Beers MH, Ouslander JG, Fingold SF, et al: Inappropriate medication prescribing in skilled nursing facilities. *Ann Intern Med* 117:684–689, 1992.

Bennett WM, Aronoff GR, Golper TA, et al: *Drug Prescribing in Renal Failure: Dosing Guidelines for Adults.* Philadelphia: American College of Physicians, 1994.

Buck JA: Psychotropic drug practice in nursing homes. *J Am Geriatr Soc* 36:409–418, 1988.

Caranasos GJ, Stewart RB, Cluff LE: Drug-induced illness leading to hospitalization. *JAMA* 288:713–717, 1974.

Cockcroft DW, Gault MH: Predictions of creatinine clearance from serum creatinine. *Nephron* 16:31–41, 1976.

Garrard J, Dunham T, Makris L, et al: Longitudinal study of psychotropic drug use by elderly nursing home residents. *J Gerontol Med Sci* 47:M183–M188, 1992.

Greenblatt DJ, Sellers EM, Shader RI: Drug therapy: Drug disposition in old age. *N Engl J Med* 306:1081–1088, 1982.

Harrington C, Tompkins C, Curtis M, Grant L: Psychotropic drug use in long-term care facilities: a review of the literature. *Gerontologist* 32:822–833, 1992.

Heerdink ER, Leufkens HG, Herings RMC, et al: NSAIDs associated with increased risk of congestive heart failure in elderly patients taking diuretics. *Arch Intern Med* 158:1108–1112, 1998.

Heston LL, Garrard J, Makris L, et al: Inadequate treatment of depressed nursing home elderly. *J Am Geriatr Soc* 40:1117–1122, 1992.

Larson EB, Kukull WA, Buchner D, et al: Adverse drug reactions associated with global cognitive impairment in elderly persons. *Ann Intern Med* 107:169–173, 1987.

Lazarou J, Pomeranz BH, Corey PN: Incidence of adverse drug reactions in hospitalized patients: a meta-analysis of prospective studies. *JAMA* 279:1200–1205, 1998.

Ouslander J, Morley J, Osterweil D: *Medical Care in the Nursing Home*, 2d ed. New York, McGraw-Hill, 1997.

Ray WA, Griffin MR, Schaffner W, et al: Psychotropic drug use and the risk of hip fracture. *N Engl J Med* 316:363–369, 1987.

Seidel LG, Thornton GF, Smith JW, et al: Studies on the epidemiology of adverse drug reactions: III. Reactions in patients on a general medical service. *Bull Johns Hopkins Hosp* 119:299–315, 1966.

Steel K, Gertman PM, Crescenzi Anderson J: Iatrogenic illness on a general medical service at a university hospital. *N Engl J Med* 304:638–642, 1981.

Steffens DC, Krishnan KRR: Metabolism, bioavailability, and drug interactions. *Clin Geriatr* 14:17–32, 1998.

Teri L, Logsdon R, Yesavage J: Measuring behavior, mood, and psychiatric symptoms in Alzheimer disease. *Alzheimer Dis Assoc Disord* 11:50–59, 1997.

Williamson J, Chopin JM: Adverse reactions to prescribed drugs in the elderly: a multicentre investigation. *Age Ageing* 9:73–80, 1980.

SUGGESTED READINGS

Beers MH: Explicit criteria for determining potentially inappropriate medication use by the elderly. *Arch Intern Med* 157:1531–1536, 1997.

Board of Directors of the American Association for Geriatric Psychiatry, Clinical Practice Committee of the American Geriatrics Society, and Committee on Long-Term Care and Treatment for the Elderly: Psychotherapeutic medications in the nursing home. *J Am Geriatr Soc* 40:946–949, 1992.

Bressler R, Katz MD (eds): *Geriatric Pharmacology.* New York, McGraw-Hill, 1993.

Carlson DL, Fleming KC, Smith GE, et al: Management of dementia-related behavioral disturbances: a nonpharmacologic approach. *Mayo Clin Proc* 70:1108–1115, 1995.

Dement WC: Rational basis for the use of sleeping pills. Pharmacology 27(suppl 2):3–38, 1983/*Int Pharmacopsychiatry* 17(suppl 2):3–38, 1982.

Foley KM: The treatment of cancer pain. *N Engl J Med* 313:84–95, 1985.

Medical Letter: Drugs for psychiatric disorders. *Med Lett* 39:33–40, 1997.

Mintzer JE, Hoernig KS, Mirski DF: Treatment of agitation in patients with dementia. *Clin Geriatr Med* 14:147–175, 1998.

Ouslander JG: Drug therapy in the elderly. *Ann Intern Med* 95:711–722, 1981.

Selma TP, Beizer JL, Higbee MD: *Geriatric Dosage Handbook,* 3d ed. Hudson, OH, American Pharmaceutical Association and Lexi-Comp, 1997.

Van Scoy RE, Wilkowske CJ: Prophylactic use of antimicrobial agents in adult patients. *Mayo Clin Proc* 67:288–292, 1992.

FOURTEEN

HEALTH SERVICES

Health care for older persons consists largely of addressing the problems associated with chronic illness (Hoffman et al., 1996). However, medical care continues to be practiced as though it consisted of a series of discrete encounters. What is needed is a systematic approach to chronic care that encourages the clinician to recognize the overall course expected for each patient and to manage treatment within those parameters. The clinical glidepath approach (described in Chap. 4) is one way to encourage such practice.

Care for frail older persons has been impeded by an artificial dichotomy between medical and social interventions. This separation has been enhanced by the funding policies, such as the auspices of Medicare and Medicaid, but it also reflects the philosophies of the dominant professions. Medical practice has been driven by what may be termed a therapeutic model. The basic expectation from medical care is that it will make a difference. The difference may not always be reflected in an improvement in the patient's status. Indeed, for many chronically ill patients decline is inevitable, but good care should at least delay that decline. Because many patients do get worse over time, it may be difficult for clinicians to see the effects of their care.

Appreciating the benefits of good care may require a comparison between what happens and what would have occurred in the absence of that care. In effect, the yield from good care is the difference between what is observed and what is reasonable to expect; but without the expected value, the benefit may be hard to appreciate. Figure 14-1 provides a theoretical model of these two curves. Both trajectories show decline, but the slope associated with better care is less acute. The area between them represents the effects of good care.

The alternative model, usually associated with social services, is compensatory care. Under this concept, a person is assessed to determine deficits and a plan of care is developed to address these deficits. Good care is defined as that which fits the profile of dependencies and thereby allows the client to enjoy as normal a lifestyle as possible. Under this paradigm, good care means meeting needs without incurring any adverse consequences.

Care for the frail older patient requires a synthesis of medical and social attention. The medical care system has not facilitated that interaction. The new developments in managed care could provide a framework for achieving this coordination, but the track record so far does not suggest that the incentives are yet in place to produce this effect. A few notable programs have been able to merge funding and services for this frail population. Probably the best example of

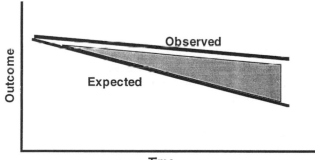

Figure 14-1 Theoretical model of observed versus expected clinical course. The area between the observed and expected outcomes represents the benefits of good care. Thus a patient's condition may deteriorate and still be considered to indicate good care if the rate of deterioration is less than expected.

creative integration is seen in the Program of All-inclusive Care of the Elderly (PACE), which uses pooled capitated funding from Medicare and Medicaid to provide integrated health and social services to older persons who are deemed to be eligible for nursing home care but are still living in the community (Kane et al., 1992; Branch et al., 1995; Eng et al., 1997). Another model that shows promise for demonstrating this integration is the second generation of the Social HMO (Kane et al., 1997b). Whether managed care will achieve its potential as a vehicle for improving coordination of care for older persons remains to be seen (Kane, 1998). In any event, care for older persons will require such integration and eventually some reconciliation about what constitutes the desired goals of such care.

Geriatric care thus implies team care. This concept does not mean that everyone needs to do everything. Rather, it means that some activities can be the purview of other disciplines who have special skills and training for such tasks. However, these colleagues must not be expected to operate alone. Good communication and coordination will avoid duplication of effort and lead to a better overall outcome. To play a useful role on the health care team, physicians need to appreciate what other health professions can do and know how and when to call on their skills.

LONG-TERM CARE

A proportion of older patients will require substantial long-term care. There is no uniform definition for long-term care, but the following description of the term highlights the important aspects. "A range of services that addresses the health, personal care, and social needs of individuals who lack some capacity for self-care. Services may be continuous or intermittent but are delivered for sustained periods to individuals who have a demonstrated need, usually measured by some index of functional incapacity."

This statement emphasizes the common thread of most discussions of long-term care: the dependence of an individual on the services of another for a substantial period. The definition is carefully unspecific about who provides those services or what they are. Long-term care is certainly not the exclusive purview of the medical profession; in fact, most of the long-term care in this country is not provided by professionals at all but by a host of individuals loosely referred to as

informal support. These persons may be family, friends, or neighbors. Informal care has been and remains the backbone of long-term care. In many instances, the family (and often nonrelatives) are the first line of support. The ideal program would keep older people at home, relying on family as the first line of support, and bolstering their efforts with more formal assistance to provide professional services and occasional respite care. Approximately 80% of all the care given in the community comes from this source. Surprisingly, this figure seems to remain fairly constant in countries with more generous provision of formal long-term care. Many observers have questioned whether the informal care role, which is largely performed by women, can be sustained as more women enter the labor force and are already managing several roles. Despite dire predictions about its inevitable collapse, there is yet no evidence of serious decline in informal care. It is important to bear in mind that as the age of frailty rises, the "children" of these frail older people may themselves be in their seventh and eight decades.

The best estimates suggest that about 15 percent of the elderly population need the help of another person to manage their daily lives. As shown in Fig. 14-2, the proportion of persons who have difficulty performing one or more ADLs increases with age, from

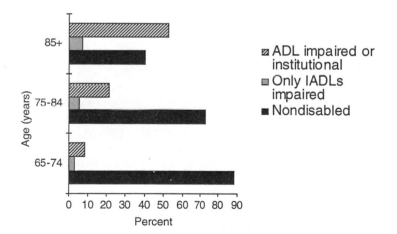

Figure 14-2 Prevalence of chronic disability in the United States, 1994. *(From Manton et al., 1997.)*

about 8 percent at age 65 to 53 percent after age 85. The prevalence of disability among older persons seems to be falling slightly since 1982 (Manton et al., 1997). If only those living in the community are examined, the proportion of persons needing help with one or more ADLs in 1991–92 was 4.1 percent of those aged 65 to 74, 9.6 percent of those 75 to 84 and 22.9 percent of those 85 and older (Kennedy et al., 1997). Recall that for each person in a nursing home today, there are between one and three equally disabled persons living in the community. Thus, first instincts are not always best. Physicians have been trained to respond to the dependent elderly person by thinking of admission to a nursing home. Nursing home placement should be the *last* resort, not the first. Table 14-1 suggests a wider array of treatment choices for various types of patients. The physician, in conjunction with other health professionals (especially social workers and nurses), can do a great deal to steer patients and their families toward these resources. Although the physician is not likely to become actively involved in specific placement decisions, the physician's suggestions and opinions about what should be considered can play a pivotal role. Moreover, the physician's medical certification of need is essential for establishing eligibility for long-term-care services under several reimbursement programs.

Why then does our system rely so heavily on the nursing home? Several reasons can be offered. First, nursing homes are available; there are more nursing home beds than acute care hospital beds in this country. Nonetheless, there is usually a waiting list to get in, especially into a relatively good home. Second, nursing home care is cheap; it is under $100 a day in most states, while a hospital day costs at least $1000 and even a good hotel room costs at least $100. Finally, and related to the first two points, the nursing home comes as an already assembled package of services. The programs to cover long-term-care services have become a complex maze of eligibility and regulations, which has not encouraged anyone to develop innovative alternatives. Particularly, as the pressure for faster discharge from hospitals has increased, the available nursing home bed is a ready recourse.

It is not altogether true to say that there have been no efforts to develop alternatives. For a period there was great effort expended trying to find less expensive ways of caring for people needing long-term care in the community. The upshot of these efforts was the recognition that community care is preferable in many cases but not

Table 14-1 Relationship between target groups and possible alternatives

Target group now in nursing home	Community alternatives		Institutional backup requirement
	Intermediate	Long-range	
Terminally ill	Home health Home hospice Homemaking Counseling	Narcotic law reform	Possibly a hospice
Those who might benefit from rehabilitation	Home health Day hospital		Rehabilitation hospital
Those requiring skilled nursing care	Home health Day hospital Meals on wheels Homemaking	Personal care attendant policy	Policy of acute care hospital service when needed
Those who are mentally ill	Halfway house Day hospital Sheltered workshops Day care	Bereavement counseling Identification of high-risk groups	Possible need for acute care hospital service
Those with social needs and minimal health problems—the frail, the very old	Sheltered housing Assisted living Day care Social programming Senior centers Primary health care	Reeducation Changed income transfer programs Employment programs	
The completely disoriented—ambulatory but needing constant supervision	Foster care		Possibility that better services can be provided through institutions

always cheaper. One of the major difficulties in controlling the cost of this care is the potential for widespread use. Because there are a large number of dependent older persons living in the community, a dependency-based eligibility system will include many people who would not opt for a nursing home. This need to control entry has stimulated great interest in case management. The continuing need to improve community care has led to some recent innovations, including new waiver programs that allow use of nursing home funds for community care if the total long-term-care budget is kept constant. As a result, there has been uneven development of community programs in different parts of the country.

The earlier emphasis on seeking community-based alternatives to nursing home care has shifted to some extent to developing other mechanisms for providing the combined housing and service functions. Among these are assisted living and adult foster care. Assisted living, in effect, renders the recipient first and foremost a tenant, who has control over her singly occupied living space (e.g., a lock on the door and determination about waking and retiring times). In addition to single occupancy, the client's autonomy is reenforced by providing modest cooking and refrigeration facilities, which allow the person to function independently without relying exclusively on the services of the institution and even to entertain modestly (Kane et al., 1993). Adult foster care homes are usually limited to a small number of clients in any home (usually no more than five). Single rooms are not required; the situation is more analogous to individuals taking clients into their own homes, with small numbers of flexibly deployed nonprofessional staff. Recent trends suggest that the historic growth in nursing home use is changing. The last few years have witnessed a decline in nursing home occupancy. At least some of this effect undoubtedly comes from the growing availability of other residential models, which consumers find more attractive.

At the same time, there is concern that a preoccupation with a search for alternatives to nursing homes may distract efforts from the sorely needed work to improve the quality of nursing home care. Even in the best situation, a substantial number of older persons will continue to need such care. One scenario for the future holds that the form of nursing homes will change. Many of the residents currently cared for in nursing homes will be treated in more flexible situations, like assisted living, which emphasize living arrangements with nursing and other services brought to the residents on a more individualized

basis. Those patients needing more intensive care will be treated in more medically oriented facilities.

PUBLIC PROGRAMS

Overview

The physician caring for elderly patients must have at least a working acquaintance with the major programs that support older people. We are accustomed to thinking about care of older people in association with Medicare. In fact, at least three parts (called *Titles*) of the Social Security Act provide important benefits for the elderly: Title XVIII (Medicare), Title XIX (Medicaid), and Social Services Block Grants (formerly Title XX). Medicare was designed to address health care, particularly acute care hospital services. The Medicare program is in flux. It was intended to deal with long-term care only to the extent that long-term care can supplant more expensive hospital care, leaving the major funding for long-term care to Medicaid. However, over the last decade the funding demarcation between acute and long-term care services has become more blurred. Especially with regard to home health care, Medicare has begun to cover more care that would be considered long-term. In 1993, approximately 60 percent of home health care visits under Medicare were delivered to persons who have received such care for at least 6 months, well beyond the traditional designation of acute care (Welch et al., 1996).

This distinction in programmatic responsibility between Medicare and Medicaid is a very important one. Whereas Medicare is an insurance-type program to which persons are entitled after contributing a certain amount, Medicaid is a welfare program, eligibility for which depends on a combination of need and poverty. Thus, to become eligible for Medicaid, a person must not only prove illness but also exhaustion of personal resources—hardly a situation conducive to restoring autonomy.

The pattern of coverage is quite different for the various services covered. Figures 14-3 and 14-4 trace spending on health care for elderly persons by Medicare and Medicaid, respectively. Medicare is a major payer of hospital and physician care but pays for only a small portion of nursing home care, whereas just the reverse applies to Medicaid.

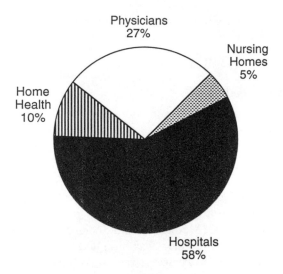

Figure 14-3 Distribution of Medicare expenditures for the aged, 1995. *(From U.S. Department of Health and Human Services, 1997a.)*

Medicare

Eligibility for Medicare differs for each of its two major parts. Part A (hospital services insurance) is available to all who are eligible for Social Security, usually by virtue of paying the Social Security tax for a sufficient number of quarters. Part B (medical services insurance) is offered for a monthly premium, paid by the individual. Almost everyone over age 65 is covered by Part A. (Federal, state, and local government employees are exceptions; until recently they were not covered by Social Security and have their own pension and medical programs.)

The introduction of prospective payment for hospitals under Medicare created a new set of problems. Hospitals are paid a fixed amount per admission according to the diagnosis-related group (DRG), to which the patient is assigned on the basis of the admitting diagnosis. The rates for DRGs are, in turn, based on expected lengths of stay and intensity of care for each condition. The incentives in such an approach run almost directly contrary to most of the goals of geriatrics. Whereas geriatrics addresses the functional result of multiple interacting problems, DRGs encourage concentration on a single problem. Extra time required to make an appropriate

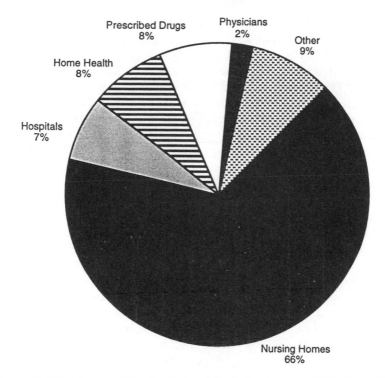

Figure 14-4 Distribution of Medicaid expenditures for the aged, 1995. *(From U.S. Department of Health and Human Services, 1997b.)*

discharge plan is discouraged. Use of ancillary personnel, such as social workers, is similarly discouraged. As a result of DRGs, hospital lengths of stay have decreased (see Fig. 2-11 in Chap. 2), leading to the phenomenon of "quicker and sicker" discharges (Kosecoff et al., 1990). Many of these former hospital patients are now cared for through home health and nursing homes. In effect, Medicare is paying for care twice: It pays for the hospital stay regardless of length and then pays for the posthospital care. The rapid rise in this latter sector has led Medicare to search for solutions. The first foray has been to propose some form of prospective payment for the different types of posthospital care akin to that used for hospitals. A more effective solution would be to combine the payment for hospital and posthospital care, although some fear that such a step would place too much control

in the hands of hospitals, which have little experience with posthospital care. The 1997 Balanced Budget Act proposes such a change. For selected DRGs, hospital discharges to post–acute care will be treated as transfers. Hospitals will receive a lower payment than the usual DRG payment if the length of stay is less than the median.

Moreover, the two payment systems now in effect create much confusion for Medicare beneficiaries. Hospitals are now paid a fixed amount per case, but the patients continue to pay under a system of deductibles. If there was ever a rationale for the copayments under Part A as a way of discouraging unnecessary stays, it has certainly disappeared with the introduction of DRGs.

All of these concerns may be rendered moot if Medicare moves aggressively to managed care. Managed care is increasingly being used as an option to traditional fee-for-service care. Under that arrangement, the managed care organizations will determine the payment arrangements and the deductibles and copayments will disappear. The Balanced Budget Act (BBA) of 1997 contains a number of provisions designed to foster the growth of Medicare managed care as well as to address some of the problems associated with it. In 1998, approximately 15 percent of Medicare beneficiaries were covered by managed care. The pricing system used by Medicare basically reflects the prices paid for fee-for-service care in each county. Managed care organizations are paid a fixed amount calculated on the basis of the average amount Medicare paid for its beneficiaries in that county. This adjusted average per capita cost (AAPCC) varies widely from one location to another (Kane et al., 1997a). The BBA calls for a shift to national pricing and provides for a minimal payment, both of which will reduce this variation. At the same time, the BBA has broadened the definition of what kinds of organizations can provide managed care to Medicare beneficiaries, removing many of the restrictions (especially financial surety bonding) that left managed care largely in the hands of insurance companies. Unlike managed care enrollees in the rest of the population, who are locked into health plans for a year, Medicare beneficiaries have the right to disenroll at any time. There is some evidence to suggest that Medicare beneficiaries may move in and out of managed care as they use up available benefits (Morgan et al., 1997).

It is not yet clear whether managed care will enhance or detract from the role of geriatrics (Lachs and Ruchlin, 1997). Ideally, managed care could provide an environment where many of the principles of

geriatrics could be implemented to the benefit of all; on the other hand, the performance to date suggests that managed care for Medicare beneficiaries has so far responded more to the incentives from favorable selection (recruiting healthy patients and getting paid average rates), discounted purchasing of services, and barriers to access than to the potential benefits from increased efficiency derived from a geriatric philosophy (Kane, 1998).

Although Medicare does pay for authorized posthospital services in nursing homes and through home health care, the payment for physicians does not encourage their active participation. For example, while a physician would be paid a regular consultation visit fee for daily rounds on a Medicare patient in a hospital, if the patient is discharged to a nursing home the following day, both the rate of physician reimbursement for a visit and the number of visits per week considered customary decrease dramatically. Although physician home visits are still a rarity, payment for these services is likewise low; however, the payment for home visits and nursing home visits has been increased substantially in recent years.

A slightly smaller proportion of the elderly population uses Part B; it is a good buy because three-quarters of the cost is subsidized, and Social Security payments were increased to allow people to purchase it. Many Medicare beneficiaries have also purchased so-called Medigap insurance. This insurance comes in a variety of forms (federal law now dictates the various components); most of this insurance covers only the gaps up to the ceilings established by Medicare (i.e., it pays deductibles and coinsurance but generally does not cover the difference between billed charges and allowable charges). An increasing number of policies cover at least some drug costs. In some cases, older persons may have purchased multiple Medigap policies under the erroneous assumption they were buying more coverage.

Medicare coverage is important but not sufficient for three basic reasons:

1. To control utilization, it mandates deductible and copayment charges for both Parts A and B.
2. It sets physician's fees by a complicated formula called the Resource-Based Relative Value Scale (RBRVS). The RBRVS is designed to pay physicians more closely according to the value of their services as determined both within a specialty and across

specialties. Theoretically, both the value of the services provided and the investment in training are considered in setting the rates. This new payment approach was intended to increase the payment for primary care relative to surgical specialties, but early reports suggest that, ironically, many geriatric assessment services have been reimbursed at a level lower than before its introduction. Under Medicare Part B physicians are generally paid less than they would usually bill for the service. [Some physicians opt to bill the patient directly for the difference but a number of states have mandated that physicians accept "assignment" of Medicare fees, i.e., they accept the fee (plus the 20 percent copayment) as payment in full.]

3. The program does not cover several services essential to patient functioning, such as drugs, eyeglasses, hearing aids, and many preventive services (although the benefits for the latter are expanding). Medicare specifically excludes services designed to provide "custodial care"—the very services often most critical to long-term care. (However, as noted above, the boundary between acute and long-term care exclusions seems to be eroding.)

As a result of these three factors, a substantial amount of the medical bill is left to the individual. In 1995, elderly persons' out-of-pocket costs for health care represented about 21 percent of their income, a figure comparable to before the passage of Medicare (Moon, 1996). In that same year, older persons paid for 39 percent of their long-term care from personal sources (Scanlon, 1998). One estimate suggests that Medicare beneficiaries' out-of-pocket expenditures are quite different for those in fee-for-service compared with managed care. The average 1997 out-of-pocket expenditure for the former was $2454 compared with $1775 for the latter (AARP Public Policy Institute et al., 1997).

Medicaid

Medicaid, in contrast, is a welfare program designed to serve the poor. It is a state-run program to which the federal government contributes (50 to 78 percent of the costs, depending on the state). In some states, persons can be covered as medically indigent even if their income is above the poverty level if their medical expenses would impoverish them. As a welfare program, Medicaid has no deductibles or coinsur-

ance (although current proposals call for modest charges to discourage excess use). It is, however, a welfare program cast in the medical model.

It is important to appreciate that the shape of the Medicaid expenditures for older people is determined largely by the gaps in Medicare. Medicaid serves primarily two distinct groups: mothers and young children under Aid to Families of Dependent Children and the elderly eligible for Old Age Assistance. (The other major route to eligibility for older people is the medically needy program, whereby eligibility is conferred when medical costs—usually nursing homes—exceed a fixed fraction of a person's income.) The former use some hospital care around birth and for the small group of severely ill children. A large portion of the Medicaid dollar goes to those things needed by the elderly but not covered by Medicare, namely, drugs, nursing home care, and custodial home care.

Because it is the major source of nursing home payments, physicians are often placed in the difficult position of being asked to certify a patient's physical limitations in order to gain the patient admittance to a nursing home for primarily social reasons (i.e., lack of social supports necessary to remain in the community).

Medicaid is the major public payer for nursing home care. (Medicare, which had formerly been an almost insignificant nursing home payer, has dramatically increased its role in the wake of Prospective Payment for hospitals. It now provides almost 10 percent of nursing home revenues.) Medicaid is thus important in shaping nursing home policies. It pays about half of the nursing costs but covers almost 70 percent of the residents. The discrepancy is explained by the policies that require residents to expend their own resources first. Thus Social Security payments, private pensions, and the like are used as primary sources of payment, and Medicaid picks up the remainder. However, it does not directly pay for most physician care in the nursing home. For elderly persons already covered by Medicaid, the welfare program will pay the Medicare Part B premium and thus reinsure through available federal funds. Medicaid would then pay the deductibles and copayments and those services not covered under Medicare.

Recently, there seems to be a change in the way Medicaid is viewed by older persons and their progeny. Whereas going on Medicaid was once seen as a great social embarrassment, associated with accepting public charity, there appears to be a growing sense among

many older persons that they are entitled to receive Medicaid help when their health care expenses, especially their long-term-care costs, are high. The stigma is displaced by the idea that they paid taxes for many years and are now entitled to reap the rewards. As a result of this shift in sentiment, at least in the states with generous levels of Medicaid eligibility, there is a burgeoning industry of financial advisers to assist older persons in preparing to become Medicaid-eligible. Because eligibility is usually based on both income and assets, such a step necessitates advance planning. Usually state laws require that assets transferred within two or more years of applying for Medicaid funds are considered to still be owned. (The situation is more complicated in the case of a married couple, where provisions have been made to allow the spouse to retain part of the family's assets.) This requirement means that older persons contemplating becoming eligible for Medicaid must be willing to divest themselves of their assets at least several years in advance of the time they expect to need such help. This step places them in a very dependent position, financially and psychologically. Much has been made of the "divestiture phenomenon" whereby older people scheme to divest themselves of their assets in order to qualify for Medicaid, but so far little evidence has been presented to suggest that this is a serious problem.

There is also growing enthusiasm for promoting various forms of private long-term-care insurance. This coverage, in effect, protects the assets of those who might otherwise be marginally eligible for Medicaid or who simply want to preserve an inheritance for their heirs. Like any insurance linked to age-related events but to a greater degree, long-term-care insurance is quite affordable when purchased at a young age (when the likelihood of needing it is very low) but becomes quite expensive as the buyer reaches age 75 or older. Thus, those most likely to consider buying it would have to pay a premium close to the average cost of long-term care itself. Only a small number of young persons have shown any interest in purchasing such coverage, especially when companies are not anxious to add it to their employee benefit packages as a free benefit. Although economic projections suggest that private long-term-care insurance is not likely to save substantial money for the Medicaid program, several states have developed programs to encourage individuals to purchase the insurance by offering linked Medicaid benefits.

Other Programs

The third part of the Social Security legislation pertinent to older persons is Title XX, now administered as Social Services Block Grants. This is also a welfare program targeted especially to those on categorical welfare programs like Aid to Families with Dependent Children and, more germane, Supplemental Security Income. The latter is a federal program, which, as the name implies, supplements Social Security benefits to provide a minimum income. Title XX funds are administered through state and local agencies, which have a substantial amount of flexibility in how they allocate the available money across a variety of stipulated services. The state also has the option of broadening the eligibility criteria to include those just above the poverty line.

The other major relevant federal program is Title III of the Older Americans Act. This program is available to all persons over age 60 regardless of income. The single largest component goes to support nutrition through congregate meal programs where elderly persons can get a subsidized hot meal, but it also provides meals-on-wheels (home-delivered meals) and a wide variety of other services. Some duplicate or supplement those covered under Social Security programs; others are unique.

Table 14-2 summarizes these four programs and their current scope. It is important to appreciate that this summary attempts to condense and simplify a complex and ever-changing set of rules and regulations. Physicians should be familiar with the broad scope and limitations of these programs but will have to rely on others, especially social workers, who are familiar with the operating details.

THE NURSING HOME

The nursing home is an important part of the health care delivery system for frail older persons. Virtually without planning, it has emerged as the touchstone of long-term care. Given its origins as the stepchild of the almshouse and the hospital, it is not surprising that it has enjoyed a poor reputation. Since the passage of the Medicaid legislation in 1965, the nursing home industry has gone through growth and transformation. As a reaction to scandals during the early years

Table 14-2 Summary of major federal programs for elderly patients

Program	Eligible population	Services covered	Deductibles and copayments
Medicare (Title XVIII of the Social Security Act) Part A: Hospital insurance	All persons eligible for Social Security and others with chronic disabilities, such as end-stage renal disease, plus voluntary enrollees 65+	Per benefit period, "reasonable cost" for 90 days of hospital care plus 60 lifetime reservation days; 100 days of skilled nursing facility (SNF); home health visits (see text); hospice care*	Full coverage for hospital care after a deductible of about 1 day for 2 days 2–60; then one-quarter day copay for days 61–90. Can use "lifetime reserve" first days thereafter. 20 SNF days fully covered; one-eight day copay for days 21–100
Part B: Supplemental medical insurance	All those covered under Part A who elect coverage; participants pay a monthly premium	80% of "reasonable cost" for physicians' services; supplies and services related to physician services; outpatient, physical, and speech therapy; diagnostic tests and radiographs; mammogram; surgical dressings; prosthetics; ambulance	Deductible and 20% copayment. (No copay after a limit reached)

| Medicaid (Title XIX of the Social Security Act) | Persons receiving Supplemental Security Income (SSI) (such as welfare) or receiving SSI and state supplement or meeting lower eligibility standards used for medical assistance criteria 1972 *or* eligible for SSI *or* were in institutions and eligible for Medicaid in 1973; medically needy who do not qualify for SSI but have high medical expenses are eligible for Medicaid in some states; eligibility criteria vary from state to state | Mandatory services for categorically needy: Inpatient hospital services; outpatient services; SNF; limited home health care; laboratory tests and radiographs; family planning; early and periodic screening, diagnosis, and treatment for children through age 20 Optional services vary from state to state: Dental care; therapies; drugs; intermediate care facilities; extended home health care; private duty nurse; eyeglasses; prostheses; personal-care services; medical transportation and home health care services. (states can limit the amount and duration of services) | None, once patient spends down to eligibility level Spend-down based on income and assets |

(*continued*)

Table 14-2 Summary of major federal programs for the elderly (*Continued*)

Program	Eligible population	Services covered	Deductibles and copayments
Social Services Block Grant (Title XX of the Social Security Act)	All recipients of Aid to Families with Dependent Children (AFDC) and SSI; optionally, those earning up to 115% of state median income and residents of specific geographic areas	Day care; substitute care; protective services; counseling; home-based services; employment, education and training; health-related services; information and referral; transportation; day services; family planning; legal services; home-delivered and congregate meals	Fees are charged to those with family incomes greater than 80% of state's median income
Title III of the Older Americans Act	All persons 60 years and older; low-income, minority, and isolated older persons are special targets	Homemaker; home-delivered meals; home health aides; transportation; legal services; counseling; information and referral plus 19 others (50% of funds must go to those listed)	Some payment may be requested

* Certified hospice providers are paid a preset amount when patient who is certified as terminal opts for this benefit in lieu of regular Medicare.

of publicly paid nursing home care, nursing homes have become heavily regulated.

Seen from one vantage point, the term *nursing home* is a misnomer. Although these institutions are better staffed and run than in the past, they remain generally somber places that offer their residents neither a great deal of real nursing care nor a very homelike environment. Most nursing home rooms are occupied by several residents. There is little privacy and few opportunities to retain control over even small parts of one's life. Fire regulations often prevent residents from bringing personal furniture into the homes. The nursing home is not a miniature hospital. Nursing homes are smaller and less well staffed than hospitals. Whereas a hospital has a ratio of over three staff for each bed, the nursing home has only about a sixth of that number, and most of those staff are aides. Nursing homes were previously divided into at least two categories: skilled and intermediate care. The distinction was based primarily on the amount of nursing care available. Nursing homes were certified as being capable of caring for patients with different needs based on these levels. In turn, patients were certified as needing a given level of care, but the criteria were vague and much was left to professional judgment.

This distinction has been officially eliminated under the regulations of the 1987 Omnibus Budget Reconciliation Act (OBRA '87), which calls for a single level of nursing facility (although it seems to persist in practice in many areas). The distinction between nursing home care and that provided in purely residential facilities with little or no nursing component has been retained.

Admission to a nursing home is very much a function of age. Figure 14-5 shows the sharp rise in the rate of nursing home use after age 85. Because this portion of the population is growing rapidly, there is great fear of being inundated with nursing home users.

The residents in nursing homes can be distinguished from older persons living in the community on several basic parameters. As shown in Table 14-3, in addition to being older, they are more likely to be white, female, and unmarried. Nursing home residents tend to have multiple chronic problems. Especially prevalent are heart disease, dementia, and urinary incontinence. About 63 percent of elderly nursing home residents exhibit disorientation or memory impairment and almost 47 percent have a diagnosis of senile dementia, an organic brain syndrome (Hing, 1987).

Nursing home users appear to have become more disabled in the last several years. Some attribute this change to the impact of DRGs,

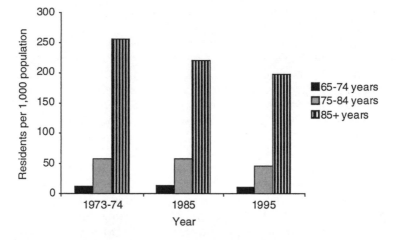

Figure 14-5 Rate of nursing home use. *(From National Center for Health Statistics, 1997.)*

but the trend had begun well in advance of that change. The contemporary nursing home user is older and more disabled than a decade ago. Figure 14-6 compares the levels of disability among nursing home residents in 1985 with those in 1995. In general there is a pattern of slightly greater levels of disability, but in one area (transferring) the pattern moves in the opposite direction. It is not clear if this represents a true effect or a statistical artifact based on the way the data were collected. In all the other cases, the level of disability has increased, but not as dramatically as anecdotes might suggest.

Any effort to describe the nursing home resident population must recognize that the nursing home plays multiple roles. It caters to a wide variety of clientele. At least five distinct groups of residents can be identified:

1. Those actively recuperating or being rehabilitated. These are largely persons discharged from hospitals and are expected to have a short course in the nursing home before returning home. This care has been called "subacute" or "transitional." The evidence of the nursing home's capacity to provide effective care of this type is mixed (Kramer et al., 1997; Kane et al., 1996).
2. Those with substantial physical dependencies. These residents need regular and usually frequent assistance during the day. Their care

Table 14-3 Comparison of nursing home residents and the noninstitutionalized population age 65+, 1995

	Percent of nursing home residents*	Percent of noninstitutionalized population[†]
Age		
65–74 years	17.5	55.9
75–84	42.3	33.2
85+	40.2	10.8
Sex		
Male	24.7	40.8
Female	75.3	59.2
Race		
White	89.5	89.6
Black	8.5	8.1
Other	2.0	2.3
Marital status		
Married	16.5	56.9
Widowed	66.0	33.2
Divorced and/or separated	5.5	5.7
Never married/single	11.1	4.2
Unknown	0.8	—

* From Dey, 1997.
[†] From U.S. Census Bureau, 1996.

could be managed in the community with sufficient formal and informal support.

3. Those with primarily severe cognitive losses. These people present special management problems because of their behavior and their propensity to wander. Some favor separate facilities for them, not necessarily because they fare better there but because such a step removes them from the environment of those who are cognitively intact. There is no evidence of improvement in the outcomes of demented residents from these "special care units" (Phillips et al., 1997).

4. Those receiving terminal care. This hospice care is directed toward making the person as comfortable as possible. Palliative care is provided but no heroic efforts are undertaken.

5. Those in a permanent vegetative state. This group includes those who are in the last stages of dementia as well as those with severe

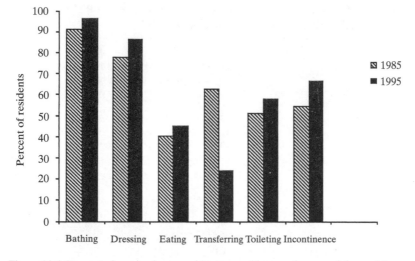

Figure 14-6 Percent of nursing home residents over 65 years of age receiving assistance with ADLs. *(From Dey, 1997, and Hing et al., 1989.)*

strokes and the like. This group is distinguished by its inability to relate to the environment. Care is primarily directed toward avoiding complications (e.g., decubitus ulcers).

It should be clear from this list that each of these subgroups will imply different treatment objectives. For those who are sensitive to their environments, quality-of-life issues will be at least as salient as traditional technical quality-of-care issues.

Especially in the wake of changing hospital practice and the rise of "subacute care," great care must be exercised in using nursing home data because of the differences in the characteristics of those entering or leaving and those resident at any point in time. The latter are more likely to have chronic problems such as dementia, whereas the former will have problems that are either rehabilitable or fatal (e.g., hip fracture and cancer). This distinction makes it tricky to talk about nursing home patients and may explain the often contradictory data presented.

For example, it is true that nursing home stays are not nearly as long as one might believe. The commonly cited statistic indicates that about half of those admitted are discharged within 3 months, but

this proportion has increased under the influence of the Prospective Payment System (PPS). A study using the 1985 National Nursing Home Survey showed that, even adjusting for episodes of care, 45 percent of residents had stays of less than 3 months, about 10 percent stayed for 6 months to a year, 17 percent for 1 to 3 years, and 9 percent stayed for 5 or more years (Spence et al., 1990). The increased use of nursing homes for posthospital care will inevitably increase the proportion of very short stays.

Payment for nursing home care has been increasing based on measures that reflect the costs of providing that care. (Although this type of payment is often called "prospective reimbursement," it is important to recognize that it is quite different from that used with hospitals. Nursing home prospective payment is calculated on a daily rate basis in contrast to the episode basis used for hospitals. Hence as a person's status changes, so does the payment.) This form of case-mix reimbursement is largely driven by the costs of the nursing personnel who provide that care. The costs are usually calculated by estimating these costs based on a set of observed times spent by different types of personnel (nurses aides, LPNs, and RNs) for different classes of residents. In some cases the time spent is self-reported by the staff; in other instances it is based on observations. These data are then used to construct models that relate the cost of professional time to the characteristics of the clients. This approach has two major problems:

1. The models generally rely on looking at what kind of care is being given rather than what sort of care is actually needed; the care is not related to outcomes obtained nor is it based on any models of especially good care.
2. The logic behind this approach to estimating payments is inherently perverse. If carried to its logical extreme, this system of payment rewards nursing homes for residents becoming more dependent instead of more independent.

The most commonly used case-mix system is the Resource Utilization Groups (RUGS). Since its development for use in New York, it has been revised several times and is now linked to a form of the MDS, which is the mandated assessment approach for nursing home care. Figure 14-7 illustrates the RUGS-III approach to classifying nursing home residents according to groups that imply different levels

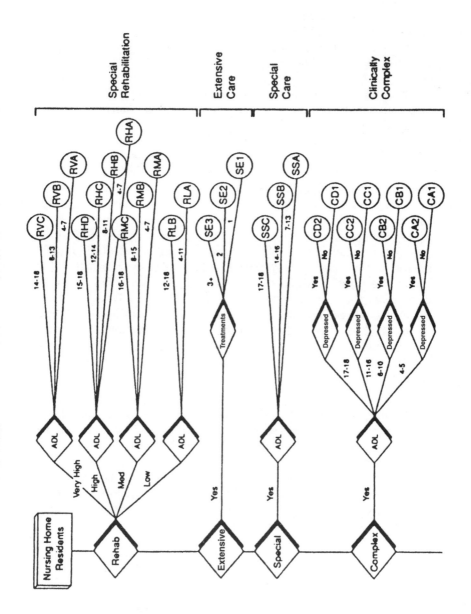

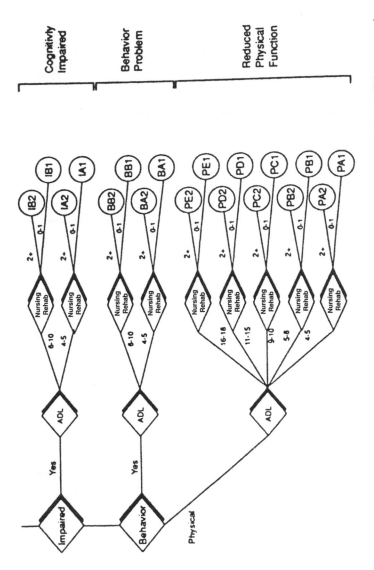

Figure 14-7 The Resource Utilization Group (RUG-III) case-mix classification system. RUGs will be generated from items in the Minimum Data Set (MDS) and used as a basis for case-mix reimbursement. (*Figures supplied by Dr. Brant Fries.*)

of staffing needs. This approach has been used by some Medicaid programs and is the basis for Medicare skilled nursing facility payments.

The physician's role in nursing home care is discussed in greater detail in Chap. 15. Suffice it to say here that the nursing home has not been an attractive place for physicians to practice. However, conditions are changing. The physician can play a critical role in setting the tone for the care of patients in the nursing home. Physicians' expectations of professional performance and their advocacy of their patients' needs can be very influential in shaping staff behavior.

New types of personnel can be used effectively to deliver primary care to nursing home patients. Nurse practitioners and physician assistants have been shown to deliver high-quality care in this setting (Kane et al., 1989, 1991a). Medicare regulations covering Part B were altered to allow greater use of physician assistants and nurse practitioners. Similarly, clinical pharmacists have proved very helpful in simplifying drug regimens and avoiding potential drug interactions.

A managed care program directed specifically at nursing home patients points to the art of the possible. Building on the prior successes of using nurse practitioners as key figures to provide primary care to nursing home residents, the EverCare program has developed Medicare managed care risk contracts specifically for long-stay nursing home patients. Under this arrangement, EverCare is responsible for all the residents' Medicare costs (both Part A and Part B) but not their nursing home costs. The underlying concept is that by providing more aggressive primary care they can prevent hospital admissions. EverCare places nurse practitioners in each participating nursing home to work with the residents' own physicians. The nurse practitioners provide closer follow up and work closely with the nursing home staff to identify problems early. In some cases EverCare will pay the nursing home extra to increase nursing attention for patients in order to treat that person in the nursing home rather than admitting her to a hospital. The theory is that the savings from avoided or shortened hospital stays will offset the added costs of more attentive primary care provided by the nurse practitioners. The apparent success of the EverCare model has spawned similar approaches.

A study by the Institute of Medicine pointed to the need for reforms, many of which were incorporated into OBRA '87. The imple-

mentation of the OBRA '87 regulations has produced a number of changes in the way nursing homes are operated. In addition to the standardized assessment mandated in the Minimum Data Set (described in Chap. 15), the emphasis in regulation has been shifted more toward addressing the outcomes of patient care; but some increases in process measures have also been introduced. For example, guidelines for the use of psychoactive drugs have been mandated. All residents admitted and already living in the nursing home must be screened to determine if they are there primarily because of chronic mental illness. If so, a specific plan of care must be developed with appropriate participation from mental health professionals. Those residents who do not require skilled care are supposed to be transferred to more appropriate care settings. More training is mandated for nurses' aides and the staffing requirements overall have been upgraded.

Regulations intended to upgrade care can also constrain care. Rather than insisting that all patients be seen on a fixed schedule, more flexibility is needed to adjust care to the patient's condition.

ASSISTED LIVING

A new form of chronic care is emerging. The traditional functions of the nursing home—housing and nursing care—can be "uncoupled," with benefits for all (Kane et al., 1991b). "Assisted living" describes a form of care for many of those who currently require nursing home care. It is designed to provide services to persons as they require them, in a setting that more closely resembles a person's home. Residents still live in institutional settings that house many people within the same facility, thus maximizing efficiency of service delivery. They use common facilities, such as a dining room, but they also retain their privacy. Basically, each resident is treated as a tenant and has control over a living unit. At a minimum, each individually occupied dwelling unit contains space for living and sleeping, a bathroom, and at least minimal cooking facilities. (The stove can be disconnected for those for whom it might pose a serious danger.) Each unit can be locked by the occupant.

Under this approach, control is shifted toward empowering the recipient of care. In contrast to the situation in a nursing home, where residents are expected to conform to the norms of the institution, in

an assisted living facility individualized care is stressed. As the tenant, the resident has control over the use of her space: care providers must be invited in; care plans must be accepted by the resident. These shifts, while subtle at one level, are fundamental at another. They imply a dramatically altered approach to care, some of which is tangible and some of which is not. The lore of nursing homes is laden with evidence of learned helplessness and enforced dependency. This approach to care is aimed at maximizing a resident's sense of self and independence as much as possible.

Especially for those chronically impaired persons who have retained an appreciation of their environment, such a philosophy of care makes great sense. Examples of such care are becoming more prevalent. They have been able to serve quite disabled persons as well as those less impaired who are most often targeted for such services. Moreover, the costs of assisted living are usually much less than comparable nursing home care.

One reason that assisted living is less expensive and more flexible is that it has thus far been spared the heavy regulatory mantle laid on nursing homes. Staffing patterns are not as intense or as professionally dictated. Staff perform multiple functions. If it is regulated in the same way, it will inevitably come to resemble nursing home care. Once again, the form of care is determined by society's willingness to accept some risks. At a minimum, those who receive the care should have an opportunity to choose what kind of care they want to get.

HOME CARE

As already noted, we have developed a backward system of long-term care in this country that focuses on the nursing home. We tend to speak of the nursing home and alternatives to it, when we should begin with the premise that elderly people belong at home and want to be cared for at home. Institutional care will be needed in some cases, when the strain on caregivers is too great, but it should not be the resource of first resort. Our system has not evolved that way, and the resources available for home care are meager, but not so underdeveloped as to be ignored. Even today, most communities have at least some home care services, and more are likely to develop.

Home care involves at least two basic types of care: home health services; and homemaking and chore services. As shown in Table 14-4, different programs provide one or both types. Most elderly people treated at home require homemaking more than home health services. Sometimes the differences between the two are purely arbitrary. If we consider that the homemaker replaces or supplements a family member, many of the tasks involved are extensions of home nursing (for example, supervising medication or giving baths). The definitions have emerged arbitrarily, often to fit the regulations governing a particular program. The physician will usually find that the home health agency is familiar with these regulations and how to deal with them.

The major problem at present is getting services. In response to political pressures, Medicare broadened its long-term-care benefit (including waiving the former requirement that a person have a prior hospital stay of at least 3 days) and moved the program from Part B to Part A, thereby removing the copayment requirement. The subsequent enormous growth in home health care under Medicare, shown in Fig. 14-8, has led to revisions in coverage that will move part of the program back under Part B. (Home health care not related to a prior 3-day hospital stay or visits after 100 if related to a stay will be covered under Part B). Despite the growth in use, some still maintain that the criteria for eligibility for these services severely restricts their use. To get home health services for a patient, a physician must certify that the patient is homebound and that intermittent skilled care is likely to produce a benefit in a reasonable time. Thus, a large number of dependent older persons who need continuing home nursing but are "custodial" are ineligible unless the physician misrepresents their situation. *Skilled service* is defined as a skilled service offered by a nurse, a physical therapist, or a speech therapist. If one of these establishing services is present, the patient may also receive the skilled services of an occupational therapist or medical social worker and/or the services of a home health aide if required by the plan. Medicare has begun to allow home health agencies to continue to serve clients who need case management, thus permitting some cases to remain open longer than the "intermittent" rule might otherwise imply. All reimbursed services must be given by a certified home health agency. (To be certified, the agency needs to offer nursing plus at least one of the five other services.) The requirement for using a certified agency greatly increases the costs of the services, although

Table 14-4 Home care provided under various federal programs

	Medicare	Medicaid	Title XX
Eligibility criteria	Must be homebound; need skilled care; need and expect benefit in a reasonable period; need certification by physician	State can use homebound criterion; not limited to skilled care; need certification by physician	Vary from state to state
Payment to provider	Reasonable costs	Varies with state	Three modes of payment possible: (1) direct provision by government agency; (2) contract with private agency; (3) independent provider
Services covered	Home health services, skilled nursing, physical or speech therapy as primary services; secondary services (social worker and home health aide) available *only* if primary service is provided; position of occupational therapy in service hierarchy ambiguous*	Limited home-health care mandatory; expanded home care optional; personal care in home optional	Wide variety of home services allowed, including home health aide, homemaker, chore worker, meal services

* Occupational therapy is considered an "extended" secondary service, which may continue if needed after primary services are discontinued.

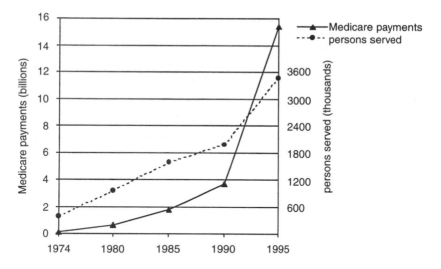

Figure 14-8 Growth in Medicare home health spending. *(From U.S. Department of Health and Human Services, 1997c.)*

the assumption is that this certification assures at least a minimal level of professional oversight. A recurring question is how much administrative overhead is affordable as the pressure on the long-term-care dollar grows.

Medicaid funds can be used to provide home health care to persons eligible for nursing home care. Until recently, Medicaid funds have not been widely used for home care. In fact, until 1980, one state (New York) accounted for almost 95 percent of the Medicaid moneys spent on home health care. (It is still by far the largest user of Medicaid home care.) Home care under Medicaid must have a physician's authorization, but the patient need not be homebound, and the care need not be "skilled." All agencies delivering home care under Medicaid must meet Medicare certification standards, but if no organized home health agencies exist in a region, a registered nurse may be reimbursed for the services. In practice, states have often modeled their Medicaid home care benefits after the medically oriented Medicare benefit and thus restricted its use.

Under Medicaid, the nursing care is a required component of home health services, and the state has the option to provide physical, occupational, and speech therapy; medical social services; and

personal-care services. Medicaid allows homemaking assistance on a more generous basis than does Medicare. Personal-care services must be prescribed by a physician and supervised by a registered nurse. These services may not be delivered by persons related to the patient. Recent changes in legislation have broadened the permissible use of Medicaid moneys to support a wide variety of long-term-care services in an effort to reduce nursing home costs. A number of states have received waivers to develop this broader package of services but most of these wavered services are limited in the numbers of "slots" they are allowed.

Despite the growth of home care under Medicaid and the growing numbers of alternative waiver programs, the large bulk of Medicaid long-term-care funds continue to flow to nursing homes. However, the relative dominance of spending on nursing home care varies widely from state to state. An analysis of 1992 data showed that the average annual long-term care expenditure per persons aged 65 and older was $935 but the range extended from $2720 (New York) to $380 (Arizona). Nursing home expenditures likewise varied widely, from $1623 in the District of Columbia to $314 in Arizona. So too did spending on home and community-based care. The average expenditure per person over age 65 was just under $200, with a range from $1180 (New York) to $30 (Mississippi) (Kane et al., 1998).

The bulk of support for homemaking services, however, continues to rest with Title III and Title XX. Title XX provides at least four methods of payment: local public agencies can provide the service directly; they can contract with agency providers (perhaps using competitive bidding); they can purchase services from agencies at negotiated prices; or they can permit the recipient to enter into agreement with independent providers, who do not work for an agency. It is possible to have all these arrangements operating in the same community. This provision for independent vendors has prompted controversy because maintaining standards is difficult in the absence of any supervisory system or institutional responsibility. Under Title XX, an employment category known as *chore worker* has emerged; although performing functions similar to the home health aide and the homemaker, chore workers do not need to be tightly supervised and cannot be reimbursed under Medicare or Medicaid.

Persons eligible for cash assistance from the state, and other persons with low incomes and unmet service needs, are eligible for Title XX as long as 50 percent of a state's annual federal allotment

is expended on those receiving cash assistance. Fees are charged to those whose family income exceeds 80 percent of the state's median income for a family of four.

Home services are one of four priority items under Title III of the Older Americans Act. This source is important because means testing (whereby eligibility is set by income) is prohibited for programs under the Older Americans Act, making it possible to target a group that cannot afford private care but is ineligible for Title XX or Medicaid. Generally speaking, the Area Agency on Aging (AAA) subcontracts for home care services rather than providing them directly. The usual pattern is that Administration on Aging dollars permit existing agencies to develop or expand a home care component. Services vary from area to area but can include personal care, homemaker service, chore service, and service for heavier jobs (e.g., minor home repairs or renovations, insect eradication, gardening, and painting). The provisions for assistance under AAA are sharply limited by their constrained budgets and the competing demands for programs.

The extent of services under these several programs is still limited at present, although enthusiasm for in-home care is growing. The total sum of public dollars spent on home care remains only a fraction of that devoted to nursing homes.

OTHER SERVICES

A number of other modes of care can be tapped on behalf of elderly patients. Table 14-5 lists some of these services. However, despite their growing availability, they are still not widely used. The most

Table 14-5 Examples of community long-term care programs

Home care (home nursing and homemaking)	Caregiver support
Adult day care	Congregate housing
Adult foster care	Home repairs
Assisted living	Meals (congregate and in-home)
Geriatric assessment	Respite care
Hospice/terminal care	Emergency alarms
Telephone reassurance	

frequently used service in that set is the senior center, a service designed for the well elderly person.

Day care can fulfill a number of needs. Most day care programs provide some combination of recreational and restorative activity. In contrast to senior centers, which are usually sponsored by recreational departments and targeted at the well elderly, day care programs serve persons with limited functional ability. Some are for cognitively impaired persons. The programs provide supervised activities, which may improve basic ADL skills and social skills. At the very least, they provide an important respite for the primary caregiver and thus may make the critical difference for allowing an impaired older person to remain at home. To increase efficiency, most programs serve any given client less than 5 days a week, usually 2 or 3 days.

Other forms of day care can include a larger medical component. Some areas have developed day hospitals for seniors, where virtually all the services of the hospital are available on an ambulatory basis. Emphasis is usually placed on rehabilitation, especially occupational and physical therapy. The adult day health center is an intermediate model, which combines day care with nursing, physical therapy, and perhaps social work. Such sites can also be used for periodic ambulatory care clinics.

A problem common to all day-care programs is transportation. It is hard to arrange, expensive, and time-consuming. Special vans are usually needed, and, to avoid excessive travel times, services are usually confined to very limited areas.

In many communities, a variety of services exist to help seniors: ombudsmen, peer counselors, mental health clinics, transportation, congregate meal sites, and meals on wheels—just to name a few. Availability varies greatly from place to place. A good source of information is the social work department in a hospital. Another resource is the Area Agency on Aging.

The physician cannot be expected to know all the resources available for geriatric patients and will have to rely on other professionals to make appropriate arrangements to take advantage of them. But a physician should have a good sense of what can be done in general and what needs to be done for any particular patient. Often knowing what is needed but not locally available can lead to its development, particularly if responsible professionals take an active role on behalf of their patients.

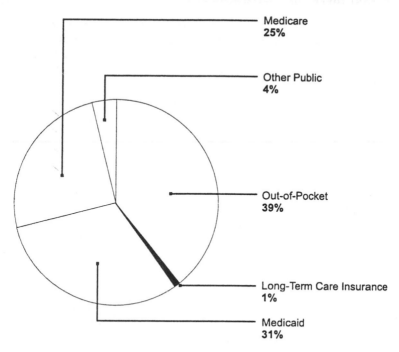

Figure 14-9 Distribution of 1995 expenditures for long-term care for older persons, by funding source. *(From Scanlon, 1998.)*

Figure 14-9 summarizes the pattern of support for long-term care services to older persons.

CASE MANAGEMENT

The growing interest in the plethora of community long-term-care services has sparked some concerns about the need to control use. A frequent answer is *case management.* This term has been widely and variably used. The basic components of case management are assessment, prescription, authorization, coordination, and monitoring. These are issues very close to activities of primary care and hence may lead to some concern about role overlap between the case manager and the primary care physician. It is possible for physicians to serve as case managers, but most do not have the interest or the

resources to perform this task. It is usually more efficient to look to other disciplines to perform this function but to recognize the important role of the physician in the overall care of the long-term-care patient. Where a full range of geriatric services is available, case management is usually included.

Regardless of discipline, the case manager faces some difficult tasks. There is often a discrepancy between responsibility and authority. It is very different to prescribe, authorize, or mandate. Case managers may or may not have the purchasing authority to pay for services they feel are necessary. Case managers may easily find themselves in the same bind as physicians. Specifically, they are expected to serve simultaneously as patient advocates and gatekeepers. The two roles are not compatible. For everyone's peace of mind, it is important to clarify at the outset who is the principal client. Because many decisions involve advocating on behalf of one group over another, this distinction is critical. It is very different to work on behalf of a client to obtain all the resources you believe they need than to work to distribute a fixed pool of resources to those who will best use them.

Another frequently heard concern about case management is the need to affix responsibility. On the one hand, the easiest way to do this is to give the case manager a budget and expect him or her to work within it to achieve the most possible. However, some have expressed anxieties that the person charged with authorizing services should be at arm's length from those providing them. Specific concerns are heard about hospital discharge planners' decisions as to when to refer patients to services owned or operated by the hospital. There is a real potential for client skimming. Similarly, if the case manager works for a caregiving agency, there is the risk that that agency may get a disproportionate share of the choicest clients. On the other hand, even when case managers are separated from direct care, they are not immune to pressure from the purveyors, just as the physician is pursued by the drug companies.

Case management has also become a mainstay of managed care. In this context, cases are usually identified on the basis of some risk indicators—either a record of heavy use of services or the presence of risk factors that imply such a pattern in the future. While some case management within managed care is patient-centered, operating on the premise that closer care can stave off costly problems (Rich

et al., 1995), much of it revolves around primarily utilization controls (Pacala et al., 1994).

REFERENCES

AARP Public Public Policy Institute, and The Lewin Group: *Out-of-Pocket Health Spending by Medicare Beneficiaries Age 65 and Older: 1997 Projections* (9705). Washington, DC, American Association of Retired Persons, 1997.

Branch LG, Coulam RF, Zimmerman YA: The PACE evaluation: Initial findings. *Gerontologist* 35:349–359, 1995.

Dey AN: *Characteristics of Elderly Nursing Home Residents: Data from the 1995 National Nursing Home Survey. Advance Data from Vital and Health Statistics* (289). Hyattsville, MD, National Center for Health Statistics, 1997.

Eng C, Pedulla J, Eleazer GP, et al: Program of All-inclusive Care for the Elderly (PACE): An innovative model of integrated geriatric care and financing. *J Am Geriatr Soc* 45:223–232, 1997.

Hing E: *Use of Nursing Homes by the Elderly: Preliminary Data from the 1985 National Nursing Home Survey. Advance Data From Vital and Health Statistics No. 135* (DHHS). Hyattsville, MD, U.S. Public Health Service, 1987.

Hing E, Sekscenski E, Strahan G: *The National Nursing Home Survey; 1985 Summary for the United States.* [Vital and Health Statistics Series 13, No. 97, DHHS Pub. No. (PHS) 89-1758.] Washington, DC, U.S. Public Health Service, 1989.

Hoffman C, Rice D, Sung H-Y: Persons with chronic conditions: Their prevalence and costs. *JAMA* 276:1473–1479, 1996.

Institute of Medicine: *Improving the Quality of Care in Nursing Homes.* Washington, DC, National Academy Press, 1986.

Kane RA, Wilson KB, *Assisted Living in the United States: A New Paradigm for Residential Care for Older Persons?* Washington, DC, American Association of Retired Persons, 1993.

Kane RL, Garrard J, Skay CL, et al: Effects of a geriaric nurse practitioner on the process and outcomes of nursing home care. *Am J Public Health* 79:1271–1277, 1989.

Kane RL, Garrard J, Buchanan JL, et al: Improving primary care in nursing homes. *J Am Geriatr Soc* 39:359–367, 1991a.

Kane RL, Kane RA: A nursing home in your future? *N Engl J Med* 324:627–629, 1991b.

Kane RL, Illston LH, Miller NA. Qualitative analysis of the Program of All-inclusive Care for the Elderly (PACE). *Gerontologist* 32:771–780, 1992.

Kane RL, Chen Q, Blewett LA, et al: Do rehabilitation nursing homes improve the outcomes of care? *J Am Geriatr Soc* 44:545–554, 1996.

Kane RL, Friedman B: State variations in Medicare expenditures. *Am J Public Health* 87:1611–1619, 1997a.

Kane RL, Kane RA, Finch M, et al: S/HMOs, the second generation: Building on the experience of the first social health maintenance organization demonstrations. *J Am Geriatr Soc* 45(1):101–107, 1997b.

Kane RL, Kane RA, Ladd RC, et al: Variation in state spending for long-term care: Factors associated with more balanced systems. *J Health Polit Policy Law* 23:363–390, 1998.

Kane RL: Managed care as a vehicle for delivering more effective chronic care for older persons. *J Am Geriatr Soc* 46:1034–1039, 1998.

Kennedy J, LaPlante MP, Kaye HS: Need for assistance in the activities of daily living. *Disabil Stat Abstr* 18:1–4, 1997.

Kosecoff J, Kahn KL, Rogers WH, et al: Prospective payment system and impairment at discharge. The "quicker-and-sicker" story revisited. 264:1980–1983, 1990.

Kramer AM, Steiner JF, Schlenker RE, et al: Outcomes and costs after hip fracture and stroke: A comparison of rehabilitation settings. *JAMA* 277:396–404, 1997.

Lachs MS, Ruchlin HS: Is managed care good or bad for geriatric medicine? *J Am Geriatr Soc* 45:1123–1127, 1997.

Manton KG, Corder L, Stallard L: Chronic disability trends in elderly United States populations: 1982–1994. *Med Sci* 94:2593–2598, 1997.

Moon M: What Medicare has meant to older Americans. *Health Care Fin Rev* 18(2):49–59, 1996.

Morgan RO, Virnig BA, DeVito CA, et al: The Medicare-HMO revolving door—The healthy go in and the sick go out. *N Engl J Med* 337:169–175, 1997.

National Center for Health Statistics: *Health, United States, 1996–97 and Injury Chartbook.* Hyattsville, MD, NCHS, 1997.

Pacala JT, Boult C, Hepburn K, et al. *Case Management of Older Adults Enrolled in Health Maintenance Organizations. Final Report of a Study Conducted Under Contract with the Robert Wood Johnson Foundation.* Minneapolis, MN: University of Minnesota, 1994.

Phillips CD, Sloane PD, Hawes C., et al: Effects of residence in Alzheimer disease special care units on functional outcomes. *JAMA* 278:1340–1344, 1997.

Rich MW, Beckham V, Wittenberg C, et al: A multidisciplinary intervention to prevent the readmission of elderly patients with congestive heart failure. *N Engl J Med* 333:1190–1195, 1995.

Scanlon WJ: *Long-Term Care: Baby Boom Generation Presents Financing Challenges (Testimony before the Special Committee on Aging. U.S. Senate)* (GAO/T-HEHS-98-107). Washington, DC, Health Financing and Systems Issues; Health, Education, and Human Services Division, 1998.

Spence DA, Wiener JM: Nursing home length of stay patterns: Results from the 1985 national nursing home survey. *Gerontologist* 30(1):16–20, 1990.

U.S. Census Bureau: *Statistical Abstract of the United States: 1996.* Washington, DC, U.S. Government Printing Office, 1996.

U.S. Department of Health and Human Services, HCFA, and Office of Research and Demonstrations: *Health Care Financing Review: Statistical Supplement, Table 16.* Baltimore, MD, USDHHS, 1997a.

U.S. Department of Health and Human Services, HCFA, and Office Research and Demonstrations: *Health Care Financing Review: Statistical Supplement, Table 88.* Baltimore, MD, USDHHS, 1997b.

U.S. Department of Health and Human Services HCFR. Growth in Medicare home health spending. *Health Care Financing Review: Statistical Supplement.* Baltimore, MD, USDHHS, 1997c.

Welch HG, Wennberg DE, Welch WP: The use of Medicare home health services. *N Engl J Med* 335:324–329, 1996.

SUGGESTED READINGS

Boult C, Boult L, Pacala JT: Systems of care for older populations of the future. *J Am Geriatr Soc* 46:499–505, 1998.

Callahan JJ, Jr, Diamond LD, Giele JZ, et al: Responsibility of families for their severely disabled elders. *Health Care Fin Rev* 1:29–73, 1980.

Kane RA, Kane RL, Ladd R: *The Heart of Long-term Care.* New York, Oxford University Press, 1998.

O'Brien CL: *Adult Day Care: A Practical Guide.* Monterey, CA, Wadsworth Health Sciences, 1982.

Pepper Commission: *A Call for Action: The Pepper Commission U.S. Bipartisan Commission on Comprehensive Health Care.* Washington, DC, U.S. Government Printing Office, 1990.

Silverstone B, Hyman HK: *You & Your Aging Parent.* New York, Pantheon, 1976.

Somers AR: Long-term care for the elderly and disabled: A new health priority. *N Engl J Med* 307:221–226, 1982.

Trager B: *Home Health Care and National Health Policy* (special issue of *Home Health Care Services Quarterly*). New York, Haworth Press, 1980.

Vladeck BG: *Unloving Care: The Nursing Home Tragedy.* New York, Basic Books, 1980.

Williams ME: *The American Geriatrics Society's Complete Guide to Aging & Health:* New York, Harmony Books, 1995.

CHAPTER FIFTEEN

NURSING HOME CARE

The focus of this chapter is the clinical care of nursing home residents. Some of the basic demographic and economic aspects of nursing home care are discussed in Chaps. 2 and 14. The term *nursing home* is somewhat of a misnomer: relatively little nursing care is provided (an average of about 70 min per day of nurses' aide care), and most facilities do not have a homelike atmosphere. Numerous reports have documented that medical care in the nursing home is often inadequate (Moss and Halamandaris, 1977; Vladek, 1980; Institute of Medicine, 1986). Physician visits are often brief and superficial, documentation in medical records is scanty, treatable conditions are under- or misdiagnosed, and psychotropic and other drugs are overused and misused in part because of the absence of mental health interventions by appropriately trained professionals (Borson et al., 1987; Beers et al., 1988; Garrard et al., 1991; Avorn et al., 1992; Heston et al., 1992).

Despite the logistic, economic, and attitudinal barriers that can foster inadequate medical care in the nursing home, many relatively straightforward principles and strategies can lead to improvements in the quality of medical care provided to nursing home residents.

Fundamental to achieving these improvements is a clear perspective on the goals of nursing home care, which are in many respects quite different from the goals of medical care in other settings and patient populations.

THE GOALS OF NURSING HOME CARE

The modern nursing home serves multiple roles. The key goals of nursing home care are listed in Table 15-1. While the prevention, identification, and treatment of chronic, subacute, and acute medical conditions are important, most of these goals focus on the functional independence, autonomy, quality of life, comfort, and dignity of the residents. Physicians who care for nursing home residents must keep these goals in perspective at the same time the more traditional goals of medical care are being addressed.

The heterogeneity of the nursing home population must also be recognized in order to focus and individualize the goals of care. This heterogeneity results in a diversity of goals for nursing home care. Nursing home residents can be subgrouped into five basic types (see Fig. 15-1). While it is not always possible to isolate these different types of residents geographically and residents often overlap or change between the types described, subgrouping nursing home residents in this manner will help the physician and interdisciplinary team to focus the care-planning process on the most critical and realistic goals for individual residents.

The underlying social contract implied by nursing home admission is quite different for each of these groups. In some cases access to

Table 15-1 Goals of nursing home care

1. Provide a safe and supportive environment for chronically ill and dependent people.
2. Restore and maintain the highest possible level of functional independence
3. Preserve individual autonomy
4. Maximize quality of life, perceived well-being, and life satisfaction
5. Provide comfort and dignity for terminally ill patients and their loved ones
6. Stabilize and delay progression, whenever possible, of chronic medical conditions
7. Prevent acute medical and iatrogenic illnesses and identify and treat them rapidly when they do occur

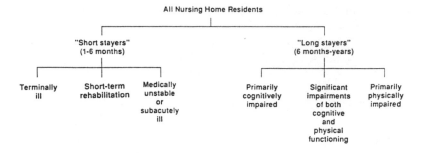

Figure 15-1 Basic types of nursing home patients.

treatment takes precedence over the living environment; in other circumstances the environment may be the most critical element of care. Those admitted to a nursing home with the intent of active treatment may be willing to accept a living situation akin to that of a hospital in the expectation that the benefit they receive from treatment will offset any discomfort or inconvenience. For terminally ill persons under the hospice model, the living environment is made as flexible and supportive as possible. Efforts are directed toward making patients comfortable and permitting them to enjoy their last days.

There is a trend to separate the cognitively impaired from those who are primarily physically impaired. There has been a growing number of special care units (SCUs) for the cognitively impaired where their care can be coordinated to maximize attention to the behavioral aspects of dementia care and to minimize the use of psychoactive drugs and restraints while maintaining a safe environment. Some see SCUs as a way of achieving better results. Others view them as controlled environments in which demented residents can be treated more humanely by staff who have chosen to concentrate on such care. Still others see the primary gain from SCUs as removing otherwise disruptive patients from the environment of those still alert enough to resent the intrusion.

Residents who are more cognitively intact may benefit from newer forms of institutional care such as assisted living (described in Chap. 14). These residents can maximize their quality of life in individual rooms that afford them privacy and a greater sense of control over their surroundings. Those residents who are, for all intents and purposes, completely out of touch with their environments (e.g., those

in permanent vegetative states or advanced dementia) may be well served by simple environments designed to maintain them safely. These individuals are the subject of increasing ethical debate (see Chap. 16).

CLINICAL ASPECTS OF CARE FOR NURSING HOME RESIDENTS

In addition to the different goals for care in the nursing home, several factors make the assessment and treatment of nursing home residents different from those in other settings (Table 15-2). Many of these factors relate to the process of care and are discussed in the following section. (For a more complete discussion of medical care in the nursing home, see Suggested Readings, Ouslander et al., 1996.) A fundamental difference in the nursing home is that medical evaluation and treatment must be complemented by an assessment and care-planning process involving staff from multiple disciplines. Data on medical conditions and their treatment are integrated with assessments of the functional, mental, and behavioral status of the resident in order to develop a comprehensive data base and individualized plan of care.

Medical evaluation and clinical decision making for nursing home residents are complicated for several reasons. Unless the physician has cared for the resident before nursing home admission, it may be difficult to obtain a comprehensive medical data base. Residents may be unable to relate their medical histories accurately or to describe their symptoms, and medical records are frequently unavailable or incomplete, especially for residents who have been transferred between nursing homes and acute-care hospitals. When acute changes in status occur, initial assessments are often performed by nursing home staff with limited skills and are transmitted to physicians by telephone. Even when the diagnoses are known or strongly suspected, many diagnostic and therapeutic procedures among nursing home residents are associated with an unacceptably high risk-to-benefit ratio. For example, a barium enema may cause dehydration or severe fecal impaction, nitrates and other cardiovascular drugs may precipitate syncope or disabling falls in frail ambulatory residents with baseline postural hypotension, and adequate control of blood sugar may be extremely difficult to achieve without a high risk for hypoglycemia

Table 15-2 Factors that make assessment and treatment in the nursing home different from that in other settings

1. The goals of care are often different (see Table 15-1)
2. Specific clinical disorders are prevalent among nursing home residents (see Table 15-3)
3. The approach to health maintenance and prevention differs (see Table 15-6)
4. Mental and functional status are just as important if not more so than medical diagnoses
5. Assessment must be interdisciplinary, including:
   Nursing
   Psychosocial
   Rehabilitation
   Nutritional
   Other (e.g., dental, pharmacy, podiatry, audiology, ophthalmology)
6. Sources of information are variable:
   Residents often cannot give a precise history
   Family members and nurses' aides with limited assessment skills may provide the most important information
   Information is often obtained over the telephone
7. Administrative procedures for record keeping in both nursing homes and acute care hospitals can result in inadequate and disjointed information
8. Clinical decision making is complicated for several reasons:
   Many diagnostic and therapeutic procedures are expensive, unavailable, or difficult to obtain and involve higher risks of iatrogenic illness and discomfort than are warranted by the potential outcome
   The potential long-term benefits of "tight" control of certain chronic illnesses (e.g., diabetes mellitus, congestive heart failure, hypertension) may be outweighed by the risks of iatrogenic illness in many very old and functionally disabled residents
   Many residents are not capable (or are questionably capable) of participating in medical decision making, and their personal preferences based on previous decisions are often unknown (see Table 15-7)
9. The appropriate site for and intensity of treatment are often difficult decisions involving medical, emotional, ethical, economic, and legal considerations that may be in conflict with each other in the nursing home setting
10. Logistic considerations, resource constraints, and restrictive reimbursement policies may limit the ability of and incentives for physicians to carry out optimal medical care of nursing home residents

among cognitively impaired diabetic residents with marginal or fluctuating nutritional intake who may not recognize or complain of hypoglycemic symptoms.

Further compounding these difficulties is the inability of many nursing home residents to participate effectively in important decisions regarding their medical care. Their previously expressed wishes are often not known, and an appropriate or legal surrogate decision maker has often not been appointed. These issues are discussed further on in this chapter and in Chap. 16.

Table 15-3 lists the most commonly encountered clinical disorders in the nursing home population. They represent a broad spectrum of chronic medical illnesses; neurologic, psychiatric, and behavioral

Table 15-3 Common clinical disorders in the nursing home population

Medical conditions
    Chronic medical illnesses
    Congestive heart failure
    Degenerative joint disease
    Diabetes mellitus
    Obstructive lung disease
    Renal failure
    Infections
        Lower respiratory tract
        Urinary tract
        Skin (pressure sores, vascular ulcers)
        Conjunctivitis
        Gastroenteritis
    Gastrointestinal disorders
        Reflux esophagitis
        Constipation
        Diarrhea

Malignancies

Neuropsychiatric conditions
    Dementia
    Behavioral disorders associated with dementia
        Wandering
        Agitation
        Aggression
        Depression

(continued)

Table 15-3 Common clinical disorders in the nursing home population *(Continued)*

Neurologic disorders other than dementia
  Stroke
  Parkinsonism
  Multiple sclerosis
  Brain or spinal cord injury

Functional disabilities necessitating rehabilitation
  Stroke
  Hip fracture
  Joint replacement
  Amputation

Geriatric problems
  Delirium
  Incontinence
  Gait disturbances, instability, falls
  Malnutrition, feeding difficulties, dehydration
  Pressure sores
  Insomnia

Chronic pain: muscoloskeletal conditions,
  neuropathies, malignancy

Iatrogenic disorders
  Adverse drug reactions
  Falls
  Nosocomial infections
  Induced disabilities
  Restraints and immobility, catheters, unnecessary
    help with basic activities of daily living

Death and dying

disorders; and problems that are especially prevalent in frail older adults (e.g., incontinence, falls, nutritional disorders, chronic pain syndromes). Recent evidence documents that pain among nursing home residents with cancer is often untreated (AGS Panel, 1998; Bernabei et al., 1998). This is clearly an area of clinical care that deserves more attention in the nursing home setting. Although the incidence of iatrogenic illnesses has not been systematically studied in nursing homes, it is likely to be as high as or higher than that in acute care hospitals (see Chap. 4). The management of many of the conditions listed in Table 15-3 is discussed in some detail in other

chapters of this text (see Table of Contents and Index regarding specific conditions).

In addition to the numerous factors already mentioned that render the medical assessment and treatment of these conditions different, the process of care in nursing homes also differs substantially from that in acute hospitals, clinics, and home care settings.

PROCESS OF CARE IN THE NURSING HOME

The process of care in nursing homes is strongly influenced by numerous state and federal regulations, the highly interdisciplinary nature of nursing home residents' problems, and the training and skills of the staff that delivers most of the hands-on care. Federal rules and regulations contained in the 1987 Omnibus Budget Reconciliation Act (OBRA) and implemented in 1991 place heavy emphasis on assessment and care planning as a means of achieving the highest practicable level of functioning for each resident (Elon and Pawlson, 1992).

Physician involvement in nursing home care and the nature of medical assessment and treatment offered to nursing home residents are often limited by logistic and economic factors. Few physicians have offices based either inside the nursing home or in close proximity to the facility. Many physicians who do visit nursing homes care for relatively small numbers of residents, often in several different facilities. Most nursing homes, therefore, have numerous physicians who make rounds once or twice per month, who are not generally present to evaluate acute changes in resident status, and who attempt to assess these changes over the telephone. Many nursing homes do not have the ready availability of laboratory, radiologic, and pharmacy services with the capability of rapid response, further compounding the logistics of evaluating and treating acute changes in medical status. Thus, nursing home residents are often sent to hospital emergency rooms, where they are evaluated by personnel who are generally not familiar with their baseline status and who frequently lack training and interest in the care of frail and dependent elderly patients.

Restrictive Medicare and Medicaid reimbursement policies may also dictate certain patterns of nursing home care. While physicians are required to visit nursing home residents only every 30 to 60 days, many residents require more frequent assessment and monitoring

of treatment—especially with the shorter acute-care hospital stays brought about by the prospective payment system (diagnosis-related groups, or DRGs). While Medicare reimbursement for physician visits in nursing homes has improved, reimbursement for a routine visit is generally not adequate for the time that is required to provide good medical care in the nursing home, including travel to and from the facility, assessment and treatment planning for residents with multiple problems, communication with members of the interdisciplinary team and the resident's family, and proper documentation in the medical record. Activities often essential to good care in the nursing home, such as attendance at interdisciplinary conferences, family meetings, complex assessments of decision-making capacity, and counseling residents and surrogate decision makers on treatment plans in the event of terminal illness are generally not reimbursable at all. Medicare intermediaries restrict reimbursement for rehabilitative services for residents not covered under Part A skilled care, thus limiting the treatment options for many residents. Although Medicaid programs vary considerably, many provide minimal coverage for ancillary services that are critical for optimum medical care, and may restrict reimbursement for several types of drugs that may be especially helpful for nursing home residents. As more and more capitated systems become involved in nursing home care, physicians and other nursing home staff will have to live within the constraints of a fixed budget. This will also be true for Medicare skilled care in nursing homes (see below). Amid these logistic and economic constraints, expectations for the care of nursing home residents are high. Table 15-4 outlines the various types of assessment generally recommended for the optimal care of nursing home residents. Physicians are responsible for completing an initial assessment within 72 h of admission and arranging for monthly visits thereafter for the next 90 days. Licensed nurses assess new residents as soon as they are admitted, on a daily basis, and generally summarize the status of each resident weekly. The nationally mandated Minimum Data Set (MDS) must be completed within 14 days of admission and updated when a major change in status occurs; several sections must be routinely updated on a quarterly basis (Morris et al., 1990). The extent of involvement of other disciplines in the assessment and care-planning process varies depending on the residents' problems, the availability of various professionals, and state regulations. Representatives from nursing, social services, dietary management, activities, and rehabilitation therapy (physical and/or

(Text continues on page 466.)

Table 15-4 Important aspects of various types of assessment in the nursing home

Type of assessment	Timing	Major objectives	Important aspects
Medical			
Initial	Within 72 h of admission	Verify medical diagnoses Document baseline physical findings, mental and functional status, vital signs, and skin condition Attempt to identify potentially remediable, previously unrecognized medical conditions Get to know the resident and family (if this is a new resident) Establish goals for the admission and a medical treatment plan	A thorough review of medical records and physical examinations is necessary Relevant medical diagnoses and baseline findings should be clearly and concisely documented in the patient's record Medication lists should be carefully reviewed and only essential medications continued Request for specific types of assessment and input from other disciplines should be made A data base should be established (see example in Fig. 15-2)
Periodic	Monthly or bimonthly	Monitor progress of active medical conditions Update medical orders Communicate with patient and nursing home staff	Progress notes should include clinical data relevant to active medical conditions and focus on changes in status Unnecessary medications, orders for care, and laboratory tests should be discontinued Mental, functional, and psychosocial status should be reviewed with nursing home staff and changes from baseline noted The medical problem list should be updated

(continued)

461

Table 15-4 Important aspects of various types of assessment in the nursing home (*Continued*)

Type of assessment	Timing	Major objectives	Important aspects
As needed	When acute changes in status occur	Identify and treat causes of acute changes	On-site clinical assessment by the physician (or nurse practitioner or physician's assistant), as opposed to telephone consultation, will result in more accurate diagnoses, more appropriate treatment, and fewer unnecessary emergency room visits and hospitalization Vital signs, food and fluid intake, and mental status often provide essential information Infection, dehydration, and adverse drug effects should be at the top of the differential diagnosis for acute changes in status
Major reassessment	Annual	Identify and document any significant changes in status and new potentially remediable conditions	Targeted physical examination and assessment of mental, functional, and psychosocial status and selected laboratory tests should be done (see Table 15-6)

| Nursing | On admission, and then routinely with monitoring of daily and weekly progress; complete Minimum Data Set (MDS) within 14 days, update when major change in status occurs and annually; update selected sections quarterly | Identify biopsychosocial and functional status strengths and weaknesses
Develop an individualized care plan
Document baseline data for ongoing assessments | Particular attention should be given to emotional state, personal preferences, and sensory function
Careful observation during the first few days of admission is important to detect effects of relocation
Potential problems related to other disciplines should be recorded and communicated to appropriate members of the interdisciplinary care team |
| Psychosocial | Withi 1–2 weeks of admission and as needed thereafter | Identify any potentially serious psychosocial signs or symptoms and refer to mental health professional if appropriate
Determine past social history, family relationships, and social resources
Become familiar with personal preferences regarding living arrangements | Getting to know the family and their preferences and concerns are critical to good nursing home care
Relevant psychosocial data should be communicated to the interdisciplinary team |

(continued)

Table 15-4 Important aspects of various types of assessment in the nursing home (*Continued*)

Type of assessment	Timing	Major objectives	Important aspects
Rehabilitation (physical and occupational therapy)	Within days of admission and daily or weekly thereafter (depending on the rehabilitation program)	Determine functional status as it relates to basic ADL Identify specific goals and time frame for improving specific areas of function Monitor progress toward goals Assess progress in relation to potential for discharge	Small gains in functional status can improve chances for discharge as well as quality of life Not all residents have areas in which they can be reasonably be expected to improve; strategies to maintain function should be developed for these residents Assessment of and recommendations for modifying the environment can be critically important for improving function and discharge planning
Nutritional	Within days of admission and then periodically thereafter	Determine nutritional status and needs Identify dietary preferences Plan an appropriate diet	Restrictive diets may not be medically necessary and can be unappetizing Weight loss should be identified and reported to nursing and medical staff
Interdisciplinary care plan	Within 1–2 weeks of admission and every 3 months thereafter	Identify interdisciplinary problems Establish goals and treatment plans Determine when maximum progress toward goals has been reached	Each discipline should prepare specific plans for communication to other team members based on their own assessment

464

Capacity for medical decision making*	Within days of admission and then whenever changes in status occur	Determine which types of medical decisions that resident is capable of participating in A resident who is still capable of making decisions independently should be encouraged to identify a surrogate decision maker in the event the resident later loses this decision-making capacity If the resident lacks capacity for many or all decisions, appropriate surrogate decision makers should be identified (if not already done)	Residents with varying degrees of dementia may still be capable of participating in many decisions regarding their medical care Attention should be given to potentially reversible factors that can interfere with decision-making capacity (e.g., depression, fear, delirium, metabolic and drug effects) Family and health professional concerns should be considered, but the resident's desires should be paramount The resident's capacity may fluctuate over time because of physical and emotional conditions
Preferences regarding treatment intensity* and nursing home routines	Within days of admission and periodically thereafter	Determine residents' wishes as to the intensity of treatment they would want in the event of acute or chronic progressive illness	Attempt to identify specific procedures the resident would or would not want This assessment is often made by ascertaining the resident's prior expressed wishes (if known), or through surrogate decision makers (legal guardian, durable power of attorney for health care, family)

* See Table 15-7 and Chap. 16.

occupational) participate in an interdisciplinary care-planning meeting. Residents are generally discussed at this meeting within 2 weeks of admission and quarterly thereafter. The product of these meetings is an interdisciplinary care plan that separately lists interdisciplinary problems (e.g., restricted mobility, incontinence, wandering, diminished food intake, poor social interaction, etc.), goals for the resident related to the problem, approaches to achieving these goals, target dates for achieving the goals, and assignment of responsibilities for working toward the goals among the various disciplines. These care plans are an important force in driving nursing staff behavior and expectations and should be reviewed by the primary physician. The MDS is intended to assist nursing home staff in identifying important clinical problems and to trigger the use of Resident Assessment Protocols (RAPs), which have been developed for 18 common clinical conditions. The MDS and the RAPs are therefore critical tools for developing individual care plans. The interdisciplinary care-planning process serves as a cornerstone for resident management in many facilities but is a difficult and time-consuming process that requires leadership and tremendous interdisciplinary (and interpersonal) cooperation. Staffing limitations in relation to the amount of time and effort required makes intensive interdisciplinary care planning and teamwork unrealistic in many nursing homes. Although physicians are seldom directly involved in the care-planning meetings in most facilities, they are generally required to review and sign the care plan and may find the team's perspective very valuable in planning subsequent medical care.

Implementation of the OBRA regulations primarily affects the activities of the nursing home staff. But some aspects of these regulations have a direct bearing on physicians who are caring for nursing home residents. Several of the RAPs require involvement of the physician in the evaluation and management of common geriatric conditions seen in nursing home residents (e.g., delirium, incontinence). The RAPs do not directly address many common medical conditions (e.g., congestive heart failure, arthritis, infections) that must be identified and managed outside the MDS/RAP paradigm. Perhaps the most direct effect on physicians relates to the specifications around the use of psychoactive medications. OBRA defines criteria for appropriate use of these medications, and requires the documentation of specific diagnoses as well as the quantitative documentation of the response of target behavioral symptoms to these

drugs. Psychoactive medications can no longer be used simply as a means to control symptoms of aggressive or disruptive behavior (i.e., as "chemical restraints"). These rules have already stimulated a re-thinking of psychoactive drug use among nursing home residents, and there is evidence that the prescription of these drugs has changed since OBRA went into effect (Llorente et al., 1998). Physician attention is also directed to the use of physical restraints. In keeping with changing attitudes about such care, the use of these restraints is generally discouraged. Restraints can be applied only upon a physician's order and only after documenting that less restrictive measures are not effective. Increasing evidence is documenting that physical restraints can be safely removed from many residents (Evans et al., 1997). Specific assessments of resident safety have been developed to assist clinicians in restraint decisions (Schnelle et al., 1994). While not all residents can be free of restraints at all times, a restraint-free environment is an appropriate goal in the nursing home setting.

The general pressure for better documentation of care and assessments should provide a welcome improvement in the quality of care for nursing home residents. These rules will inevitably mean that physicians will be asked to make more detailed clinical notes, especially with respect to indicating the underlying reasons for their actions. Although these changes may place a modest added burden on the attending physician, they do not demand a great deal of extra effort and should help to provide a better environment in which to practice.

STRATEGIES TO IMPROVE MEDICAL CARE IN NURSING HOMES

Several strategies might improve the process of medical care delivered to nursing home residents. Four strategies will be briefly described: (1) the use of improved documentation practices; (2) a systematic approach to screening, health maintenance, and preventive practices for the frail, dependent nursing home population; (3) the use of nurse practitioners or physicians' assistants; and (4) utilization of practice guidelines and related quality improvement activities.

In addition to these strategies, strong leadership of a medical director who is appropriately trained and dedicated to improving the facilities' quality of medical care is essential in order to develop,

implement, and monitor policies and procedures for medical services. The role of the medical director in nursing homes is discussed in detail elsewhere (see Suggested Readings). The medical director should set standards for medical care and serve as an example to the medical staff by caring for some of the residents in the facility. The medical director should also be involved in various committees (pharmacy, infection control, quality assurance) and should involve interested medical staff in these committees as well as educational efforts through formal in-service presentations, teaching rounds, and appropriate documentation procedures.

The federal government's approach to improving the quality of care in nursing homes is based on the OBRA rules and the MDS and RAPs in particular. Computerized MDS data, which will be available for all nursing home residents, can be used to generate selected quality indicators and to identify outlier facilities that may require targeted evaluation (Zimmerman et al., 1995). While some data suggest that various aspects of nursing home care have improved since the implementation of the OBRA rules and regulations, many caveats about these early data have been voiced (Ouslander, 1997). Other approaches to improving quality will be necessary to complement the OBRA rules and regulations (Kane, 1998).

Documentation Practices

Nursing home residents often have multiple coexisting medical problems and long previous medical histories. Residents often cannot relate their medical histories, and their previous medical records are frequently unavailable or incomplete. There is also a danger in perpetuating old diagnoses that are inaccurate. This is especially true for psychiatric diagnoses but may also occur for other medical diagnoses such as congestive heart failure and stroke. Thus, it is difficult and sometimes impossible to obtain a comprehensive medical data base. The effort should, however, be invested and not wasted. Critical aspects of the medical data base should be recorded on one page or face sheet of the medical record. An example of a format for a face sheet is shown in Fig. 15-2. Additional standardized documentation should contain social information, such as individuals to contact at critical times and information about the resident's treatment status in the event of acute illness. These data are essential to the care of the resident and should be readily available in one place in the record,

MEDICAL FACE SHEET

ACTIVE MEDICAL PROBLEMS

1. _____
2. _____
3. _____
4. _____
5. _____
6. _____
7. _____
8. _____

NEUROPSYCHIATRIC STATUS

A. Dementia ___Absent ___Present
  If present:

  ___Alzheimer's ___Mixed
  ___Multi-infarct ___Uncertain/other

B. Psychiatric/behavioral disorders
  1. _____
  2. _____

PAST HISTORY

A. Acute hospitalizations since admission to JHA

Diagnoses	Month/Year
1. _____	___/___
2. _____	___/___
3. _____	___/___
4. _____	___/___

C. Usual mental status
  ___Alert, oriented, follows simple instructions
  ___Alert, disoriented, but *can* follow simple directions
  ___Alert, disoriented, *cannot* follow simple directions
  ___Not alert (lethargic, comatose)

D. Most recent Mini Mental State Score
  ___/30 (Date ___/___/___)

FUNCTIONAL STATUS

B. Major surgical procedures *before* admission to JHA

Procedure	Year
1. _____	_____
2. _____	_____
3. _____	_____
4. _____	_____

A. Ambulation
  ___Unassisted
  ___With cane
  ___With walker
  ___Unable
  Transfer: ___Ind ___Dep

B. Continence

	Cont	Inc
Urine	—	—
Stool	—	—

C. Basic ADL

	Ind	Dep
Bathing	—	—
Dressing	—	—
Grooming	—	—
Feeding	—	—

D. Vision
  ___Adequate for regular print
  ___Impaired-can see large print
  ___Highly impaired-but can get around
  ___Severely impaired-has difficulty getting around

E. Hearing
  ___Adequate
  ___Minimal difficulty
  ___Hears only w/amplifier
  Highly impaired-no useful hearing

C. Allergies
  1. _____
  2. _____

TREATMENT STATUS (See treatment Status Sheet Note Date ___/___/___)

___Full code   ___DNR   ___DNR, do not hospitalize   ___No tube feeding

This form completed by _____ Date ___/___/___

Figure 15-2 Example of a face sheet for a nursing home medical record.

so that when emergencies arise, when medical consultants see the resident, or when members of the interdisciplinary team need an overall perspective, they will be easy to locate. The face sheet should be copied and sent to the hospital or other health care facilities to which the resident might be transferred. Time and effort will be required in order to keep the face sheet updated. For facilities with access to computers and/or word processing, incorporating the face

sheet into a data base should be relatively easy and facilitate its rapid completion and periodic updating.

Medical documentation in progress notes for routine visits and assessments of acute changes is frequently scanty and/or illegible. Statements such as "Stable" or "No change" are too frequently the only documentation for routine visits. While time constraints may preclude extensive notes, certain standard information should be documented. The SOAP (*s*ubjective, *o*bjective, *a*ssessment, *p*lan) format for charting routine notes is especially appropriate for nursing home residents (Table 15-5). Simple data bases with word-processing capabilities can be used to enable physicians to efficiently produce legible, concise, yet comprehensive progress notes. Another tool for documenting change in residents over time is the benchmark approach utilizing flow sheets (see Chap. 4).

Another area in which medical documentation is often inadequate relates to the residents' decision-making capacity and treatment pref-

Table 15-5 SOAP format for medical progress notes on nursing home residents

Subjective	New complaints
	Symptoms related to active medical conditions
Objective	General appearance and mood
	Weight
	Vital signs
	Physical findings relevent to new complaints and active medical conditions
	Laboratory data
	Reports from nursing staff
	Progress in rehabilitative therapy (if applicable)
	Reports of other interdisciplinary team members
	Consultant reports
Assessment	Presumptive diagnosis(es) for new complaints or changes in status
	Stability of active medical conditions
	Responses to psychotropic medications (if applicable)
Plans	Changes in medications or diet
	Nursing interventions (e.g., monitoring of vital signs, skin care)
	Assessments by other disciplines
	Consultants
	Laboratory studies
	Discharge planning (if relevant)

erences. These issues are discussed briefly at the end of this chapter as well as in Chap. 16. In addition to placing critical information in a standardized format in readily accessible locations, it is essential that physicians thoroughly and legibly document all discussions they have had with the resident, family, legal guardians; they must also document any durable power of attorney for health care about these issues. Failure to do so may result not only in poor communication and inappropriate treatment but also in substantial legal liability. Notes about these issues should not be removed from the medical record and are probably best kept on a separate page behind the face sheet.

Screening, Health Maintenance, and Preventive Practices

A second approach to improving medical care in nursing homes is the development and implementation of selected screening, health maintenance, and preventive practices. Table 15-6 lists examples of such practices. With few exceptions, the efficacy of these practices has not been well studied in the nursing home setting. In addition, not all the practices listed in Table 15-6 are relevant for every nursing home resident. For example, some of the annual screening examinations are not appropriate for short-stayers or for many long-staying residents with end-stage dementia (Fig. 15-1). Thus, the practices outlined in Table 15-6 must be tailored to the specific nursing home population as well as the individual resident and must be creatively incorporated into routine care procedures as much as possible in order to be time-efficient, cost-effective, and reimbursable by Medicare.

Nurse Practitioners and Physician Assistants

A third strategy that may help to improve medical care in nursing homes is the use of nurse practitioners and physician assistants. This approach appears to be cost-effective in both managed care and fee-for-service settings (Polich et al., 1990; Malone et al., 1993; Burl et al., 1998; Ackerman and Kemle, 1998), and these health professionals may be especially helpful in carrying out specific functions in the nursing home setting (Kane et al., 1989). Physician assistants and nurse practitioners can bill for services under fee-for-service Medicare; moreover, several states will reimburse their services, and individual facilities and/or physician groups can hire them on a salaried basis. Although there is substantial overlap in training and skills, nurse

(Text continues on page 477.)

Table 15-6 Screening, health maintenance, and preventive practices in the nursing home

Practice	Recommended frequency*	Comment
		Screening
History and physical examination	Yearly	Focused exam including rectal, breast, and, in some women, pelvic exam
Weight	Monthly	Generally required Persistent weight loss should prompt a search for treatable medical, psychiatric, and functional conditions
Functional status assessment, including gait and mental status testing and screening for depression[†]	Yearly	Functional status assessed periodically by nursing staff using the minimum data set (MDS) Systematic global functional assessment done at least yearly using MDS to detect potentially treatable conditions (or prevent complications) such as early dementia, depression, gait disturbances, urinary incontinence
Visual screening	Yearly	Assess acuity, intraocular pressure, identify correctable problems
Auditory	Yearly	Identify correctable problems
Dental	Yearly	Assess status of any remaining teeth, fit of dentures, and identify any pathology
Podiatry	Yearly	More frequently in diabetics and residents with peripheral vascular disease Identify correctable problems and ensure appropriateness of shoes
Tuberculosis	On admission and yearly	All residents and staff should be tested Booster testing recommended for nursing home residents (see text)

Laboratory tests Stool for occult blood Complete blood count Fasting glucose Electrolytes Renal function tests Albumin, calcium, phosphorous Thyroid function tests (including TSH level)	Yearly	These tests have reasonable yield in the nursing home population

Monitoring in selected residents

All residents Vital signs, including weight	Monthly	More often if unstable or subacutely ill
Diabetics Fasting and postprandial glucose, glycosylated hemoglobin	Every 1–2 months when stable	Fingerstick tests may be useful if staff can perform reliably
Residents on diuretics or with renal insufficiency (creatinine >2 or BUN >35); Electrolytes, BUN, creatinine	Every 2–3 months	Nursing home residents are more prone to dehydration, azotemia, hyponatremia, and hypokalemia
Anemic residents who are on iron replacement or who have hemoglobin <10: Hemoglobin/hematocrit	Monthly until stable, then every 2–3 months	Iron replacement should be discontinued once hemoglobin value stabilizes

(continued)

473

Table 15-6 Screening, health maintenance, and preventive practices in the nursing home (*Continued*)

Practice	Recommended frequency*	Comment
		Monitoring in selected residents
Blood level of drug for residents on specific drugs, e.g.: Carbamazepine Digoxin Dilantin Lithium Theophylline Nortriptyline	Every 3–6 months	More frequently if drug treatment has just been initiated
	Prevention	
Influenza Vaccine	Yearly	All residents and staff with close resident contact should be vaccinated
Amantadine	Within 24–48 h of outbreak of suspected influenza A	Dose should be reduced to 100 mg per day in older adults; further reduction if renal failure present Unvaccinated residents and staff should be treated throughout outbreak; vaccinated can be treated until their symptoms resolve
Pneumococcal/pneumonia bacteremia Pneumococcal vaccine	Once	
Tetanus booster	Every 10 years, or every 5 years with tetanus-prone wounds	Many older people have not received primary vaccinations; they require tetanus toxoid, 250–500 units of tetanus immune globulin, and completion of the immunization series with toxoid injection 4–6 weeks later and then 6–12 months after the second injection

Tuberculosis Isoniazid 300 mg per day for 9–12 months	Skin-test conversion in selected residents	Residents with abnormal chest film (more than granuloma), diabetes, end-stage renal disease, hematologic malignancies, steroid or immunosuppressive therapy or malnutrition should be treated
Antimicrobial prophylaxis for residents at risk‡	Generally recommended for dental procedures, genitourinary procedures, and most operative procedures	Chronically catheterized residents should not be treated with continuous prophylaxis (see Chap. 7)
Body positioning and range of motion for immobile residents	Ongoing	Frequent turning of very immobile residents is necessary to prevent pressure sores Semiupright position is necessary for residents with swallowing disorders or enteral feeding to help prevent aspiration Range of motion to immobile limbs and joints is necessary to prevent contractures
Infection-control procedures and surveillance	Ongoing	Policies and protocols should be in effect in all nursing homes Surveillance of all infections should be continuous to identify outbreaks and resistance patterns
Environmental safety	Ongoing	Appropriate lighting, colors, and the removal of hazards for falling are essential in order to prevent accidents Routine monitoring of potential safety hazards and accidents may lead to alterations that may prevent further accidents

* Frequency may vary depending on resident's condition.
† The MDS can be supplemental by various standardized tools (see Chap. 3 and Appendix).
‡ See Chap. 3.

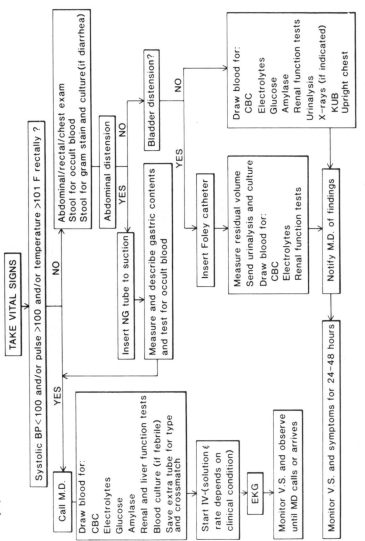

ACUTE ABDOMINAL PAIN

Symptoms: Sudden onset of diffuse or localized pain with or without nausea, vomiting, diarrhea

TAKE VITAL SIGNS

Systolic BP < 100 and/or pulse >100 and/or temperature >101 F rectally ?

YES → Call M.D.

Draw blood for:
CBC
Electrolytes
Glucose
Amylase
Renal and liver function tests
Blood culture (if febrile)
Save extra tube for type and crossmatch

Start IV–(solution & rate depends on clinical condition)

EKG

Monitor V.S. and observe until MD calls or arrives

NO → Abdominal/rectal/chest exam
Stool for occult blood
Stool for gram stain and culture (if diarrhea)

Abdominal distension

YES → Insert NG tube to suction

Measure and describe gastric contents and test for occult blood

NO → Bladder distension?

YES → Insert Foley catheter

Measure residual volume
Send urinalysis and culture
Draw blood for:
CBC
Electrolytes
Renal function tests

NO → Draw blood for:
CBC
Electrolytes
Glucose
Amylase
Renal function tests
Urinalysis
X–rays (if indicated)
KUB
Upright chest

Notify M.D. of findings

Monitor V.S. and symptoms for 24–48 hours

Figure 15-3 Example of an algorithm protocol for the management of acute abdominal pain in the nursing home by a nurse practitioner or physician's assistant.

practitioners may have an especially helpful perspective in interacting with nursing staff about the nonmedical aspects of care for nursing home residents. On the other hand, physicians' assistants may be especially helpful in facilities where there is a high concentration of subacutely ill patients who require frequent medical assessment and intervention. Both can be very helpful in implementing some of the screening, monitoring, and preventive practices outlined in Table 15-6 and in communicating with interdisciplinary staff, families, and residents at times when the physician is not in the facility. One of the most appropriate roles for nurse practitioners and physicians' assistants is in the initial assessment of acute or subacute changes in resident status. They can perform a focused history and physical examination and order appropriate diagnostic studies. Several algorithms have been developed for this purpose, one of which is shown in Fig. 15-3. This strategy enables the on-site assessment of acute change, the detection and treatment of new problems early in their course, more appropriate utilization of acute care hospital emergency rooms, and the rapid identification of residents who need to be hospitalized.

Clinical Practice Guidelines and Quality Improvement Activities

Several clinical practice guidelines relevant to nursing home care have been developed by the Agency for Health Care Policy and Research (AHCPR) and other organizations. The American Medical Directors Association (AMDA) has developed and published several that are specific to nursing homes. In addition, the 18 RAPs are, in fact, basically clinical practice guidelines. While these guidelines are largely based on expert opinion rather than on controlled clinical trials, they are helpful as a basis for standards of practice that will improve care. Implementation and maintenance of practice guidelines can be difficult (Schnelle et al., 1997). One of the AMDA guidelines specifically addresses issues concerning the implementation of practice guidelines (see Suggested Readings).

Clinical practice guidelines can be useful tools in an overall quality improvement program. Nursing homes are required to have an ongoing quality assurance committee. The most effective approaches are probably those ones based on principles of total quality management (TQM) or continuous quality improvement (CQI) (Schnelle et al.,

1993). These approaches utilize front-line staff to monitor objective outcomes (such as the frequency of falls, severity of incontinence, adverse drug reactions, skin problems, etc.) and to identify work processes that can be modified to continuously improve these outcomes. Effective CQI activities will require the further development of software such as that which has been utilized for incontinence care (Schnelle et al., 1995). Nursing home administrators, directors of nursing, and medical directors must create an environment that provides incentives for ongoing CQI activities in order to maintain these programs over time.

SUBACUTE CARE AND THE NURSING HOME–ACUTE CARE HOSPITAL INTERFACE

As economic pressure continues to be placed on the health care system, lengths of acute hospital stays continue to decline. Many Medicare risk HMOs admit patients with acute but relatively stable conditions (e.g., deep vein thrombosis, cellulitis) directly to nursing homes without an acute hospital stay. As a result, nursing homes are providing more and more postacute or subacute care. The term *subacute care* has many connotations; for the purposes of this chapter, it refers to skilled care reimbursed by Medicare Part A (or by a capitated system) in a free-standing nursing home. Recent studies have begun to examine the outcomes of such care in nursing homes as opposed to other settings (Kane et al., 1996; Kramer et al., 1997). Subacute care is also discussed in Chap. 14, and more detail is provided in the Suggested Readings.

Caring for subacutely ill patients in a free-standing nursing home intensifies many of the challenges already alluded to in this chapter (see Table 15-2). This level of care requires greater involvement of physicians, nurse practitioners, and physician assistants; nursing staff trained for more acute patients; ready availability of ancillary services such as lab, x-ray, physical, and respiratory therapy; and more intensive discharge planning. Moreover, Medicare reimbursement for Part A services is being "bundled," so that nursing homes will be at financial risk for services that are ordered by medical staff. This reimbursement structure will require unprecedented cooperation between physicians and nursing home administrators in order to make this form of subacute care economically viable.

As a result of the increasing acuity and frailty of the nursing home resident population, transfer back and forth between the nursing home and one or more acute care hospitals is common. The major reasons for transfer include infection and the need for parenteral antimicrobials and hydration as well as acute cardiovascular conditions and hip fractures (Kayser-Jones et al., 1989). Transfer to an acute care hospital is often a disruptive process for a chronically or subacutely ill nursing home resident. In addition to the effects of the acute illness, nursing home residents are subject to acute mental status changes and a myriad of potential iatrogenic problems (see Chap. 4). Probably the most prevalent of these iatrogenic problems are related to immobility, including deconditioning, difficulty regaining ambulation and/or transfer capabilities, and the development of pressure sores.

Because of the risks of acute care hospitalization, the decision to hospitalize a nursing home resident must carefully weigh a number of factors. A variety of medical, administrative, logistic, economic, and ethical issues can influence decisions to hospitalize nursing home residents (Rubenstein et al., 1988; Ouslander, 1988; Zimmer et al., 1988). Decisions regarding hospitalization often boil down to the capabilities of the physician and the nursing home staff to provide services in the nursing home, the preferences of the resident and the family, and the logistic and administrative arrangements for acute hospital care. If, for example, the nursing home staff has been trained and has the personnel to institute intravenous therapy without detracting from the care of the other residents or has arranged for an outside agency to oversee intravenous therapy and there is a nurse practitioner or physician's assistant to perform follow-up assessments, the resident with an acute infection who is otherwise medically stable may best be managed in the nursing home.

ETHICAL ISSUES IN NURSING HOME CARE

Ethical issues arise as much or more in the day-to-day care of nursing home residents as in the care of patients in any other setting. Several of the most common ethical dilemmas that occur in the nursing home are outlined in Table 15-7. Although most attention has been directed toward those marginally able to express their preferences, important daily ethical dilemmas also face those who are capable of decision making. These more subtle problems are easily overlooked (Kane et

Table 15-7 Common ethical issues in the nursing home*

Ethical issue	Examples
Preservation of autonomy	Choices in many areas are limited in most nursing homes (e.g., mealtimes, sleeping hours) Families, physicians, and nursing home staff tend to be paternalistic
Decision-making capacity	Many nursing home residents are incapable or are questionably capable of participating in decisions about their care There are no standard methods of assessing decision-making capacity in this population
Surrogate decision making	Many nursing home residents have not clearly stated their preferences or appointed a surrogate before becoming unable to decide for themselves Family members may be in conflict, have hidden agendas, or be incapable of or unwilling to make decisions
Quality of life	This concept is often entered into decision making, but it is difficult to measure, especially among those with dementia Ageist biases can influence perceptions of nursing home residents' quality of life
Intensity of treatment	A range of options must be considered, including cardiopulmonary resuscitation and mechanical ventilation, hospitalization, treatment of specific conditions (e.g., infection) in the nursing home without hospitalization, enteral feeding, comfort or supportive care only

* See also Chap. 16.

al., 1997). Nursing homes do care for an extraordinarily high concentration of individuals who are unable or questionably capable of participating in decisions concerning their current and future health care. It is among these same individuals that severe functional disabilities and terminal illnesses are prevalent. Thus, questions regarding individual autonomy, decision-making capacity, surrogate decision makers, and the intensity of treatment that should be given at the end of life arise on a daily basis. These questions are both troublesome and complex but must be dealt with in a straightforward and systematic manner in order to provide optimal medical care to nursing home

residents within the context of ethical principles and state and federal laws. Nursing homes should be encouraged to develop their own ethics committees or to participate in a local existing committee in another facility. Ethics committees can be helpful in educating staff; developing, implementing, and monitoring policies and procedures; and in providing consultation in difficult cases. Some practical methods of approaching ethical issues are discussed in Chap. 16. In addition, several helpful references are provided in the Suggested Readings sections of the bibliography at the end of this chapter as well as in Chap. 16.

REFERENCES

Ackerman RJ, Kemle KA: The effect of a physician assistant on the hospitalization of nursing home residents. *J Am Geriatr Soc* 46:610–614, 1998.

AGS Panel on Chronic Pain in Older Persons: The management of chronic pain in older persons. *J Am Geriatr Soc* 46:635–651, 1998.

Avorn J, Soumerai SB, Everitt DE, et al: A randomized trial of a program to reduce the use of psychoactive drugs in nursing homes. *N Engl J Med* 327:168–173, 1992.

Beers M, Avorn J, Soumerai SB, Everitt DE: Psychoactive medication use in intermediate care facility residents. *JAMA* 260:3016–3020, 1988.

Berg L, Buckwalter KC, Chafetz PF, et al: Special care units for persons with dementia. *J Am Geriatr Soc* 39:1229–1236, 1991.

Bernabei R, Gambassi G, Lapane K, et al: Management of pain in elderly patients with cancer. *JAMA* 279:1877–1882, 1998.

Borson S, Liptzin B, Nininger J, et al: Psychiatry in the nursing home. *Am J Psychiatr* 144:1412–1418, 1987.

Burl JB, Bonner A, Rao M, Khan AM: Geriatric nurse practitioners in long-term care: demonstration of effectiveness in managed care. *J Am Geriatr Soc* 46:506–510, 1998.

Elon R, Pawlson L: The impact of OBRA on medical practice within nursing facilities. *J Am Geriatr Soc* 40:958–963, 1992.

Evans LK, Strumpf NE, Allen-Taylor SL, et al: A clinical trial to reduce restraints in nursing homes. *J Am Geriatr Soc* 45:675–681, 1997.

Garrard J, Makris L, Dunham T, et al: Evaluation of neuroleptic drug use by nursing home elderly under proposed Medicare and Medicaid regulations. *JAMA* 265:463–467, 1991.

Heston LL, Garrard J, Makris L, et al: Inadequate treatment of depressed nursing home elderly. *J Am Geriatr Soc* 40:1117–1122, 1992.

Institute of Medicine: *Improving the Quality of Care in Nursing Homes*. National Academy Press, 1986.

Kane RL, Garrard J, Skay CL, et al: Effects of a geriatric nurse practitioner on process and outcome of nursing home care. *Am J Public Health* 79:1271–1277, 1989.

Kane RL, Chen Q, Blewett LA, et al: Do rehabilitative nursing homes improve the outcomes of care? *J Am Geriatr Soc* 44:545–554, 1996.

Kane RL: Assuring quality in nursing home care. *J Am Geriatr Soc* 46:232–237, 1998.

Kayser-Jones JS, Wiener CL, Barbaccia JC: Factors contributing to the hospitalization of nursing home residents. *Gerontologist* 29:502–510, 1989.

Kramer AJ, Steiner JF, Schlenker RE, et al: Outcomes and costs after hip fracture and stroke: a comparison of rehabilitation settings. *JAMA* 277(5):396–404, 1997.

Levenson S (ed): *Medical Direction in Long Term Care.* Owings Mills, MD, National Health Publishing, 1988.

Llorente MD, Olsen EJ, Leyva O, et al: Use of antipsychotic drugs in nursing homes: current compliance with OBRA regulations. *J Am Geriatr Soc* 46:198–201, 1998.

Malone JK, Chase D, Bayard JL: Caring for nursing home residents. *J Health Care Benefits* January/February:51–54, 1993.

Morris JN, Hawes C, Fries BE, et al: Designing the national resident assessment instrument for nursing homes. *Gerontologist* 30:293–307, 1990.

Moss FE, Halamandaris VJ: *Too Old, Too Sick, Too Bad: Nursing Homes in America.* Germantown, PA, Aspen Systems, 1977.

Ouslander JG: Reducing the hospitalization of nursing home residents. *J Am Geriatr Soc* 36:171–173, 1988.

Ouslander JG: The resident assessment instrument (RAI): Promise and pitfalls. *J Am Geriatr Soc* 45:975–976, 1997.

Polich CL, Bayard J, Jacobson RA, et al: A nurse-run business to improve health care for nursing home residents. *Nurs Econ* 8(2):96–101, 1990.

Rubenstein LZ, Ouslander JG, Wieland D: Dynamics and clinical implications of the nursing home-hospital interface. *Clin Geriatr Med* 4:471–492, 1988.

Schnelle JF, Ouslander JG, Osterweil D, Blumenthal S: Total quality management: administrative and clinical applications in nursing homes. *J Am Geriatr Soc* 41:1259–1266, 1993.

Schnelle JF, MacRae PG, Simmons SF, et al: Safety assessment for the frail elderly: a comparison of restrained and unrestrained nursing home residents. *J Am Geriatr Soc* 42:586–592, 1994.

Schnelle JF, McNees P, Crook V, et al: The use of a computer-based model to implement an incontinence management program. *Gerontologist* 36:656–665, 1995.

Schnelle J, et al: Policy with technology: a barrier to improving nursing home care. *The Gerontologist* 37(4):527–532, 1997.

Vladek B: *Unloving Care: The Nursing Home Tragedy.* New York, Basic Books, 1980.

Zimmer JG, Eggert GM, Treat A, et al: Nursing homes as acute care providers: a pilot study of incentives to reduce hospitalizations. *J Am Geriatr Soc* 36:124–129, 1988.

Zimmerman DR, Karon SL, et al: Development and testing of nursing home quality indicators. *Health Care Fin Rev* 16(4):107–127, 1995.

SUGGESTED READINGS

Nursing Home Care (General)

Aiken LH, Mezey MD, Lynaugh JE, et al: Teaching nursing homes: prospects for improving long-term care. *J Am Geriatr Soc* 33:196–201, 1985.

Avorn J, Langer E: Induced disability in nursing home patients: a controlled trial. *J Am Geriatr Soc* 30:397–400, 1982.

Cohen-Mansfield J, Billig N: Agitated behaviors in the elderly: I. A conceptual review. *J Am Geriatr Soc* 34:711–721, 1986.

Fabiszewski KJ, Volicer B, Volicer L: Effect of antibiotic treatment on outcome of fevers in institutionalized Alzheimer patients. *JAMA* 263:3168–3172, 1990.

Harvell J: Subacute care: its role and the assurance of quality. *Annu Rev of Gerontol Geriatr* 16:37–59, 1996.

Levenson SA (ed.): *Medical Direction in Long Term Care: A Guidebook for the Future,* 2d ed. Durham, NC, Carolina Academic Press, 1993.

Levenson SA: *Subacute and Transitional Care Handbook.* St. Louis, Beverly Cracom, 1996.

Ouslander J, Osterweil D: Physician evaluation and management of nursing home residents. *Ann Intern Med* 121:584–592, 1994.

Ouslander J, Osterweil D, Morley J: *Medical Care in the Nursing Home.* 2d ed. New York, McGraw-Hill, 1996.

Smith PW, Rusnak PG: Infection prevention and control in the long-term-care facility. *Infect Control Hosp Epidemiol* 18:831–849, 1997.

Smith RL, Osterweil D: The medical director in hospital-based transitional care units. *Med Dir Long Term Care* 11:373–389, 1995.

Zweibel NR, Cassel CK (eds): Clinical and policy issues in care of the nursing home patient. *Clin Geriatr Med,* Vol. 4, No. 3, 1988.

Ethical Issues in Nursing Homes

Besdine RW: Decisions to withhold treatment from nursing home residents. *J Am Geriatr Soc* 30:602–606, 1983.

Brown NK, Thompson DJ: Nontreatment of fever in extended-care facilities. *N Engl J Med* 300:1246–1250, 1979.

Hilfiker D: Allowing the debilitated to die. *N Engl J Med* 308:716–719, 1983.

Lo B, Dornbrand L: Guiding the hand that feeds: Caring for the demented elderly. *N Engl J Med* 311:402–404, 1984.

Lynn J: Dying and dementia. *JAMA* 256:2244–2245, 1986.

Steinbrook R, Lo B: Artificial feeding—Solid ground, not a slipping slope. *N Engl J Med* 318:286–290, 1988.

Uhlman RF, Clark H, Pearlman RA, et al: Medical management decisions in nursing home patients: principles and policy recommendations. *Ann Intern Med* 106:879–885, 1987.

Volicer L, Rheaume Y, Brown J, et al: Hospice approach to the treatment of patients with advanced dementia of the Alzheimer's type. *JAMA* 256:2210–2213, 1986.

SIXTEEN

ETHICAL ISSUES IN THE CARE OF OLDER PERSONS

Ethics is a fundamental part of geriatrics. While ethical dilemmas are central to the practice of medicine itself, the dependent nature of the geriatric patient raises special concerns. Discussions of ethics and aging seem to focus on the roles of autonomy and rationing. In many instances, the former may be used as basis for the latter. Ironically, the greatest ethical attention is focused on the group who are least able to express a preference: those in some form of vegetative state. There has been great pressure (including federal regulations) to encourage older persons to indicate their preferences in advance for how they would wish to be treated in the event that they are too incapacitated to express their wishes. This advocacy has been viewed as sparing unnecessary suffering. However, it is also conveniently directed at cost control. Thus, there is a danger that compassion can be used to disguise economy. Despite a growing enthusiasm for these advanced directives among many health professionals and policy makers, recent studies have raised serious questions about older patients' enthusiasm for curtailing efforts to prolong their lives (Tsevat et al., 1998). This report is consistent with earlier findings that people's fears of developing a given chronic illness are much greater than the

enthusiasm of those with such illnesses to get rid of the same problem (Torrance, 1987).

The issues that tend to attract the greatest attention are those affecting life-and-death decisions: Should one withhold or withdraw treatment? Do you resuscitate? What about tube feeding? These are each important and taxing questions posed in the context of real people. However, they arise much less often than do the less heralded ethical dilemmas that confront us each day as we decide about discharge from hospital, arrange placement in a nursing home, or recommend therapies. Consideration of the ethics of geriatric care must address the full spectrum of these issues.

AUTONOMY AND BENEFICENCE

Table 16-1 provides a framework for discussing ethical issues. Two principal components to ethical discussions are the concepts of autonomy and beneficence. *Autonomy* refers to one's right to control one's destiny, to exert one's will. Obviously there are limits to how freely such control can be expressed, but for geriatric purposes the principal issue revolves around whether the patient is able to assess the situation

Table 16-1 Major ethical principles

Beneficence
    The obligation to do good

Nonmaleficence
    The obligation to avoid harm

Autonomy
    Duty to respect persons and their right to independent self-determination
        regarding the course of their lives and issues concerning the integrity of their
        bodies and minds

Justice
    Nondiscrimination: duty to treat individuals fairly; not to discriminate on the basis
        of irrelevant characteristics
    Distribution: duty to distribute resources fairly, nonarbitrarily,
        and noncapriciously

Fidelity
    Duty to keep promises

and make a rational decision independently. This raises the second concept. The term *beneficence* refers to the duty to do good for others, to help them directly and in avoiding harm. This idea comes very close to paternalism, where one becomes the agent of another to make decisions as a father might do for a child. Such action directly conflicts with the principle of autonomy.

Physicians face a difficult set of choices in practice when they seek to walk these often fine lines. As Meier and Cassel (1986) note:

> Although the medical community has frequently been attacked for its paternalistic attitude toward patients, it is usually conceded that paternalism can be justified if certain criteria are met: if the dangers averted or benefits gained for the person outweigh the loss of autonomy resulting from the intervention; if the person is too ill to choose freely; and if other persons in similar circumstances would likely choose the same intervention.

The challenge then comes down to several fundamental issues:

1. Is the patient capable of understanding the dilemma?
2. Is the patient able to express a preference?
3. Has the patient received accurate information about the benefits and risks?
4. Are there clear options? Have they been made clear?
5. What happens when the patient's preferences are contrary to the physician's or the patient's family's?

COMPETENCE AND INFORMED CONSENT

In the case of elderly persons, much of the concern is directed toward the issue of understanding and expressing opinions. The two most extreme cases are the comatose patient, who clearly cannot communicate, and the aphasic patient, who may not be able to communicate effectively. In the former case, we must look for other ways to preserve autonomy. In the latter, we must be very careful to assess and separate areas of communication from reasoning.

There is an important difference between the concepts of competence and decision-making capability. The former is a legal term that refers to a person's ability to act reasonably after understanding the

nature of the situation being faced. Someone not competent to act on his or her own behalf requires an agent to act *for* the person. In the case of dementia, persons may or may not be capable of understanding and interpreting complex situations and making a rational decision. Intellectual deficits are spotty. A person may get lost easily or forget things but still be able to make decisions. A good example is the classic absent-minded professor. The presence of a formal diagnosis of dementia, even by type, may not be a sufficient indicator of the individual's ability to comprehend and express a meaningful preference. Just as it is wrong to infantilize such patients by directing questions to others more quick to respond, so, too, might it be inappropriate to prejudge their ability to participate in decisions about their own care.

Determining cognitive ability and decision-making capacity is not easy. One must distinguish memory from understanding. Physicians' judgments about patients' capacity to consent were much better for cognitively intact patients than for mildly demented patients (Marson et al., 1997). It is important to separate executive intellectual function from simple verbal recall ability (Marson et al., 1997). Younger age and more education were predictors of understanding informed consents, but simplifying the form did not consistently improve understanding (Taub et al., 1986). Varying the mode of presentation of information was not very helpful (Tymchuk et al., 1986). However, major deficits in short-term memory or verbal knowledge were associated with reduced understanding. Neither study attempted any form assistance such as reminders or prompts. Patients with memory deficits may need special help in recalling the components of the issue, but once reminded, they can often express a clear, sensible opinion.

One criterion for decision making, often presented with regard to informed consent, is the confirmation of the decision after a period of time during which the patient can consider the issues at hand. Clearly, memory is an important ingredient in such an approach. Its feasibility will vary greatly with circumstances. The pressures of contemporary funding sadly prohibit such a reasonable approach to many crucial decisions. Contrast the situation for deciding about post-hospital placement with that about discontinuing treatment or pursuing a high-risk treatment. The former decision is typically made under great duress, with utilization review looming. Choices are frequently poorly described and the consequences of the alternatives, when such are even presented, are not well defined.

The other side of the coin is the question of how information is presented. In order to make a rational decision, we all need a clear sense of the alternatives, including their benefits and risks. Ideally, a person making a care decision would have full information about the full range of options and the risks and benefits associated with each option. The decision-making process would be structured to allow the individual (and perhaps the family) to identify which outcomes (from a large menu) they are most keen to assure. The physician is a major source of this information. More often than not, the range of alternatives is foreshortened to emphasize those deemed most appropriate. Rarely are patients given the full description of the benefits and risks. In some instances this is appropriate, since the entire list of all possible risks may be excessive, and a discussion of very serious yet very rare conditions may inappropriately frighten a patient. When decisions about nursing home entry are made, they are not given the same level of serious attention accorded those about surgery. In many cases physicians may not know all the risks and benefits, but they never will until they are forced to address them.

When patients face decisions about entering a nursing home, for example, they need to understand the options at several levels. First, is a nursing home the best answer? What are the trade-offs between safety, privacy, and loss of autonomy? What other service configurations might work? At what cost, financial and otherwise? Next, they need to choose among nursing homes. Which one offers the social environment that suits their lifestyles as well as having available resources to meet their physical needs? In too many cases, patients do not get to choose in either category. Decisions, especially decisions made in hospitals, are made under great time pressure. Availability often takes precedence. A physician was heard to remark that a good discharge plan was one where patients knew where they were going. Surely something better than that should be expected.

ADVANCE DIRECTIVES

One way of trying to deal with the situation when the patient cannot express a preference is to encourage the development of advance directives, in which persons indicate what they want done under such circumstances (High, 1987). Federal law requires that all persons entering a hospital or a nursing home be offered the opportunity to

indicate advance directives. Too often this exercise means that older persons are confronted with long lists of possible procedures and asked to choose which ones they would want to have if the occasion arose. Done poorly, the experience can provoke anxiety unnecessarily and lead to poor decisions that may be regretted later. The two most common forms of these advance directives are living wills and durable powers of attorney. The former indicates in as much detail as possible what actions should or should not be taken under specific circumstances. These living wills have been criticized as being too vague or too specific, and some research shows that a person's intentions and preferences change with circumstances. People usually are more anxious to avoid a bad condition than to get rid of it once it occurs. Similarly, it is difficult to know for certain how you would feel if you were faced with a certain life-threatening choice.

Living wills most often address the issue of extraordinary actions to sustain life, generally the question of resuscitation, but they can also cover such things as hospitalization, use of life-sustaining therapies including parenteral and tube feeding, and even the use of antibiotics. They provide a means to indicate whether the patient prefers that heroic measures not be undertaken. In one sense, the more specific are such orders the better. Under what conditions? What constitutes a heroic measure? Another class of extraordinary measures is the use of artificial life supports. Again there is a need for specificity. Is a feeding tube the equivalent of a respirator? Some would argue that it is (Steinbrook et al., 1988).

Forgoing heroic measures need not mean abrogating all interest in surviving. One terrible anecdote is told about a nursing home staff that allowed a patient to choke to death on aspirated food because he had signed a "do not resuscitate" (DNR) request. Does not wanting cardiopulmonary resuscitation mean that the patient does not want to have his or her pneumonia treated? DNR is not synonymous with "do not care."

Although there is a desire for specificity, both ethical and practical considerations enter into the picture. Few persons are prepared to sit down with a list of circumstances and actions to indicate in a calm, rational way if this occurs, this is what I want done or not done. At best, one may get a sense of a person's priorities and feelings about active efforts. Despite the requirement that advance directives be solicited whenever an older person is admitted to a health care institution, some suggest that it is unrealistic to expect that persons can

make clear, thoughtful determinations at such a time of high stress. The danger of not building the decision into the admission routine, or at least the admission data collection process, is that it goes unattended. If the decision is best postponed until a calmer time after a period of adjustment, it should not be forgotten.

There are standard forms available to guide you in making choices and indicating preferences, but filling out such a list may be disconcerting. More than two-thirds of the states have some form of living will legislation, but the precise nature of those laws varies greatly in terms of what must be specified and under what conditions the delineated preferences can be followed.

An alternative to the living will approach of prespecification is the designation of a proxy, who is authorized to act on the patient's behalf if that person is unable to communicate. This designation can be done by using a durable power of attorney, previously used to transfer control of property. States must specifically extend their durable power of attorney statutes to cover medical decisions. Under this approach one can specify both the person one wishes to act as agent and the conditions under which such a proxy should be exercised. The components of a durable power of attorney for health care are shown in Table 16-2.

With both the living will and the durable power of attorney, there is some potential for misuse. Decisions once made can be difficult to revoke. What is the test of mental competence that allows one to change one's mind about a decision to not use life-support systems? Stories are told about families who followed the patient's instructions even when the patient appeared to have a change of mind.

In the absence of any specification of actions or agents, someone must be identified to act for a person who is unable to act on his or her own behalf. There are legal procedures to accomplish this, which vary from state to state. In general, the two major classes of legally empowered agents are conservators and guardians. The latter usually have greater powers. A formal legal decision is needed to establish such a condition.

A critical question is, who is the person best qualified to assume that responsibility? Common wisdom suggests that it is the next of kin, but the ethical community argues that it should be the person most familiar with the patient's preferences, the person who can most closely estimate what the patient would have wanted. A rarely seen relative might know much less about the patient's wishes or lifestyle

Table 16-2 Components of a durable power of attorney for health care*

Creation of durable power of attorney for health care
Statement that gives intention and refers to statute(s) authorizing such

Designation of health care agent
Statement naming and facilitating access to (address, telephone number) agent, state laws will vary as to who may serve as agent—some states preclude providers of health care or employees of institutions where care is given; person designated as agent should have agreed to assume this role

General statement of authority granted
Statement about circumstances under which the agent is granted power and indications of the power the agent will have in that event (usually a general statement about right to consent or refuse or withdraw consent for care, treatment, service or procedure, or release of information subject to any specific provisions and limitations indicated)

Statement of desires, special provisions, and limitations
Opportunity to indicate general preferences (e.g., wish not to have life prolonged if burdens outweigh benefits; wish for life-sustaining treatment unless in coma that physicians believe to be irreversible, then no such efforts; wish for all possible efforts regardless of prognosis); opportunity for specific types of things wanted done or not done and indications for such actions

Signatures
Individual dated signature
Witnesses (better notarized): witnesses cannot be those named as agents, providers of health care, or employees of facilities giving such care

Conditions
Form should have place where person signing indicates awareness of rights, including the right to revoke the document and the conditions under which the document comes into force; some states require a mandatory maximum period such a document can be valid without renewal

---

* A copy of a basic form of a durable power of attorney for health care can be obtained from many state medical associations.

than might a close friend, clergyman, or even the attending physician. The choice should rest on the level of knowledge possessed. Where there are multiple contenders for the role, the courts may have to decide who is best positioned to know the patient's preferences. In cases where there is no one appropriate, the court may appoint a public guardian.

Agents, whether designated by durable power of attorney or chosen as the best available person, are vulnerable to pursuing their own interests rather than the patient's. At best, they must make inferences about the patient's wishes from their knowledge of the patient or the choice indicated in the durable power document. Surrogates' decisions may not be congruent with the wishes of the individuals they represent. They can be sincerely torn between acting in what they perceive to be the individual's wishes and best interests, two different perspectives on the issue.

Recent court decisions suggest that families and physicians may not have the last word in decisions about the care of incompetent persons. In the case of a demented woman with a legal guardian, the court ordered that a state ombudsman had to become involved in the decision to prevent premature discontinuation of tube feeding (Lo and Dornbrand, 1986).

Substantial controversy surrounds end-of-life care. On the one side are those who argue that in our effort to avoid confronting the reality of death, we engage in a great deal of futile and expensive care (Lynn, 1986). Others counter that much of the claims for substantial potential savings from eliminating such care are spurious (Emanuel and Emanuel, 1994; Emanuel, 1996).

A study looking at a large group of older patients thought to be in terminal condition who were receiving intensive care has raised a number of questions about how the health professionals handle end-of-life situations. The original goal of the study was to make care teams more comfortable with such care and encourage them to forgo dramatic and traumatic therapeutic interventions where they seemed futile. Despite active training efforts the study team achieved only modest changes in clinician behavior (SUPPORT Principal Investigators, 1995). They interpreted this lack of effect as a treatment failure but an alternative interpretation would suggest that the absence of a response was because the clinicians were not comfortable terminating care. This behavior is supported by a study from the same effort that indicated that many frail older persons were not anxious to give up years of life even if it meant becoming disease free (Tsevat et al., 1998).

These findings raise serious questions about the ethical basis for the prevalent enthusiasm for advance directives. Some observers see this effort as a means of implementing rationing sub rosa. When prominent ethicists have called for overt rationing on the basis of age (Callahan, 1987), gerontologists have risen up to cry "ageism."

However, some of these same defenders of older persons' rights see in advance directives an opportunity for autonomy.

THE PHYSICIAN'S ROLE

The physician may feel under great pressure. At times the physician's preferences will differ from those of the patient or the patient's agent. Nor are there only two poles to work between. Especially in the care of dependent older persons, family may exert strong influences to pursue what they perceive as the best interests of the patient or for other reasons. The physician must keep in mind who is the client.

One important issue is how actively should physician preferences be voiced. Physicians have an obligation to provide patients with a full set of information: the alternatives and the risks and benefits associated with each option, and to be sure that the patient appreciates that information. It is difficult to be fully objective in many instances. Few physicians have enough information to present information on the range of options and their associated risks and benefits; even fewer are capable of estimating the effects of competing risks from other conditions if the immediate problem is alleviated (Welch et al., 1996). Values may unconsciously distort the way options are portrayed; risks may be minimized or even overlooked. Some physicians prefer to think of themselves as simply conduits of information, but others believe strongly that their opinions should be counted. They argue that the physician is often the most knowledgeable person involved and has a duty to guide and at least suggest a course of therapy. In some cases, patients may specifically ask for advice or even indicate that they want the doctor to make the decision. Despite efforts to maintain a shared decision-making relationship, physicians will often find themselves unequal partners because of their authoritarian position. This deference is especially true with the current group of geriatric patients who were raised with a much more respectful set of beliefs about physicians than is currently the case among younger generations. The contemporary geriatrician must struggle hard to encourage the maximum autonomy from patients.

In an era of litigation, many physicians are understandably wary of taking charge (Kapp, 1992). Fearful of being held responsible, they may wash their hands of the decision. Physicians find themselves smack in the middle of the pulls between autonomy and beneficence.

Physicians who want to do what is best for their patients will offer their opinions and give their reasons. But in the end, they cannot override the patient. If they find themselves in strong disagreement, they can assist patients to find new sources of care, but they cannot abandon a patient because of a difference of opinion. Physicians and hospitals facing patients who want to act in a way different from their convictions have often worked very hard to transfer the locus of care, but until that transfer is accomplished, they are stuck with dealing with patients on their terms or going to court. A recent court decision affirmed that "competent patients have the right to decline life-prolonging treatment, even if physicians disagree because of conscience or ethics." Moreover, the hospitals and physicians involved would not be criminally or civilly liable if they carried out the patient's wishes in these matters (Lo and Dornbrand, 1986).

A difficult problem for most physicians is when to introduce the topic of the patient's need to consider some form of advance directive. Speaking about such topics may seem like conceding defeat, but it represents a significant service to the patient, who needs to plan for the future appropriately. A legal vehicle designating who has legal responsibility can save much heartache later, even when it may not be legally binding.

The physician's role has come under special scrutiny with regard to end-of-life care because of the actions of certain physicians who have openly practiced assisted suicide (Sachs et al, 1995). In a 1996 national survey of physicians, 11 percent of respondents said that they would be willing to prescribe medications to hasten a patient's death and 7 percent would use lethal injections. These proportions rose to 36 percent and 24 percent, respectively, if such practices were to be made legal (Meier et al., 1998). The appropriate role of physicians in participating in this activity has been a topic of active debate. Many physicians and ethicists hold that a physician cannot and should not be responsible for fostering both life and death (Bachman et al., 1996). A few states have passed legislation permitting such physician-assisted suicides, but even in those places many physicians are reluctant to participate for fear of reprisal.

SPECIAL PROBLEMS WITH NURSING HOME RESIDENTS

Nursing home residents present some special problems. Patients are usually admitted to nursing homes because of a reduced capacity to

cope. Many suffer from some degree of cognitive impairment. In one sense they are subject to a cruel paradox: because the quality of their daily lives may be so miserable, their lives are seen to have less value. It is easier to justify inattention or withholding extensive care (Brown and Thompson, 1979).

Table 16-3 lists four areas where clinical decisions in treating long-term-care patients may pose the greatest ethical dilemmas. As noted in Chap. 15, beyond the usually considered question of resuscitation, the physician faces difficult decisions in determining when it is appropriate to transfer a patient from a nursing home to a hospital or when to intervene aggressively to treat changes in physiologic status from fluid imbalance or infection. Perhaps one of the most perplexing areas is when to pursue heroic measures to maintain nutritional supports. Especially with the tremendous growth in technology for establishing effective but expensive nutritional regimens in persons incapable of eating on their own for sustained periods, this issue is faced with increasing frequency. Artificial feeding decisions seem to arouse more controversy than other life-sustaining treatment issues. The growing consensus seems to favor the view that tube and intravenous feedings are more akin to a medical intervention than to routine nursing care or comfort care (Steinbrook and Lo, 1988).

Physicians must be diligent in working to preserve the patient's personhood. Essentially nursing home residents should not lose any of their rights as people just because they enter a nursing home. They should be eligible to participate in a full range of activities and to make choices about their lives and their health care. They should be the first ones consulted about changes in their condition or therapy. Visits to a nursing home should be more like home calls or office visits than hospital visits.

In practice, this freedom is often not allowed. One set of arguments for constraining nursing home resident choice is the limitations

Table 16-3 Major topics for clinical ethical decisions about nursing home residents

Resuscitation
Transfer to more intensive level of care
Treatment of infections and other intercurrent physiological derangements
Nutrition and hydration

Source: Lynn, 1986.

imposed by any institution. Just as college students must eat at certain times and choose from a menu, so, too, must nursing home residents. But the similarity breaks down when one appreciates the limited options available to the residents. They cannot easily order in a pizza or go out for a beer. Again part of the restriction is imposed by their medical status. Pizza and beer may be prohibited from their diet. Often this medicalization represents its own set of ethical dilemmas. When is dietary control a greater good than culinary pleasure? But too often medical orders become excuses for not individualizing regimens. Few conditions are aggravated by different hours of going to bed. In fact, sleeping medications might be prescribed less often if there were more flexibility in bedtimes. Similarly, participation in activities or the right to privacy become major issues in a world shrunk to nursing home proportions. How much say should a resident have in the choice of a roommate? Some would argue that single rooms should be the norm. The same people who would not deign to share a hotel room with a stranger for a single night seem to have no problem committing nursing home residents to roommates for years. An often repressed subject is the nursing home resident's rights to sexual privacy. Neither age nor dependency means a need to abrogate all rights to a sexual life. Sexual intimacy requires privacy. Too often nursing home staffs are insensitive and intolerant to these needs (McCartney et al., 1987).

There is a danger that the physician will treat the staff's needs rather than the patient's. Care should be exercised to avoid prescribing "as needed" restraints or sedatives to offer easy ways for staff to deal with behaviors they find disruptive. Too available recourse to such orders strips the patient of personhood and makes the patient simply an object to be controlled.

Decisions about advance directives take on special meaning in the nursing home context. Because the likelihood of survival is quite low, the value of cardiopulmonary resuscitation (CPR) must be carefully evaluated (Applebaum et al., 1990; Wanzer et al., 1989; Murphy, 1988). However, one cannot assume that all nursing residents have elected to forego active care (O'Brien et al., 1995).

Because nursing home residents are vulnerable, special care is needed to protect their rights. Uhlmann and colleagues have developed an excellent set of principles and practices for this purpose (Uhlmann et al., 1987). The general goal is to maximize the resident's autonomy in making decisions about treatment. Several ombudsman groups have created a parallel set of concerns in the form of a resi-

dent's bill of rights, which outlines the choices that should be available and the protections that can be sought. The Institute of Medicine study of nursing home quality took special pains to emphasize the need to integrate quality-of-life considerations with quality of care (Institute of Medicine, 1986). The former is an essential component of the latter. As such, it is the responsibility of the physician to see that these elements are addressed as part of basic care. The implementation of that report, the Nursing Home Reform Act of 1987 [part of the Omnibus Budget Reconciliation Act of 1987 (OBRA 1987)] did not succeed in enforcing this tenet. Although attention was directed to issues around quality of care, no specific mechanism for assessing this aspect was prescribed. Instead, attention was directed to observable behaviors that led to inferences about quality of life.

The same act did create major reforms in the way nursing home residents are managed. The prescriptions for avoiding physical restraints led to dramatic reductions in their use (Kane et al., 1993). Likewise, requirements for closer attention to the use of psychoactive medications greatly reduced their use as well.

One useful approach to buffer the relations between the nursing home, outside investigators and practitioners, and the residents is to establish an ethics committee composed of persons within and without the home (Glasser et al., 1988). Traditionally such committees began with the major charge of overseeing research activities, but they have increasingly begun to take responsibility for reviewing and facilitating standards for other aspects of the institution's activities and for serving as resources to establish guidelines for managing decision making around ethically difficult areas. Such committees are especially useful when they operate in a proactive manner, exploring issues in advance rather than assessing actions already taken. In many instances, they offer a disinterested forum where these very sensitive matters can be discussed with maximum dispassion and all sides of an issue aired.

SPECIAL CASE OF DEMENTIA

The wishes of patients with dementia may be ignored or undervalued. Although a diagnosis of dementia does not necessarily imply an inability to state preferences (Freedman et al., 1991), as noted earlier, physicians have more difficulty assessing competence to make decisions among such patients. Because dementia effectively robs individ-

uals of personality as well as memory, it can be very difficult to assess the quality of lives and hence the extent of effort appropriate to prolong them (Rango, 1985; Volicer et al., 1986; Lynn, 1986; Callahan, 1995). As already noted, the loss of cognitive function makes patient participation in decision making very difficult. Those left to act as agents for the demented patient must struggle with the difficult issue of when the loss of self-awareness and ability to maintain relationships constitutes substantial suffering. The loss of intellect is perhaps the most serious loss experienced by people. In one effort to explore the value of alternative outcomes among nursing home residents, if the resident was described as having loss of cognitive ability, all outcomes were substantially lower rated by a variety of persons, including care providers, family, policy makers, and the general public (Kane et al., 1986).

The management of demented patients poses additional problems. Demented persons are frequently intrusive. They threaten the privacy of those cognitively intact residents who must live with them. It does not seem right to diminish the quality of life for the latter in the name of efficiency or in some hope that they will stimulate the demented. Separate programs or units seem much more humane and sensible. Some have expressed concern about the burden on staff, but this anxiety does not seem to be borne out by experience. The separation allows more appropriate programming and facility design. In fact, the basic plans for facilities for the physically impaired and the cognitively impaired are also diametrically opposed. The former need ready access to nursing stations and short distances to walk, whereas the latter are best left to wander unimpeded in an eventually enclosed area with as much space as possible. In the continuum of special care facilities for the demented, we are now seeing the extension of the principles of hospice care to this group and their families (Volicer et al., 1986).

POLICY ISSUES

Older people are prime targets for rationing efforts because they consume disproportionately large amounts of medical care and because they are seen as having already lived their lives (Scitovsky and Capron, 1986). They have less to offer future generations. Given the difficulty of launching a frontal attack to curtail spending on older

people, more devious approaches have been used. Some of these are cloaked in ethical concepts. The concern expressed over the reports of withholding services like renal dialysis in the United Kingdom's National Health Service (Aaron and Schwartz, 1984) suggests that our country is uncomfortable with such an approach, but it has been proposed (Callahan, 1987). At a more subtle level, measures of program effectiveness tend to use something equivalent to the quality-adjusted life year (QALY). This term implies that valuable life is that lived free of dependency. Gerontologic researchers have called it *active life expectancy* (Katz et al., 1983). Such proxies for program effectiveness incorporate ethical components subtly. We have not established the base on which to put a value on life lived at some level of dependency. To assume that it has no value, as is implied by active life years, appears to contradict the very purpose for geriatrics, which treats primarily dependent older people. Many older people would actively challenge the tenet that disability implies an absence of quality of life. Severely disabled persons at various ages can continue to enjoy pleasant and productive lives. As advocates for their patients, geriatricians must be extremely vigilant to how such terms are used both in everyday speech and in analyses. It is important to bear in mind that any measure that uses life expectancy will tend to be biased against the elderly (Avorn, 1984). One that relies on dependency as the primary outcome implies that those who are dependent no longer count; by such logic disability is equivalent to death. At a time when there is an effort to pit one generation against another, care must be taken to avoid setting the terms of the debate such that the outcome is inevitable.

An important ethical issue closely linked to long-term-care policy concerns the appropriate role of caregivers. In Chap. 14 we noted the central role played by informal caregivers, who constitute the backbone of long-term care. The question then is, how much of such care should they be expected to provide? What is the nature of the obligation of one generation to another, or even to spouses and siblings from the same generation? A substantial portion of informal care is undoubtedly provided out of love and compassion. This approach works well when it is left up to the family to decide how much care they can give, but what happens when such care becomes mandated? Pressure to control public costs of long-term care could easily lead to demands to require care from families or to require that families pay directly for a certain amount of that care. Concerns

have already been expressed about the possibility that older persons are manipulating their assets to become unfairly eligible for Medicaid coverage. Although there is little substantiation for these claims of divestiture, advertisements for seminars on how to do it create an image of exploitation. Policies of familial responsibility would undoubtedly create a new demand for private long-term-care insurance, because preservation of older persons' assets primarily benefits the heirs.

The emergence of managed care as a major health care force affecting older persons raises its own set of ethical issues. Here too the goal of rationing care may be played out in a different arena. Whereas managed care offers older persons some attractive advantages, its propensity to reduce access to care can be a major threat. By hiding behind a complex bureaucracy, managed care companies can effectively thwart consumer feedback while claiming that the majority of their older customers are satisfied with the care they receive. Sometimes only dogged efforts, even to the point of litigation, are needed to generate a systemic response to a complaint. Medicare has determined that the benefits and costs will be set in the context of those for fee-for-service. In effect, the consumer has been removed from the loop until the time of enrollment.

SUMMARY

Ethical issues around care of older people are played out at all levels. Policy issues largely address questions of access and coverage, but these can be influenced too by individual clinician beliefs about what elements of care are "appropriate" for older people. These beliefs in turn can reflect stereotypes. Microethical issues occur at the bedside when decisions about initiating or continuing treatment are made. These decisions, too, are based on beliefs about appropriateness, including who should have the ultimate word about how much and what kind of care is rendered. Some of these decisions are couched as ethical issues because the requisite facts are not known. Once evidence is presented about the efficacy of a therapy for older persons, the tenor of the discussion changes. Often other factors than age are much better predictors of who will likely benefit from a given type of treatment. Great care must be taken to avoid couching rationing

decisions as ethical dilemmas. Measures that discount older or frail people will inevitably lead to decisions against treating older persons. Elderly patients should not lose their rights to full consideration of options and participation in the decisions that affect their care. The principles of autonomy and beneficence, which form a central part of the ethics of medicine in general, are strained with dependent older persons because the temptation toward paternalism is greater in the presence of the tendency to infantilize frail elderly patients, especially when they cannot readily communicate. Concerns about how to make decisions for persons unable to express their own preferences are often couched in terms of fear of litigation, but the growing body of experience suggests that carefully pursued efforts to establish agency and act accordingly will not put physicians or institutions at great risk of lawsuits. Finally, it is important to recognize that the life of dependent older persons, especially those in nursing homes, is composed of many little incidents. The daily loss of dignity, privacy, and self-respect may be too readily ignored. To be truly the patient's advocate, the physician must be vigilant to these small but critical ethical insults. It would be the greatest irony if geriatric patients were daily abused while living, only to become the subject of profound ethical analysis about dying. This is precisely the kind of behavior geriatrics is in business to prevent.

REFERENCES

Aaron HJ, Schwartz WB, *The Painful Prescription: Rationing Hospital Care.* Washington, DC, Brookings Institution, 1984.

Applebaum GE, King JE, Finucane TE: The outcome of CPR initiated in nursing homes. *J Am Geriatr Soc* 38:197–200, 1990.

Avorn J: Benefit and cost analysis in geriatric care: turning age discrimination into health policy. *N Engl J Med* 310:1294–1301, 1984.

Bachman JG, Alcser KH, Doukas DJ, et al: Attitudes of Michigan physicians and the public toward legalizing physician-assisted suicide and voluntary euthanasia. *N Engl J Med* 334:303–309, 1996.

Brown NK, Thompson DJ: Nontreatment of fevers in extended-care facilities. *N Engl J Med* 300:1248–1250, 1979.

Callahan D: *Setting Limits: Medical Goals in an Aging Society.* New York, Simon and Schuster, 1987.

Callahan D: Terminating life-sustaining treatment of the demented. *Hastings Center Rep* 25 (6):25–31, 1995.

Emanuel EJ: Cost savings at the end of life. *JAMA* 275:1907–1914, 1996.

Emanuel EJ, Emanuel LL: The economics of dying: The illusion of cost savings at the end of life. *N Engl J Med* 330:540–544, 1994.

Freedman M, Stuss DT, Gordon M: Assessment of competency: The role of neurobehavioral deficits. *Ann Intern Med* 15:203–208, 1991.

Glasser G, Zweibel NR, Cassel CK: The ethics committee in the nursing home: Results of a national survey. *J Am Geriatr Soc* 36:150–156, 1988.

High DM: Planning for decisional incapacity: A neglected area in ethics and aging. *J Am Geriatr Soc* 35:814–820, 1987.

Institute of Medicine: *Improving the Quality of Care in Nursing Homes.* Washington, DC: National Academy Press.

Kane RL, Bell RM, Riegler SZ: Value preferences for nursing-home outcomes. *Gerontologist* 26:303–308, 1986.

Kane RL, Williams CC, Williams TF, et al: Restraining restraints: Changes in a standard of care. *Annu Rev Public Health* 14:545–584, 1993.

Kapp MB: Our hands are tied: Legally induced moral tensions in health care delivery. *J Gen Intern Med* 6:345–348, 1991.

Katz K, Branch LG, Branson MH, et al: Active life expectancy. *N Engl J Med* 309:1218–1224, 1983.

Lo B, Dornbrand L: The case of Claire Conroy: Will administrative review safeguard incompetent patients? *Ann Intern Med* 106:869–873, 1986.

Lynn J: Dying and dementia, *JAMA* 256:2210–2213, 1986.

Marson DC, Hawkins L, McInturff B, et al. Cognitive models that predict physician judgments of capacity to consent in mild Alzheimer's disease. *J Am Geriatr Soc* 45:458–464, 1998.

Marson DC, McInturff B, Hawkins L, et al: Consistency of physician judgments of capacity to consent in mild Alzheimer's disease. *J Am Geriatr Soc* 45:453–457, 1997.

McCartney JR, Izeman H, Rogers D, et al: Sexuality and the institutionalized elderly. *J Am Geriatr Soc* 35:331–333, 1987.

Meier DE, Cassel CK: Nursing home placement and the demented patient: A case presentation and ethical analysis. *Ann Intern Med* 104:98–105, 1986.

Meier DE, Emmons CA, Wallenstein S, et al: A national survey of physician-assisted suicide and euthanasia in the United States. *N Engl J Med* 338:1193–1201, 1998.

Murphy DJ: Do-not-resuscitate orders: Time for reappraisal in long-term care institutions. *JAMA* 260:2098–2101, 1988.

O'Brien LA, Grisso JA, Maislin G, et al: Nursing home residents' preferences for life-sustaining treatments. *JAMA* 274:1775–1779, 1995.

Rango N: The nursing home resident with dementia: Clinical care, ethics and policy implications. *Ann Intern Med* 102:835–841, 1985.

Sachs GA, Ahronheim JC, Rhymes JA, et al: Good care of dying patients: The alternative to physician-assisted suicide and euthanasia. *J Am Geriatr Soc* 43:577–578, 1995.

Scitovsky AA, Capron AM: Medical care at the end of life: The interaction of economics and ethics. *Annu Rev Public Health* 7:59–75, 1986.

Steinbrook R, Lo B: Artificial feeding—Solid ground, not a slippery slope. *N Engl J Med* 318:286–290, 1988.

SUPPORT Principal Investigators: A controlled trial to improve care for seriously ill hospitalized patients: The study to understand prognoses and preferences for outcomes and risks of treatments (SUPPORT). *JAMA* 274:1591–1598, 1995.

Taub HA, Baker MT, Sturr JF: Informed consent for research: Effects of readibility, patient age, and education. *J Am Geriatr Soc* 34:601–606, 1986.

Torrance GW: Utility approach to measuring health-related quality of life. *J Chronic Dis* 40:593–600, 1987.

Tsevat J, Dawson NV, Wu AW, et al: Health values of hospitalized patients 80 years or older. *JAMA* 279:371–375, 1998.

Tymchuk AJ, Ouslander JG, Rader N: Informing the elderly: A comparison of four methods. *J Am Geriatr Soc* 34:818–822, 1986.

Uhlmann RF, Clark H, Pearlman RA: Medical management decisions in nursing home patients. *Ann Intern Med* 106:879–885, 1987.

Volicer L, Rheaume Y, Brown J, et al: Hospice approach to the treatment of patients with advanced dementia of the Alzheimer type. *JAMA* 256: 2244–2245, 1986.

Wanzer SH, Federman DD, Adelstein SJ, et al: The physician's responsibility toward hopelessly ill patients. A second look. *N Engl J Med* 320:844–849, 1989.

Welch HG, Albertsen PC, Nease RF, et al: Estimating treatment benefits for the elderly: The effect of competing risks. *Ann Intern Med* 124:577–584, 1996.

SUGGESTED READINGS

Beauchamp TL, Childress JF: *Principles of Biomedical Ethics.* New York, Oxford University Press, 1979.

Cassel CK, Meier DE, Traines ML: Selected bibliography of recent articles in ethics and geriatrics. *J Am Geriatr Soc* 34:399–409, 1986.

Ciocon JG, Silverstone FA, Graver LM, et al: Tube feedings in elderly patients: Indications, benefits and complications. *Arch Intern Med* 148:429–433, 1988.

Elford RJ: *Medical Ethics and Elderly People.* Edinburgh, Churchill Livingstone, 1987.

Emanuel EJ: A review of the ethical and legal aspects of terminating medical care. *Am J Med* 84:291–301, 1988.

Jonsen AR, Siegler M, Winslade WJ: *Clinical Ethics.* New York, Macmillan, 1982.

Lynn J: *By No Extraordinary Means. The Choice to Forgo Life-Sustaining Food and Water.* Bloomington, IN, Indiana University Press, 1986.

Lynn J: Measuring quality of care at the end of life: a statement of principles. *J Am Geriatr Soc* 45:526–527, 1997.

Meier DE, Morrison RS, Cassel CK: Improving palliative care. *Ann Intern Med* 127:225–230, 1997.

APPENDIX

SUGGESTED GERIATRIC
MEDICAL FORMS

KATZ INDEX OF INDEPENDENCE IN ACTIVITIES OF DAILY LIVING (ADL)

The index of independence in activities of daily living is based on an evaluation of the functional independence or dependence of patients in bathing, dressing, going to the toilet, transferring, continence, and feeding. Specific definitions of functional independence and dependence appear below the index.

A.	Independent in feeding, continence, transferring, toileting, dressing and bathing
B.	Independent in all but one of these functions
C.	Independent in all but bathing and one additional function
D.	Independent in all but bathing, dressing, and one additional function
E.	Independent in all but bathing, dressing, toileting, and one additional function
F.	Independent in all but bathing, dressing, toileting, transferring, and one additional function
G.	Dependent in all six functions
Other	Dependent in at least two functions, but not classifiable as C, D, E, or F. Independence means without supervision, direction, or active personal assistance, except as specifically noted below. This is based on actual status and not on ability. Patients who refuse to perform a function are considered as not performing the funtion, even though they are deemed able.

Bathing (sponge, shower, or tub)
Independent: needs assistance only in bathing a single part (as back or disabled extremity) or bathes self completely
Dependent: needs assistance in bathing more than one part of the body and in getting in or out of tub or does not bath self

Transfer
Independent: moves in and out of bed independently and moves in and out of chair independently (may or may not be using mechanical supports)
Dependent: assistance in moving in or out of bed and/ or chair; does not perform one or more transfers

Dressing

Independent: gets clothes from closets and drawers; puts on clothes, outer garments, braces; manages fasteners; act of tying shoes excluded

Dependent: does not dress self or remains partly undressed

Toileting

Independent: gets to toilet; gets on and off toilet; arranges clothes; cleans organs of excretion (may manage own bedpan used at night only and may not be using mechanical supports)

Dependent: uses bedpan or commode or receives assistance in getting to and using toilet

Continence

Independent: urination and defecation entirely self-controlled

Dependent: partial or total incontinence in urination or defecation; partial or total control by enemas, catheters, or regulated use of urinals and/or bedpans

Independent: gets food from plate or its equivalent into mouth (precutting of meat and preparation of food, as buttering bread, are excluded from evaluation)

Dependent: assistance in act of feeding (see above); does not eat all or parenteral feeding

MAIN COMPONENTS OF THE TINETTI FALL RISK SCALE

Balance Assessment
- Sitting balance (in a hard, straight-backed chair)
- Arising from chair
- Immediate standing balance (first 3–5 seconds)
- Standing balance
- Balance with eyes closed (with feet as close together as possible)
- Turning balance (360°)
- Nudge on sternum (patient standing with feet as close together as possible, examiner pushes with light even pressure over sternum 3 times; reflects ability to withstand displacement)
- Neck turning (patient asked to turn head sideways and look up while standing with feet as close together as possible)
- One leg standing balance
- Back extension (ask patient to lean back as far as possible, without holding onto object if possible)
- Reaching up (have patient attempt to remove an object from a shelf high enough to require stretching or standing on toes)
- Bending down (patient is asked to pick up small objects, such as a pen, from the floor)

Gait Assessment (Patient stands with examiner at end of obstacle-free hallway. Patient uses usual walking aid. Examiner asks patient to walk down hallway at usual pace. Examiner observes one component of gait at a time. For some components the examiner walks behind the patient; for other components, the examiner walks next to the patient. May require several trips to complete.)

- Initiation of gait (patient is asked to begin walking down hallway)
- Step height (begin observing after first few steps; observe one foot, then the other; observe from side)
- Step length (observe distance between toe of stance foot and heel of swing foot; observe from side; do not judge first few or last few steps; observe one side at a time)
- Step symmetry (observe the middle part of the patch, not the first or last steps; observe from side; observe distance between heel of each swing foot and toe of each stance)
- Step continuity
- Path deviation [observe from behind; observe one foot over several strides; observe in relation to line on floor (e.g., tiles) if possible; difficult to assess if patient uses walker]
- Trunk stability (observe from behind; side to side motion of trunk may be a normal gait pattern, need to differentiate this from instability)
- Walk stance (observe from behind)
- Turning while walking

Source: Tinetti ME (1986). Performance-oriented assessment of mobility problems in elderly patients. *J Am Geriatr Soc* 34:119–126.

REUBEN'S PHYSICAL PERFORMANCE TEST

	Time, seconds*	Scoring	Score
1. Write a sentence (The whale lives in the blue ocean)	——	$\leq$10 s = 4 10.5–5 s = 3 15.5–20 s = 2 >20 s = 1 Unable = 0	——
2. Simulate eating	——	$\leq$10 s = 4 10.5–5 s = 3 15.5–20 s = 2 >20 s = 1 Unable = 0	——
3. Lift a book and put it on a shelf	——	$\leq$2 s = 4 2.5–4 s = 3 4.5–6 s = 2 Unable = 0	——
4. Put on and remove a jacket	——	$\leq$10 s = 4 10.5–5 s = 3 15.0–20 s = 3 >20 s = 1	——

5. Pick up penny from floor	_____	≤ 2 s = 4
		2.5–4 s = 3
		4.5–6 s = 2
		Unable = 0
6. Turn 360°	Discontinuous steps	0
	Continuous steps	2
	Unsteady (grabs, staggers)	0
	Steady	2
7. 50-ft-walk test	_____	≤ 15 s = 4
		15.5–20 s = 3
		20.5–25 s = 2
		>25 s = 1
		Unable = 0
8. Climb one flight of stairs[†]	_____	≤ 5 s = 4
		5.5–10 s = 3
		10.5–15 s = 2
		>15 s = 1
		Unable = 0
9. Climb stairs[†]	Number of flights of stairs up and down (maximum four)	

TOTAL SCORE (maximum 36 for 9-item test, 28 for 7-item test) _____ 9 items _____ 7 items

* Round time off to nearest 0.5 seconds.
† Omit for 7-item test.

Note: For details of administering the test, see Reuben DB, Siu AL: An objective measure of physical function of elderly persons: The physical performance test. *J Am Geriatr Soc* 38:1105–1112, 1990.

FOLSTEIN MINI-MENTAL STATE EXAMINATION: THE GERIATRIC DEPRESSION SCALE

Choose the best answer for how you felt the past week:

1.	Are you basically satisfied with your life?	Yes	No*
2.	Have you dropped many of your activities and interests?	Yes*	No
3.	Do you feel that your life is empty?	Yes*	No
4.	Do you often get bored?	Yes*	No
5.	Are you hopeful about the future?	Yes	No*
6.	Are you bothered by thoughts you can't get out of our head?	Yes*	No
7.	Are you in good spirits most of the time?	Yes	No*
8.	Are you afraid that something bad is going to happen to you?	Yes*	No
9.	Do you feel happy most of the time?	Yes	No*
10.	Do you often feel helpless?	Yes*	No
11.	Do you often get restless and fidgety?	Yes*	No
12.	Do you prefer to stay at home rather than going out and doing new things?	Yes*	No
13.	Do you frequently worry about the future?	Yes*	No
14.	Do you feel you have more problems with memory than most?	Yes*	No
15.	Do you think it is wonderful to be alive now?	Yes	No*
16.	Do you often feel downhearted and blue?	Yes*	No
17.	Do you feel pretty worthless the way you are now?	Yes*	No
18.	Do you worry a lot about the past?	Yes*	No
19.	Do you find life very exciting?	Yes	No*
20.	Is it hard for you to get started on new projects?	Yes*	No
21.	Do you feel full of energy?	Yes	No*
22.	Do you feel that your situation is hopeless?	Yes	No
23.	Do you think that most people are better off than you are?	Yes*	No
24.	Do you frequently get upset over little things?	Yes*	No
25.	Do you frequently feel like crying?	Yes*	No
26.	Do you have trouble concentrating?	Yes*	No
27.	Do you enjoy getting up in the morning?	Yes	No*
28.	Do you prefer to avoid social gatherings?	Yes*	No
29.	Is it easy for you to make decisions?	Yes	No*
30.	Is your mind as clear as it used to be?	Yes	No*

Note: Each answer indicated by an asterisk counts 1 point. Scores between 15 and 22 suggest mild depression; scores above 22 suggest severe depression. The 15-item short form includes questions 1–4, 7–10, 12, 14, 15, 17, and 21–23. On the short form, scores between 5 and 9 suggest depression; scores above 9 generally indicate depression.

Source: Yesavage and Brink, *J Psychiatr Res* 17:37–49, 1983.

COMPREHENSIVE MEDICAL HISTORY AND PHYSICAL ASSESSMENT

A. Medical History

1. Patient's major complaint(s) (in patient's own or caregiver's language)

_____

2. Prior surgery

   Date   Surgical procedure

   ___/___/___   _____

   ___/___/___   _____

   ___/___/___   _____

3. Other hospitalizations

   Date   Hospital   Diagnoses

   ___/___/___   _____   _____

   ___/___/___   _____   _____

4. Health maintenance

   a. TB test status _____

   b. Immunization status _____

      1. Pneumococcal _____

      2. Tetanus _____

      3. Influenza _____

   c. Last dental visit _____

   d. Last Papanicolaou (Pap) test _____

   e. Last mammogram _____

5. Allergies: _____

6. Habits   No   Yes

   a. Smoking   ___   ___

   b. Alcohol consumption   ___   ___

      If yes, specify amount and duration _____

   c. Diet _____

   d. Exercise _____

(continued)

A. Medical History (*continued*)

7. Current medications

Prescribed drugs   Dosage and frequency

_____   _____

_____   _____

_____   _____

Over-the-counter drugs   Dosage and frequency

_____   _____

_____   _____

_____   _____

8. Symptom review

a. Patient's overall rating of own health

_____ Excellent   _____ Very good   _____ Good   _____ Fair   _____ Poor

b. Selected symptom review (enter C for chronic, N for new).

If positive, describe briefly.

_____ Anorexia

_____ Fatigue

_____ Weight loss (10 lb in 6 months)

_____ Insomnia

_____ Pain (describe)

_____ Headache

_____ Visual impairment

_____ Hearing impairment

_____ Dental/denture discomfort

_____ Cough or wheezing

_____ Dyspnea

_____ Exertional chest discomfort

_____ Orthopnea

_____ Edema

— Claudication
— Dizziness/unsteadiness
— Falls
— Syncope
— Dysphagia
— Abdominal pain
— Change in bowel habit or constipation
— Blood in stool
— Urinary frequency and/or urgency
— Nocturia
— Hesitancy, straining, or intermittent stream
— Incontinence
— Foot problems
— Focal weakness or sensory loss
— Transient visual disturbance
— Forgetfulness
— Depression
— Disruptive behavior/ wandering

9. Depression screen

For the following question, which description comes closest to the way you have been feeling *during the past month?*

All the time	Most of the time	Some of the time	A little of the time	None of the time

How much of the time, *during the past month,* have you felt downhearted and blue?

Answer of "all the time" or "most of the time" should raise suspicion of depression, and a full depression scale should be administered.

(continued)

A. Medical History (*continued*)

10. Functional status

a. Instrumental and basic activities of daily living

	Fully independent	Needs some human assistance (including supervision)	Totally independent
IADLs			
Preparing meals	___	___	___
Managing money	___	___	___
Managing medications	___	___	___
Using telephone	___	___	___
BADLs			
Bathing	___	___	___
Ambulation	___	___	___
Transfer	___	___	___
Dressing	___	___	___
Personal grooming	___	___	___
Toileting	___	___	___
Eating	___	___	___

b. Functional limitations

For how long (if at all) has your health limited you in each of the following activities? (Check the category which is the best description.)

	Limited for more than 3 months	Limited for 3 months or less	Not limited at all
The kinds or amounts of *vigorous* activities you can do, like lifting heavy objects, running, or participating in strenuous sports	___	___	___
The kinds or amounts of *moderate* activities you can do, like moving a table or carrying groceries	___	___	___
The kinds of work or housework you can do around your home	___	___	___
Working at a job			
Walking uphill or climbing stairs			
Bending, lifting, or stooping			
Walking one block	___	___	___
Eating, dressing, bathing, or using the toilet	___	___	___

B. Physical Examination

1. Vital signs

	Supine	Sitting	Standing
Blood pressure	__/__	__/__	__/__
Pulse (per minute)			
Respiratory rate (per minute)			

Weight (lb) _____ Height _____

Weight last examination (lb) _____

(date of last examination ____/____/____)

2. Skin

_____ Excessive dryness

_____ Rash (Describe: _____)

_____ Lesions—suspected malignant (Location: _____)

_____ Pressure sores

Location	Size (cm)	Stage (I–IV)
_____	_____	_____
_____	_____	_____
_____	_____	_____

3. Hearing

_____ Hears normal voice

_____ Hears whispered voice

_____ Hears 1024-Hz tuning fork

_____ Impaired

_____ Wears hearing aid

_____ Cerumen impacted in ear canals

Frequency threshold at 40 dB _____

4. Vision

Able to read newsprint

_____ With corrective lenses   _____ Without corrective lenses

(continued)

517

B. Physical Examination (*continued*)

Visual acuity

	Reading	Distance
Right	____ / ____ /	____ //
Left	____ / ____ /	____ //

Cataract present: ____ Right ____ Left

Funduscopic findings

	Normal	Abnormal (describe)	Unable to visualize
Right	____	____	____
Left	____	____	____

5. Mouth

____ Poor oral hygiene

Dentures

____ None ____ Good fit ____ Poor fit

____ Sores under dentures ____ Other lesion (describe)

6. Neck

	Normal	Abnormal
Range of motion	____	____

Thyroid

____ Thyroid scar

____ Mass (describe)

7. Lymph nodes

____ No lymphadenopathy

____ Enlarged nodes (Describe: _____)

8. Breasts

Mass present? ____ Yes ____ No

If yes: ____ Right ____ Left (Describe: _____)

Other abnormality _____

9. Lungs

	No	Yes		No	Yes
Crackles	___	___	Bronchospasm	___	___
Rhonchi	___	___	Other (specify)	___	___

If yes, describe: _____

10. Cardiovascular

a. Heart

	No	Yes
Irregular rhythm	___	___
Murmur	___	___
S_3	___	___
S_4	___	___
Other (specify)	___	___

If yes, describe: _____

b. Bruits

_____ None

	Right	Left
Carotid	___	___
Femoral	___	___

c. Distal pulses

	Present	Absent
Right dorsalis pedis	___	___
Right posterior tibial	___	___
Left dorsalis pedis	___	___
Left posterior tibial	___	___

d. Edema

	None	1+	2+	3+	4+
Pedal	___	___	___	___	___
Tibial	___	___	___	___	___
Sacral	___	___	___	___	___

(continued)

B. Physical Examination (*continued*)

11. Abdomen

Liver size ——— cm

Abdominal masses ——— None ——— Pulsatile ——— Other

Bruits ——— Yes ——— No

Tenderness ——— Yes ——— No

Describe positive findings:

12. Rectal

——— Diminished/absent sphincter tone

——— Enlarged prostate (Describe: _____)

——— Prostate mass

——— Rectal mass

——— Fecal impaction

Occult blood ——— Negative ——— Positive

13. Genital/pelvic

a. Men

——— Normal

——— Abnormal (Describe: _____)

b. Women

——— Normal

——— Abnormal (Describe: _____)

——— Vaginal atrophy ——— Mass

——— Atrophic vaginitis ——— Tenderness

——— Pelvic prolapse ——— Other

Pap test done ——— Yes ——— No

14. Musculoskeletal

	None	Spine	Shoulders	Elbows	Hands	Hips	Knees	Feet
Deformity		———	———	———	———	———	———	———
Limited range of motion		———	———	———	———	———	———	———
Tenderness		———	———	———	———	———	———	———
Prominent swelling or inflammation		———	———	———	———	———	———	———

Description of deformity or limited range of motion: _____

15. Neurologic
a. Mental status

	Intact	Impaired
Orientation		
Person	___	___
Place	___	___
Time	___	___
Situation	___	___
Memory		
Remote	___	___
Recent	___	___
Object recall after 5 min	___	___
Immediate (repetition)	___	___

(If dementia is suspected, further assessment should be undertaken. See "Dementia Assessment" on the following pages.)

b. Mood/affect:

  ___ Appropriate   ___ Labile   ___ Depressed

  ___ Agitated   ___ Anxious

c. General

	Normal	Abnormal (describe)
Cranial nerves	___	___
Motor		
Strength	___	___
Tone	___	___
Sensation		
Pin	___	___
Touch	___	___
Vibration	___	___
Reflexes	___	___
Cerebellar		
Finger to nose	___	___
Heel to shin	___	___
Romberg	___	___

(continued)

B. Physical Examination (*continued*)

Gait _____

Description of abnormal findings: _____

d. Other signs	Absent	Present (describe)
Resting tremor	_____	
Cogwheel rigidity	_____	
Bradykinesia	_____	
Intention tremor	_____	
Involuntary movements	_____	
Pathologic reflexes	_____	

Description of findings present: _____

C. Laboratory Data

Test/procedure	Date	Normal	Abnormal (describe)
_____	__/__/__		
_____	__/__/__		
_____	__/__/__		

D. Problem List

Medical problems
_____

Functional status problems
_____

Psychosocial problems
_____

DEMENTIA ASSESSMENT

A. History

1. Active medical conditions

   _____
   _____
   _____

2. Medications

   _____
   _____
   _____

3. History of (describe):
   ___ Hypertension
   ___ Stroke
   ___ Transient ischemic attack
   ___ Depression
   ___ Other psychiatric disorder

4. Current symptoms (complaints of patient or family)
   ___ Memory loss
   ___ Forgets recent events
   ___ Forgets things just said
   ___ Forgets names of people
   ___ Forgets words
   ___ Gets lost
   ___ Asks questions or tells stories repeatedly

(continued)

A. History *(continued)*

     _____ Confused about date or place
     _____ Can't do simple calculations
     _____ Can't understand what is read or said
     _____ Impairment of other cognitive functions
     _____ Anxiety/agitation
     _____ Paranoia
     _____ Delusions/hallucination
     _____ Wandering
     _____ Disruptive behavior
     _____ Incontinence

5. Onset of symptoms
     _____ Recent (days to few weeks)
     _____ Longer duration (months)
     _____ Uncertain

6. Progression of symptoms
     _____ Rapid
     _____ Gradual
     _____ Stepwise (irregular, stuttering deteriorations)
     _____ Uncertain

7. Activities of daily living (ADL)
Does the impairment of cognitive function interfere with instrumental ADL?
     _____ Yes   _____ No
If yes, which ones? _____
Basic ADL? _____ Yes   _____ No _____
If yes, which ones? _____

B. Physical Examination

1. General appearance
   ____ Normal
   ____ Abnormal (Describe: _____)

2. Blood pressure
   Right arm ____ / ____
   Left arm ____ / ____

	Normal	Abnormal
3. Hearing		
Normal voice	____	____
Audioscopic screening	____	____

	No	Yes
4. Orientation		
Person	____	____
Place	____	____
Time	____	____
Situation	____	____

	Normal	Impaired
5. Memory function		
Remote	____	____
Recent (object recall after 5 min)	____	____
Immediate (digit repetition)	____	____

6. Mini-Mental State Exam Score ____ / 30

	Normal	Impaired
7. Other cognitive functions		
General fund of knowledge	____	____
Simple calculations	____	____
Ability to write name	____	____
Interpretations of proverbs	____	____
Naming common objects	____	____
Name animals (12 in 1 min is normal)	____	____
Insight	____	____
Judgment	____	____

(continued)

B. Physical Examination *(continued)*

Ability to follow simple verbal commands
(e.g., "Touch your left ear with your right hand") _____

8. Thought content
   ____ Normal
   ____ Delusions
   ____ Paranoid ideation
   ____ Other (Describe: _____)

9. Mood/affect (standardized screening tests are available)
   ____ Appropriate   ____ Depressed   ____ Labile   ____ Agitated
   ____ Other (Describe: _____)

10. Behavior during examinations   Yes   No
    Good attention and concentration   ____ ____
    Good effort to answer questions and perform tasks   ____ ____
    Many "don't know" answers   ____ ____

11. Remainder of neurologic examination
    ____ Focal neurologic signs (Describe: _____)

    ____ Signs of parkinsonism (Describe: _____)

    Pathological reflexes:
    ____ Babinski
    ____ Hoffman
    ____ Grasp
    ____ Palmomental

    Gait:
    ____ Normal
    ____ Abnormal (Describe: _____)
    ____ Other abnormality (Describe: _____)

Sensory examination:

_____ Normal

_____ Abnormal (Describe: _____)

12. Hachinski ischemia score

Characteristic	Point score
Abrupt onset	2
Stepwise deterioration	1
Somatic complaints	1
Emotional incontinence	1
History or presence of hypertension	1
History of strokes	2
Focal neurologic symptoms	2
Focal neurologic signs	2

Total score: _____

(Score of 4 or more suggests multi-infarct dementia.)

C. Diagnostic Studies

	Normal	Abnormal
Blood:		
CBC	_____	_____
Sedimentation rate	_____	_____
Glucose	_____	_____
BUN	_____	_____
Electrolytes	_____	_____
Calcium	_____	_____
Liver function tests	_____	_____
Free thyroxine index	_____	_____
TSH	_____	_____

(continued)

C. Diagnostic Studies (*continued*)

VDRL	_____
Vitamin B$_{12}$	_____
Folate	_____
Radiographic:	
Chest film	_____
CT or MRI scan	_____
Other:	
Urinalysis	_____
ECG	_____
EEG	_____

D. Clinical Diagnosis

_____ Probable primary degenerative dementia (Alzheimer's type)

_____ Multi-infarct dementia

_____ Dementia with Lewy bodies

_____ Mixed

_____ Uncertain

_____ Depression

_____ Other potentially reversible cause of dementia (describe)

INCONTINENCE

I. Assessment of Acute Incontinence and Reversible Factors

If incontinence is of recent onset (within a few days) and/or associated with an acute illness, check for any of the following:

_____ Acute urinary tract infection

_____ Fecal impaction

_____ Acute confusion (delirium)[a]

_____ Immobility[a]

_____ Drug effects (e.g., excessive sedation, polyuria caused by diuretics, urinary retention, other autonomic effects)

_____ Metabolic abnormality with polyuria (e.g., hyperglycemia, hypercalcemia)

If incontinence persists despite management of any of these conditions and/or resolution of an acute illness, further assessment (as shown in Part II) should be pursued.

II. Assessment of Persistent Incontinence

A. History

1. Do you ever leak urine when you don't want to? _____ No, never _____ Yes

2. Do you ever have trouble getting to the toilet on time or have accidents getting your clothes or bed wet? _____ No, never _____ Yes

   Do you every wear any pads to protect yourself from leakage? _____ No, never _____ Yes

3. How long have you had a problem with urinary leakage?

   _____ Less than 1 week

   _____ 1 to 4 weeks

   _____ 1 to 3 months

   _____ 4 to 12 months

   _____ 1 to 5 years

   _____ Longer than 5 years

(continued)

529

A. History *(continued)*

4. How often do you leak urine?
   _____ Less than once per week
   _____ More than once per week, but less than once per day
   _____ About once per day
   _____ More than once per day
   _____ Continual leakage
   _____ Variable

5. Does the leakage occur
   _____ Mainly during the day
   _____ Mainly at night
   _____ Both night and day

6. When you leak urine, how much leaks?
   _____ Just a few drops
   _____ More than a few drops but less than a cupful
   _____ More than a cupful (enough to wet clothes and/or bed linens)
   _____ Variable
   _____ Unknown

7. Do any of the following cause you to leak urine?
   _____ Coughing
   _____ Laughing
   _____ Exercise or other forms of straining
   _____ Inability to get to the toilet in time

8. How often do you normally urinate?
   _____ Every 6 to 8 h or less often
   _____ About every 3 to 5 h
   _____ About every 1 to 2 h
   _____ At least every hour or more often
   _____ Frequency varies
   _____ Unknown

9. Do you wake up at night to urinate?
_____ Never or rarely
_____ Yes, usually once
_____ Yes, two or three times per night
_____ Yes, four or more times per night
_____ Yes, but frequency varies

10. Once your bladder feels full, how long can you hold your urine?
_____ As long as you want (several minutes at least)
_____ Just a few minutes
_____ Less than a minute or two
_____ Not at all
_____ Cannot tell when bladder is full

11. Do you have any of the following when you urinate?
_____ Difficulty in getting the urine started
_____ Very slow stream or dribbling
_____ Straining to finish
_____ Discomfort or pain
_____ Burning
_____ Blood in the urine

12. Have you had any previous evaluation or treatment for the incontinence?
_____ No
_____ Yes (Describe: _____)

13. Are you currently using any of the following to help with the urinary leakage?
_____ Bed or furniture pads
_____ Sanitary napkins[b]
_____ Other types of pads in your underwear[b]
_____ Special undergarments[b]
_____ Medication
_____ Bedside commode
_____ Urinal
_____ Other (Describe: _____)

14. Is the urinary leakage enough of a problem that you consider surgery for it?
_____ Yes _____ Possibly _____ No

(continued)

A. History (continued)

15. Are you constipated?

    _____ No _____ Yes _____ Average # BM/week

16. Do you ever have uncontrolled loss of stool?

    _____ No, never _____ Yes

17. Relevant medical history

    _____ Stroke
    _____ Dementia
    _____ Parkinson's disease
    _____ Prior CNS trauma/surgery
    _____ Other neurologic disorder
    _____ Diabetes
    _____ Congestive heart failure
    _____ Other (Specify: _____)

18. Prior genitourinary history

    _____ Multiple vaginal deliveries
    _____ Cesarean section(s)
    _____ Abdominal hysterectomy
    _____ Vaginal hysterectomy
    _____ Bladder suspension or sling
    _____ Periuretral injection
    _____ TURP (transurethral prostatectomy)
    _____ Suprapubic prostatectomy
    _____ Urethral stricture/dilatation
    _____ Bladder tumor
    _____ Pelvic irradiation
    _____ Recurrent urinary tract infections

19. Medications

    Diuretic _____
    Antihypertensive _____
    Other drugs that affect the autonomic nervous system _____
    Psychotropics _____

Estrogen _____

Other _____

B. Physical Examination

1. Mental status
   _____ Normal
   _____ Mild/moderate cognitive impairment
   _____ Severe cognitive impairment (unaware of toileting needs)

2. Mobility
   _____ Ambulates independently, with adequate speed
   _____ Ambulates independently, but slowly (so that ability to get to a toilet is impaired)
   _____ Not independently ambulatory, but able to use urinal, bedpan, or bedside commode independently
   _____ Chair- or bed-bound, but able to use urinal or bedpan independently
   _____ Dependent on others for toileting

3. Abdominal examination
   _____ Bladder enlarged and palpable
   _____ Bladder not palpable
   _____ Suprapubic tenderness

4. Neurologic examination of lower extremities
   _____ Normal
   _____ Evidence of upper motor neuron lesion
   _____ Evidence of lower motor neuron lesion
   _____ Peripheral neuropathy

5. Rectal examination
   _____ Decreased resting rectal sphincter tone
   _____ Decreased perianal sensation
   _____ Absent bulbocavernosus reflex
   _____ Prostate enlarged
   _____ Prostate cancer suspected

(continued)

B. Physical Examination (*continued*)

6. Voluntary contraction of rectal sphincter
   ____ Good
   ____ Fair
   ____ Poor
   ____ Unable
7. External genitalia
   ____ Skin irritation
   ____ Diminished sensation
   ____ Abnormal (Describe: _____)
8. Vaginal examination
   ____ Atrophic vaginitis
   ____ Mild prolapse
   ____ Moderate/severe prolapse
   ____ Rectocele
   ____ Adenexal or uterine mass
   ____ Stress incontinence (supine)

C. Diagnostic Studies

1. Cough test with full bladder for stress incontinence (standing)
   ____ No leakage
   ____ Leakage, small amount
   ____ Leakage, large amount
   ____ Delayed leakage
2. Voided volume
   ____ Unable ____ mL
3. Postvoid residual
   ____ mL (or volume in bladder ____ mL)

4. Urinalysis

    _____ Normal

    _____ Hematuria (or positive heme and dipstick)

    _____ Pyuria (or positive leukocyte esterase)

    _____ Bacteriuria (or positive nitrite)

D. Management

    _____ Treatment reversible factors (describe)

    _____ Treat for urge incontinence

    _____ Treat for stress incontinence

    _____ Treat for mixed incontinence

    _____ Manage supportively

    _____ Refer for further evaluation

    _____ Reason: _____

List specific treatment program

_____

_____

_____

_____

[a] Such that ability to get to a toilet (or toilet substitute) is impaired.

[b] Describe type and number used per 24-h period

535

Numeric Identifier _____

MINIMUM DATA SET (MDS) — *VERSION 2.0*
FOR NURSING HOME RESIDENT ASSESSMENT AND CARE SCREENING

BASIC ASSESSMENT TRACKING FORM

GENERAL INSTRUCTIONS

Complete this information for submission with all full and quarterly assessments (Admission, Annual, Significant Change, State or Medicare required assessments, or Quarterly Reviews, etc.)

SECTION AA. IDENTIFICATION INFORMATION

1.	RESIDENT NAME[a]				
	a. (First)	b. (Middle Initial)	c. (Last)	d. (Jr/Sr)	
2.	GENDER[b]	1. Male 2. Female			
3.	BIRTHDATE[c]	Month — Day — Year			
4.	RACE/ ETHNICITY	1. American Indian/Alaskan Native 2. Asian/Pacific Islander 3. Black, not of Hispanic origin 4. Hispanic 5. White, not of Hispanic origin			
5.	SOCIAL SECURITY[d] AND MEDICARE NUMBERS[e] [C in 1st box if non med. no.]	a. Social Security Number b. Medicare number (or comparable railroad insurance number)			
6.	FACILITY PROVIDER NO.[f]	a. State No. b. Federal No.			
7.	MEDICAID NO. ["+" if pending, "N" if not a Medicaid recipient]				

536

8.	REASONS FOR ASSESS- MENT	[Note—Other codes do not apply to this form]

a. Primary reason for assessment
1. Admission assessment (required by day 14)
2. Annual assessment
3. Significant change in status assessment
4. Significant correction of prior full assessment
5. Quarterly review assessment
10. Significant correction of prior quarterly assessment
0. *NONE OF ABOVE*

b. Codes for assessments required for Medicare PPS or the State
1. *Medicare 5 day assessment*
2. *Medicare 30 day assessment*
3. *Medicare 60 day assessment*
4. *Medicare 90 day assessment*
5. *Medicare readmission/return assessment*
6. *Other state required assessment*
7. *Medicare 14 day assessment*
8. *Other Medicare required assessment*

9.	SIGNATURES OF PERSONS COMPLETING THESE ITEMS:

	Title	Date
a. Signatures		
b.		

⊙ = Key items for computerized resident tracking

☐ = When box blank, must enter number or letter   a. = When letter in box, check if condition applies

537

MINIMUM DATA SET (MDS) — *VERSION 2.0*
FOR NURSING HOME RESIDENT ASSESSMENT AND CARE SCREENING
BACKGROUND (FACE SHEET) INFORMATION AT ADMISSION

SECTION AB. DEMOGRAPHIC INFORMATION

1.	DATE OF ENTRY	*Date the stay began. Note — Does not include readmission if record was closed at time of temporary discharge to hospital, etc. In such cases, use prior admission date*

Month — Day — Year

2.	ADMITTED FROM (AT ENTRY)	1. Private home/apt. with no home health services 2. Private home/apt. with home health services 3. Board and care/assisted living/group home 4. Nursing home 5. Acute care hospital 6. Psychiatric hospital, MR/DD facility 7. Rehabilitation hospital 8. Other

3.	LIVED ALONE (PRIOR TO ENTRY)	0. No 1. Yes 2. In other facility

4.	ZIP CODE OF PRIOR PRIMARY RESIDENCE	

5.	RESIDENTIAL HISTORY 5 YEARS PRIOR TO ENTRY	*(Check all settings resident lived in during 5 years prior to date of entry given in item AB1 above)*

Prior stay at this nursing home — a.
Stay in other nursing home — b.
Other residential facility—board and care home, assisted living, group home — c.
MH/psychiatric setting — d.
MR/DD setting — e.
NONE OF ABOVE — f.

6.	LIFETIME OCCUPATION(S) [Put "/" between two occupations]	

SECTION AC. CUSTOMARY ROUTINE

1.	CUSTOMARY ROUTINE	*(Check all that apply. If all information UNKNOWN, check last box only.)*
	(In year prior to DATE OF ENTRY to this nursing home, or year last in community if now being admitted from another nursing home)	**CYCLE OF DAILY EVENTS**

Stays up late at night (e.g., after 9 pm) — a.
Naps regularly during day (at least 1 hour) — b.
Goes out 1+ days a week — c.
Stays busy with hobbies, reading, or fixed daily routine — d.
Spends most of time alone or watching TV — e.
Moves independently indoors (with appliances, if used) — f.
Use of tobacco products at least daily — g.
NONE OF ABOVE — h.

EATING PATTERNS

Distinct food preferences — i.
Eats between meals all or most days — j.
Use of alcoholic beverage(s) at least weekly — k.
NONE OF ABOVE — l.

ADL PATTERNS

In bedclothes much of day — m.
Wakens to toilet all or most nights — n.
Has irregular bowel movement pattern — o.
Showers for bathing — p.
Bathing in PM — q.
NONE OF ABOVE — r.

INVOLVEMENT PATTERNS

Daily contact with relatives/close friends	s.
Usually attends church, temple, synagogue (etc.)	t.
Finds strength in faith	u.
Daily animal companion/presence	v.
Involved in group activities	w.
NONE OF ABOVE	x.
UNKNOWN—Resident/family unable to provide information	y.

7.	EDUCATION (Highest Level Completed)	1. No schooling 2. 8th grade/less 3. 9-11 grades 4. High school 5. Technical or trade school 6. Some college 7. Bachelor's degree 8. Graduate degree
8.	LANGUAGE	(Code for correct response) a. Primary Language 0. English 1. Spanish 2. French 3. Other b. If other, specify
9.	MENTAL HEALTH HISTORY	Does resident's RECORD indicate any history of mental retardation, mental illness, or developmental disability problem? 0. No 1. Yes
10.	CONDITIONS RELATED TO MR/DD STATUS	*(Check all conditions that are related to MR/DD status that were manifested before age 22, and are likely to continue indefinitely)* Not applicable—no MR/DD (Skip to AB11) a. MR/DD with organic condition Down's syndrome b. Autism c. Epilepsy d. Other organic condition related to MR/DD e. MR/DD with no organic condition f.
11.	DATE BACKGROUND INFORMATION COMPLETED	Month — Day — Year

SECTION AD. FACE SHEET SIGNATURES

SIGNATURES OF PERSONS COMPLETING FACE SHEET:

a.	Signature of RN Assessment Coordinator		Date
b. Signatures	Title	Sections	Date
c.			Date
d.			Date
e.			Date
f.			Date
g.			Date

MDS 2.0 01/30/98

☐ = When box blank, must enter number or letter   [a.] = When letter in box, check if condition applies

Resident _____   Numeric Identifier _____

MINIMUM DATA SET (MDS) — *VERSION 2.0*
FOR NURSING HOME RESIDENT ASSESSMENT AND CARE SCREENING
FULL ASSESSMENT FORM

(Status in last 7 days, unless other time frame indicated)

SECTION A. IDENTIFICATION AND BACKGROUND INFORMATION

1.	**RESIDENT NAME**	a. (First)	b. (Middle Initial)	c. (Last)	d. (Jr/Sr)
2.	**ROOM NUMBER**				
3.	**ASSESS-MENT REFERENCE DATE**	a. *Last day of MDS observation period* Month — Day — Year b. Original (0) or corrected copy of form (enter number of correction)			
4a.	**DATE OF REENTRY**	Date of reentry from most recent temporary discharge to a hospital in last 90 days (or since last assessment or admission if less than 90 days) Month — Day — Year			
5.	**MARITAL STATUS**	1. Never married 2. Married 3. Widowed 4. Separated 5. Divorced			
6.	**MEDICAL RECORD NO.**				
7.	**CURRENT PAYMENT SOURCES FOR N.H. STAY**	*(Billing Office to indicate; check all that apply in last 30 days)* a. Medicaid per diem f. VA per diem b. Medicare per diem g. Self or family pays for full per diem c. Medicare ancillary part A h. Medicaid resident liability or Medicare co-payment d. Medicare ancillary part B i. Private insurance per diem (including co-payment) e. CHAMPUS per diem j. Other per diem			
8.	**REASONS FOR ASSESS-MENT**	a. Primary reason for assessment 1. Admission assessment (required by day 14) 2. Annual assessment 3. Significant change in status assessment 4. Significant correction of prior full assessment			

3.	**MEMORY/ RECALL ABILITY**	*(Check all that resident was normally able to recall during last 7 days)* a. Current season d. That he/she is in a nursing home b. Location of own room e. NONE OF ABOVE are recalled c. Staff names/faces	
4.	**COGNITIVE SKILLS FOR DAILY DECISION-MAKING**	*(Made decisions regarding tasks of daily life)* 0. INDEPENDENT—decisions consistent/reasonable 1. MODIFIED INDEPENDENCE—some difficulty in new situations only 2. MODERATELY IMPAIRED—decisions poor; cues/supervision required 3. SEVERELY IMPAIRED—never/rarely made decisions	
5.	**INDICATORS OF DELIRIUM— PERIODIC DISOR- DERED THINKING/ AWARENESS**	*(Code for behavior in the last 7 days.)* [Note: Accurate assessment requires conversations with staff and family who have direct knowledge of resident's behavior over this time]. 0. Behavior not present 1. Behavior present, not of recent onset 2. Behavior present, over last 7 days appears different from resident's usual functioning (e.g., new onset or worsening) a. EASILY DISTRACTED—(e.g., difficulty paying attention; gets sidetracked) b. PERIODS OF ALTERED PERCEPTION OR AWARENESS OF SURROUNDINGS—(e.g., moves lips or talks to someone not present; believes he/she is somewhere else; confuses night and day) c. EPISODES OF DISORGANIZED SPEECH—(e.g., speech is incoherent, nonsensical, irrelevant, or rambling from subject to subject; loses train of thought) d. PERIODS OF RESTLESSNESS—(e.g., fidgeting or picking at skin, clothing, napkins, etc; frequent position changes; repetitive physical movements or calling out) e. PERIODS OF LETHARGY—(e.g., sluggishness; staring into space; difficult to arouse; little body movement) f. MENTAL FUNCTION VARIES OVER THE COURSE OF THE DAY—(e.g., sometimes better, sometimes worse; behaviors sometimes present, sometimes not)	
6.	**CHANGE IN COGNITIVE STATUS**	Resident's cognitive status, skills, or abilities have changed as compared to status of **90 days ago** (or since last assessment if less than 90 days) 0. No change 1. Improved 2. Deteriorated	

540

[Note—If this is a discharge or reentry assessment, only a limited subset of MDS items need be completed]

5. Quarterly review assessment
6. Discharged—return not anticipated
7. Discharged—return anticipated
8. Discharged prior to completing initial assessment
9. Reentry
10. Significant correction of prior quarterly assessment
0. NONE OF ABOVE

b. Codes for assessments required for Medicare PPS or the State
1. Medicare 5 day assessment
2. Medicare 30 day assessment
3. Medicare 60 day assessment
4. Medicare 90 day assessment
5. Medicare readmission/return assessment
6. Other state required assessment
7. Medicare 14 day assessment
8. Other Medicare required assessment

9. RESPONSI-BILITY/ LEGAL GUARDIAN	(Check all that apply)	
a. Legal guardian	d. Durable power attorney/financial	
b. Other legal oversight	e. Family member responsible	
c. Durable power of attorney/health care	f. Patient responsible for self	
	g. NONE OF ABOVE	

10. ADVANCED DIRECTIVES	(For those items with supporting documentation in the medical record, check all that apply)	
a. Living will	f. Feeding restrictions	
b. Do not resuscitate	g. Medication restrictions	
c. Do not hospitalize	h. Other treatment restrictions	
d. Organ donation	i. NONE OF ABOVE	
e. Autopsy request		

SECTION B. COGNITIVE PATTERNS

1. COMATOSE	(Persistent vegetative state/no discernible consciousness)
	0. No 1. Yes (If yes, skip to Section G)

2. MEMORY	(Recall of what was learned or known)
	a. Short-term memory OK—seems/appears to recall after 5 minutes
	0. Memory OK 1. Memory problem
	b. Long-term memory OK—seems/appears to recall long past
	0. Memory OK 1. Memory problem

SECTION C. COMMUNICATION/HEARING PATTERNS

1. HEARING	(With hearing appliance, if used)	
	0. HEARS ADEQUATELY—normal talk, TV, phone	
	1. MINIMAL DIFFICULTY when not in quiet setting	
	2. HEARS IN SPECIAL SITUATIONS ONLY—speaker has to adjust tonal quality and speak distinctly	
	3. HIGHLY IMPAIRED/absence of useful hearing	

2. COMMUNI-CATION DEVICES/ TECH-NIQUES	(Check all that apply during last 7 days)	
	Hearing aid, present and used	a.
	Hearing aid, present and not used regularly	b.
	Other receptive comm. techniques used (e.g., lip reading)	c.
	NONE OF ABOVE	d.

3. MODES OF EXPRESSION	(Check all used by resident to make needs known)		
	Speech	a. Signs/gestures/sounds	d.
	Writing messages to express or clarify needs	b. Communication board	e.
	American sign language or Braille	Other	f.
		c. NONE OF ABOVE	g.

4. MAKING SELF UNDER-STOOD	(Expressing information content—however able)	
	0. UNDERSTOOD	
	1. USUALLY UNDERSTOOD—difficulty finding words or finishing thoughts	
	2. SOMETIMES UNDERSTOOD—ability is limited to making concrete requests	
	3. RARELY/NEVER UNDERSTOOD	

5. SPEECH CLARITY	(Code for speech in the last 7 days)	
	0. CLEAR SPEECH—distinct, intelligible words	
	1. UNCLEAR SPEECH—slurred, mumbled words	
	2. NO SPEECH—absence of spoken words	

6. ABILITY TO UNDER-STAND OTHERS	(Understanding verbal information content—however able)	
	0. UNDERSTANDS	
	1. USUALLY UNDERSTANDS—may miss some part/intent of message	
	2. SOMETIMES UNDERSTANDS—responds adequately to simple, direct communication	
	3. RARELY/NEVER UNDERSTANDS	

7. CHANGE IN COMMUNI-CATION/ HEARING	Resident's ability to express, understand, or hear information has changed as compared to status of 90 days ago (or since last assessment if less than 90 days)	
	0. No change 1. Improved 2. Deteriorated	

MDS 2.0 01/30/98

☐ = When box blank, must enter number or letter   [a.] = When letter in box, check if condition applies

SECTION D. VISION PATTERNS

1.	VISION	*(Ability to see in adequate light and with glasses if used)* 0. ADEQUATE—sees fine detail, including regular print in newspapers/books 1. IMPAIRED—sees large print, but not regular print in newspapers/books 2. MODERATELY IMPAIRED—limited vision; not able to see newspaper headlines, but can identify objects 3. HIGHLY IMPAIRED—object identification in question, but eyes appear to follow objects 4. SEVERELY IMPAIRED—no vision or sees only light, colors, or shapes; eyes do not appear to follow objects	
2.	VISUAL LIMITATIONS/ DIFFICULTIES	Side vision problems—decreased peripheral vision (e.g., leaves food on one side of tray, difficulty traveling, bumps into people and objects, misjudges placement of chair when seating self)	a.
		Experiences any of following: sees halos or rings around lights; sees flashes of light; sees "curtains" over eyes	b.
		NONE OF ABOVE	c.
3.	VISUAL APPLIANCES	Glasses; contact lenses; magnifying glass 0. No 1. Yes	

SECTION E. MOOD AND BEHAVIOR PATTERNS

1.	INDICATORS OF DEPRES- SION, ANXIETY, SAD MOOD	*(Code for indicators observed in last 30 days, irrespective of the assumed cause)* 0. Indicator not exhibited in last 30 days 1. Indicator of this type exhibited up to five days a week 2. Indicator of this type exhibited daily or almost daily (6, 7 days a week)
		VERBAL EXPRESSIONS OF DISTRESS
		a. Resident made negative statements—e.g., *Nothing matters; Would rather be dead; What's the use; Regrets having lived so long; Let me die*
		b. Repetitive questions—e.g., *"Where do I go; What do I do?"*
		c. Repetitive verbalizations— e.g., calling out for help, (*"God help me"*)
		h. Repetitive health complaints—e.g., persistently seeks medical attention, obsessive concern with body functions
		i. Repetitive anxious complaints/concerns (non-health related) e.g., persistently seeks attention/ reassurance regarding schedules, meals, laundry, clothing, relationship issues
		SLEEP-CYCLE ISSUES
		j. Unpleasant mood in morning

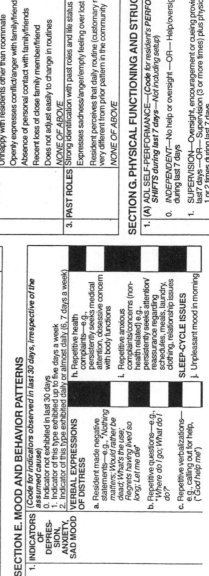

| 5. | CHANGE IN BEHAVIORAL SYMPTOMS | Resident's behavior status has changed as compared to **status of 90 days ago** (or since last assessment if less than 90 days)
0. No change 1. Improved 2. Deteriorated | |

SECTION F. PSYCHOSOCIAL WELL-BEING

1.	SENSE OF INITIATIVE/ INVOLVE- MENT	At ease interacting with others	a.
		At ease doing planned or structured activities	b.
		At ease doing self-initiated activities	c.
		Establishes own goals	d.
		Pursues involvement in life of facility (e.g., makes/keeps friends; involved in group activities; responds positively to new activities; assists at religious services)	e.
		Accepts invitations into most group activities	f.
		NONE OF ABOVE	g.
2.	UNSETTLED RELATION- SHIPS	Covert/open conflict with or repeated criticism of staff	a.
		Unhappy with roommate	b.
		Unhappy with residents other than roommate	c.
		Openly expresses conflict/anger with family/friends	d.
		Absence of personal contact with family/friends	e.
		Recent loss of close family member/friend	f.
		Does not adjust easily to change in routines	g.
		NONE OF ABOVE	h.
3.	PAST ROLES	Strong identification with past roles and life status	a.
		Expresses sadness/anger/empty feeling over lost roles/status	b.
		Resident perceives that daily routine (customary routine, activities) is very different from prior pattern in the community	c.
		NONE OF ABOVE	d.

SECTION G. PHYSICAL FUNCTIONING AND STRUCTURAL PROBLEMS

1. (A) ADL SELF-PERFORMANCE—*(Code for resident's PERFORMANCE OVER ALL SHIFTS during last 7 days—Not including setup)*

0. INDEPENDENT—No help or oversight —OR— Help/oversight provided only 1 or 2 times during last 7 days

1. SUPERVISION—Oversight, encouragement or cueing provided 3 or more times during last 7 days —OR— Supervision (3 or more times) plus physical assistance provided only 1 or 2 times during last 7 days

MDS 2.0 01/30/98

Mood (continued)

d. Persistent anger with self or others—e.g., easily annoyed, anger at placement in nursing home; anger at care received

e. Self deprecation—e.g., "I am nothing; I am of no use to anyone"

f. Expressions of what appear to be unrealistic fears—e.g., fear of being abandoned, left alone, being with others

g. Recurrent statements that something terrible is about to happen—e.g., believes he or she is about to die, have a heart attack

k. Insomnia/change in usual sleep pattern

SAD, APATHETIC, ANXIOUS APPEARANCE

l. Sad, pained, worried facial expressions—e.g., furrowed brows

m. Crying, tearfulness

n. Repetitive physical movements—e.g., pacing, hand wringing, restlessness, fidgeting, picking

LOSS OF INTEREST

o. Withdrawal from activities of interest—e.g., no interest in long standing activities or being with family/friends

p. Reduced social interaction

2. MOOD PERSISTENCE — One or more indicators of depressed, sad or anxious mood were not easily altered by attempts to "cheer up", console, or reassure the resident over last 7 days
0. No mood indicators
1. Indicators present, easily altered
2. Indicators present, not easily altered

3. CHANGE IN MOOD — Resident's mood status has changed as compared to status of 90 days ago (or since last assessment if less than 90 days)
0. No change
1. Improved
2. Deteriorated

4. BEHAVIORAL SYMPTOMS — (A) *Behavioral symptom frequency in last 7 days*
0. Behavior not exhibited in last 7 days
1. Behavior of this type occurred 1 to 3 days in last 7 days
2. Behavior of this type occurred 4 to 6 days, but less than daily
3. Behavior of this type occurred daily

(B) *Behavioral symptom alterability in last 7 days*
0. Behavior not present OR behavior was easily altered
1. Behavior was not easily altered

(A) (B)

a. WANDERING (moved with no rational purpose, seemingly oblivious to needs or safety)

b. VERBALLY ABUSIVE BEHAVIORAL SYMPTOMS (others were threatened, screamed at, cursed at)

c. PHYSICALLY ABUSIVE BEHAVIORAL SYMPTOMS (others were hit, shoved, scratched, sexually abused)

d. SOCIALLY INAPPROPRIATE/DISRUPTIVE BEHAVIORAL SYMPTOMS (made disruptive sounds, noisiness, screaming, self-abusive acts, sexual behavior or disrobing in public, smeared/threw food/feces, hoarding, rummaged through others' belongings)

e. RESISTS CARE (resisted taking medications/injections, ADL assistance, or eating)

---

2. LIMITED ASSISTANCE—Resident highly involved in activity; received physical help in guided maneuvering of limbs or other nonweight bearing assistance 3 or more times — OR—More help provided only 1 or 2 times during last 7 days

3. EXTENSIVE ASSISTANCE—While resident performed part of activity, over last 7-day period, help of following type(s) provided 3 or more times:
— Weight-bearing support
— Full staff performance during part (but not all) of last 7 days

4. TOTAL DEPENDENCE—Full staff performance of activity during entire 7 days

8. ACTIVITY DID NOT OCCUR during entire 7 days

(B) ADL SUPPORT PROVIDED—(Code for MOST SUPPORT PROVIDED OVER ALL SHIFTS during last 7 days; code regardless of resident's self-performance classification)
0. No setup or physical help from staff
1. Setup help only
2. One person physical assist
3. Two+ persons physical assist
8. ADL activity itself did not occur during entire 7 days

(A) SELF-PERF | (B) SUPPORT

a. **BED MOBILITY** — How resident moves to and from lying position, turns side to side, and positions body while in bed

b. **TRANSFER** — How resident moves between surfaces—to/from: bed, chair, wheelchair, standing position (EXCLUDE to/from bath/toilet)

c. **WALK IN ROOM** — How resident walks between locations in his/her room

d. **WALK IN CORRIDOR** — How resident walks in corridor on unit

e. **LOCOMOTION ON UNIT** — How resident moves between locations in his/her room and adjacent corridor on same floor. If in wheelchair, self-sufficiency once in chair

f. **LOCOMOTION OFF UNIT** — How resident moves to and returns from off unit locations (e.g., areas set aside for dining, activities, or treatments). If facility has only one floor, how resident moves to and from distant areas on the floor. If in wheelchair, self-sufficiency once in chair

g. **DRESSING** — How resident puts on, fastens, and takes off all items of street clothing, including donning/removing prosthesis

h. **EATING** — How resident eats and drinks (regardless of skill). Includes intake of nourishment by other means (e.g., tube feeding, total parenteral nutrition)

i. **TOILET USE** — How resident uses the toilet room (or commode, bedpan, urinal); transfer on/off toilet, cleanses, changes pad, manages ostomy or catheter, adjusts clothes

j. **PERSONAL HYGIENE** — How resident maintains personal hygiene, including combing hair, brushing teeth, shaving, applying makeup, washing/drying face, hands, and perineum (EXCLUDE baths and showers)

Resident ___

2	BATHING	How resident takes full-body bath/shower, sponge bath, and transfers in/out of tub/shower (EXCLUDE washing of back and hair.) *Code for most dependent in self-performance and support.* (A) BATHING SELF-PERFORMANCE codes appear below	(A)	(B)
		0. Independent—No help provided		
		1. Supervision—Oversight help only		
		2. Physical help limited to transfer only		
		3. Physical help in part of bathing activity		
		4. Total dependence		
		8. Activity itself did not occur during entire 7 days		
		(Bathing support codes are as defined in Item 1, code B above)		

3	TEST FOR BALANCE (see training manual)	*(Code for ability during test in the last 7 days)*	
		0. Maintained position as required in test	
		1. Unsteady, but able to rebalance self without physical support	
		2. Partial physical support during test; or stands (sits) but does not follow directions for test	
		3. Not able to attempt test without physical help	
		a. Balance while standing	
		b. Balance while sitting—position, trunk control	

4	FUNCTIONAL LIMITATION IN RANGE OF MOTION (see training manual)	*(Code for limitations during last 7 days that interfered with daily functions or placed resident at risk of injury)* (A) RANGE OF MOTION	(B) VOLUNTARY MOVEMENT	(A)	(B)
		0. No limitation	0. No loss		
		1. Limitation on one side	1. Partial loss		
		2. Limitation on both sides	2. Full loss		
		a. Neck			
		b. Arm—Including shoulder or elbow			
		c. Hand—Including wrist or fingers			
		d. Leg—Including hip or knee			
		e. Foot—Including ankle or toes			
		f. Other limitation or loss			

5	MODES OF LOCOMOTION	*(Check all that apply during last 7 days)*		
		a. Cane/walker/crutch	Wheelchair primary mode of locomotion	d.
		b. Wheeled self		
		c. Other person wheeled	NONE OF ABOVE	e.

6	MODES OF TRANSFER	*(Check all that apply during last 7 days)*		
		a. Bedfast all or most of time	Lifted mechanically	d.
		b. Bed rails used for bed mobility or transfer	Transfer aid (e.g., slide board, trapeze, cane, walker, brace)	e.
		c. Lifted manually	NONE OF ABOVE	f.

3	APPLIANCES AND PROGRAMS	Any scheduled toileting plan	a.	Did not use toilet room/commode/urinal	f.
		Bladder retraining program	b.	Pads/briefs used	g.
		External (condom) catheter	c.	Enemas/irrigation	h.
		Indwelling catheter	d.	Ostomy present	i.
		Intermittent catheter	e.	NONE OF ABOVE	j.

4	CHANGE IN URINARY CONTINENCE	Resident's urinary continence has changed as compared to status of 90 days ago (or since last assessment if less than 90 days)
		0. No change 1. Improved 2. Deteriorated

SECTION I. DISEASE DIAGNOSES

Check only those diseases that have a **relationship** to current ADL status, cognitive status, mood and behavior status, medical treatments, nursing monitoring, or risk of death. (Do not list inactive diagnoses)

1	DISEASES	*(If none apply, CHECK the NONE OF ABOVE box)*			
		ENDOCRINE/METABOLIC/NUTRITIONAL		Hemiplegia/Hemiparesis	v.
				Multiple sclerosis	w.
		Diabetes mellitus	a.	Paraplegia	x.
		Hyperthyroidism	b.	Parkinson's disease	y.
		Hypothyroidism	c.	Quadriplegia	z.
		HEART/CIRCULATION		Seizure disorder	aa.
		Arteriosclerotic heart disease (ASHD)	d.	Transient ischemic attack (TIA)	bb.
		Cardiac dysrhythmias	e.	Traumatic brain injury	cc.
		Congestive heart failure	f.	**PSYCHIATRIC/MOOD**	
		Deep vein thrombosis	g.	Anxiety disorder	dd.
		Hypertension	h.	Depression	ee.
		Hypotension	i.	Manic depression (bipolar disease)	ff.
		Peripheral vascular disease	j.	Schizophrenia	gg.
		Other cardiovascular disease	k.	**PULMONARY**	
		MUSCULOSKELETAL		Asthma	hh.
		Arthritis	l.	Emphysema/COPD	ii.
		Hip fracture	m.	**SENSORY**	
		Missing limb (e.g., amputation)	n.	Cataracts	jj.
		Osteoporosis	o.	Diabetic retinopathy	kk.
		Pathological bone fracture	p.	Glaucoma	ll.

7.	TASK SEGMENTA-TION	Some or all of ADL activities were broken into subtasks during last 7 days so that resident could perform them 0. No 1. Yes	
8.	ADL FUNCTIONAL REHABILITA-TION POTENTIAL	Resident believes he/she is capable of increased independence in at least some ADLs	a.
		Direct care staff believe resident is capable of increased independence in at least some ADLs	b.
		Resident able to perform tasks/activity but is very slow	c.
		Difference in ADL Self-Performance or ADL Support, comparing mornings to evenings	d.
		NONE OF ABOVE	e.
9.	CHANGE IN ADL FUNCTION	Resident's ADL self-performance status has changed as compared to status of 90 days ago (or since last assessment if less than 90 days) 0. No change 1. Improved 2. Deteriorated	

SECTION H. CONTINENCE IN LAST 14 DAYS

1.	CONTINENCE SELF-CONTROL CATEGORIES *(Code for resident's PERFORMANCE OVER ALL SHIFTS)*
	0. *CONTINENT—Complete control [includes use of indwelling urinary catheter or ostomy device that does not leak urine or stool]*
	1. *USUALLY CONTINENT—BLADDER, incontinent episodes once a week or less; BOWEL, less than weekly*
	2. *OCCASIONALLY INCONTINENT—BLADDER, 2 or more times a week but not daily; BOWEL, once a week*
	3. *FREQUENTLY INCONTINENT—BLADDER, tended to be incontinent daily, but some control present (e.g., on day shift); BOWEL, 2-3 times a week*
	4. *INCONTINENT—Had inadequate control BLADDER, multiple daily episodes; BOWEL, all (or almost all) of the time*

a.	BOWEL CONTI-NENCE	Control of bowel movement, with appliance or bowel continence programs, if employed	
b.	BLADDER CONTI-NENCE	Control of urinary bladder function (if dribbles, volume insufficient to soak through underpants), with appliances (e.g., foley) or continence programs, if employed	

2.	BOWEL ELIMINATION PATTERN	Bowel elimination pattern regular—at least one movement every three days	a.	Diarrhea	c.
				Fecal impaction	d.
		Constipation	b.	NONE OF ABOVE	e.

MDS 2.0 01/30/98

NEUROLOGICAL

Alzheimer's disease		Macular degeneration	mm.
Aphasia		OTHER	
Cerebral palsy		Allergies	nn.
Cerebrovascular accident (stroke)		Anemia	oo.
		Cancer	pp.
Dementia other than Alzheimer's disease		Renal failure	qq.
		NONE OF ABOVE	rr.

2.	INFECTIONS	*(If none apply, CHECK the NONE OF ABOVE box)*	
		Antibiotic resistant infection (e.g., Methicillin resistant staph)	a.
		Septicemia	g.
		Sexually transmitted diseases	h.
		Clostridium difficile (c. diff.)	b.
		Tuberculosis	i.
		Conjunctivitis	c.
		Urinary tract infection in last 30 days	j.
		HIV infection	d.
		Viral hepatitis	k.
		Pneumonia	e.
		Wound infection	l.
		Respiratory infection	f.
		NONE OF ABOVE	m.

3.	OTHER CURRENT OR MORE DETAILED DIAGNOSES AND ICD-9 CODES	a.	•
		b.	•
		c.	•
		d.	•
		e.	•

SECTION J. HEALTH CONDITIONS

1.	PROBLEM CONDITIONS	*(Check all problems present in last 7 days unless other time frame is indicated)*	
		INDICATORS OF FLUID STATUS	
		Weight gain or loss of 3 or more pounds within a 7 day period	a.
		Inability to lie flat due to shortness of breath	b.
		Dehydrated; output exceeds input	c.
		Insufficient fluid; did NOT consume all/almost all liquids provided during last 3 days	d.
		OTHER	
		Delusions	e.
		Dizziness/Vertigo	f.
		Edema	g.
		Fever	h.
		Hallucinations	i.
		Internal bleeding	j.
		Recurrent lung aspirations in last 90 days	k.
		Shortness of breath	l.
		Syncope (fainting)	m.
		Unsteady gait	n.
		Vomiting	o.
		NONE OF ABOVE	p.

Numeric Identifier _____

SECTION M. SKIN CONDITION

			Number at Stage
1.	ULCERS (Due to any cause)	*(Record the number of ulcers at each ulcer stage—regardless of cause. If none present at a stage, record "0" (zero). Code all that apply during last 7 days. Code 9 = 9 or more.) [Requires full body exam.]*	
		a. Stage 1. A persistent area of skin redness (without a break in the skin) that does not disappear when pressure is relieved.	
		b. Stage 2. A partial thickness loss of skin layers that presents clinically as an abrasion, blister, or shallow crater.	
		c. Stage 3. A full thickness of skin is lost, exposing the subcutaneous tissues - presents as a deep crater with or without undermining adjacent tissue.	
		d. Stage 4. A full thickness of skin and subcutaneous tissue is lost, exposing muscle or bone.	
2.	TYPE OF ULCER	*(For each type of ulcer, code for the highest stage in the last 7 days using scale in item M1—i.e., 0=none; stages 1, 2, 3, 4)*	
		a. Pressure ulcer—any lesion caused by pressure resulting in damage of underlying tissue	
		b. Stasis ulcer—open lesion caused by poor circulation in the lower extremities	
3.	HISTORY OF RESOLVED ULCERS	Resident had an ulcer that was resolved or cured in **LAST 90 DAYS** 0. No 1. Yes	
4.	OTHER SKIN PROBLEMS OR LESIONS PRESENT	*(Check all that apply during last 7 days)*	
		Abrasions, bruises	a.
		Burns (second or third degree)	b.
		Open lesions other than ulcers, rashes, cuts (e.g., cancer lesions)	c.
		Rashes—e.g., intertrigo, eczema, drug rash, heat rash, herpes zoster	d.
		Skin desensitized to pain or pressure	e.
		Skin tears or cuts (other than surgery)	f.
		Surgical wounds	g.
		NONE OF ABOVE	h.
5.	SKIN TREATMENTS	*(Check all that apply during last 7 days)*	
		Pressure relieving device(s) for chair	a.
		Pressure relieving device(s) for bed	b.
		Turning/repositioning program	c.
		Nutrition or hydration intervention to manage skin problems	d.
		Ulcer care	e.
		Surgical wound care	f.

2.	PAIN SYMPTOMS	*(Code the highest level of pain present in the last 7 days)*		
		a. FREQUENCY with which resident complains or shows evidence of pain 0. No pain *(skip to J4)* 1. Pain less than daily 2. Pain daily	b. INTENSITY of pain 1. Mild pain 2. Moderate pain 3. Times when pain is horrible or excruciating	
3.	PAIN SITE	*(If pain present, check all sites that apply in last 7 days)*		
		a. Back pain	f. Incisional pain	
		b. Bone pain	g. Joint pain (other than hip)	
		c. Chest pain while doing usual activities	h. Soft tissue pain (e.g., lesion, muscle)	
		d. Headache	i. Stomach pain	
		e. Hip pain	j. Other	
4.	ACCIDENTS	*(Check all that apply)*		
		a. Fell in past 30 days	c. Hip fracture in last 180 days	
		b. Fell in past 31-180 days	d. Other fracture in last 180 days	
			e. NONE OF ABOVE	
5.	STABILITY OF CONDITIONS	Conditions/diseases make resident's cognitive, ADL, mood or behavior patterns unstable—(fluctuating, precarious, or deteriorating)		a.
		Resident experiencing an acute episode or a flare-up of a recurrent or chronic problem		b.
		End-stage disease, 6 or fewer months to live		c.
		NONE OF ABOVE		d.

SECTION K. ORAL/NUTRITIONAL STATUS

1.	ORAL PROBLEMS	Chewing problem	a.
		Swallowing problem	b.
		Mouth pain	c.
		NONE OF ABOVE	d.
2.	HEIGHT AND WEIGHT	Record *(a.) height in inches and (b.) weight in pounds. Base weight on most recent measure in last 30 days; measure weight consistently in accord with standard facility practice—e.g., in a.m. after voiding, before meal, with shoes off, and in nightclothes*	a. HT (in.) [ ] b. WT (lb.) [ ]

3. WEIGHT CHANGE
a. Weight loss—5 % or more in last 30 days; or 10 % or more in last 180 days
 0. No   1. Yes
b. Weight gain—5 % or more in last 30 days; or 10 % or more in last 180 days
 0. No   1. Yes

4. NUTRITIONAL PROBLEMS

Complains about the taste of many foods	a.
Regular or repetitive complaints of hunger	b.
Leaves 25% or more of food uneaten at most meals	c.
NONE OF ABOVE	d.

5. NUTRITIONAL APPROACHES
(Check all that apply in last 7 days)

Parenteral/IV	a.
Feeding tube	b.
Mechanically altered diet	c.
Syringe (oral feeding)	d.
Therapeutic diet	e.
Dietary supplement between meals	f.
Plate guard, stabilized built-up utensil, etc.	g.
On a planned weight change program	h.
NONE OF ABOVE	i.

6. PARENTERAL OR ENTERAL INTAKE (Skip to Section L if neither 5a nor 5b is checked)
a. Code the proportion of total calories the resident received through parenteral or tube feedings in the last 7 days
 0. None   3. 51% to 75%
 1. 1% to 25%   4. 76% to 100%
 2. 26% to 50%
b. Code the average fluid intake per day by IV or tube in last 7 days
 0. None   3. 1001 to 1500 cc/day
 1. 1 to 500 cc/day   4. 1501 to 2000 cc/day
 2. 501 to 1000 cc/day   5. 2001 or more cc/day

SECTION L. ORAL/DENTAL STATUS

1. ORAL STATUS AND DISEASE PREVENTION

Debris (soft, easily movable substances) present in mouth prior to going to bed at night	a.
Has dentures or removable bridge	b.
Some/all natural teeth lost—does not have or does not use dentures (or partial plates)	c.
Broken, loose, or carious teeth	d.
Inflamed gums (gingiva);swollen or bleeding gums; oral abscesses; ulcers or rashes	e.
Daily cleaning of teeth/dentures or daily mouth care—by resident or staff	f.
NONE OF ABOVE	g.

---

6. FOOT PROBLEMS AND CARE
(Check all that apply during last 7 days)

Resident has one or more foot problems—e.g., corns, callouses, bunions, hammer toes, overlapping toes, pain, structural problems	a.
Infection of the foot—e.g., cellulitis, purulent drainage	b.
Open lesions on the foot	c.
Nails/calluses trimmed during last 90 days	d.
Received preventative or protective foot care (e.g., used special shoes, inserts, pads, toe separators)	e.
Application of dressings (with or without topical medications)	f.
NONE OF ABOVE	g.

(continued from above — items a.–j.)

Application of dressings (with or without topical medications) other than to feet	g.
Application of ointments/medications (other than to feet)	h.
Other preventative or protective skin care (other than to feet)	i.
NONE OF ABOVE	j.

SECTION N. ACTIVITY PURSUIT PATTERNS

1. TIME AWAKE
(Check appropriate time periods over last 7 days)
Resident awake all or most of time (i.e., naps no more than one hour per time period) in the:

Morning	a.	Evening	c.
Afternoon	b.	NONE OF ABOVE	d.

(If resident is comatose, skip to Section O)

2. AVERAGE TIME INVOLVED IN ACTIVITIES
(When awake and not receiving treatments or ADL care)
 0. Most—more than 2/3 of time   2. Little—less than 1/3 of time
 1. Some—from 1/3 to 2/3 of time 3. None

3. PREFERRED ACTIVITY SETTINGS
(Check all settings in which activities are preferred)

Own room	a.	Outside facility	d.
Day/activity room	b.	NONE OF ABOVE	e.
Inside NH/off unit	c.		

4. GENERAL ACTIVITY PREFERENCES (adapted to resident's current abilities)
(Check all PREFERENCES whether or not activity is currently available to resident)

Cards/other games	a.	Trips/shopping	g.
Crafts/arts	b.	Walking/wheeling outdoors	h.
Exercise/sports	c.	Watching TV	i.
Music	d.	Gardening or plants	j.
Reading/writing	e.	Talking or conversing	k.
Spiritual/religious activities	f.	Helping others	l.
		NONE OF ABOVE	m.

MDS 2.0 01/30/98

547

5.	PREFERS CHANGE IN DAILY ROUTINE	Code for resident preferences in daily routines. 0. No change 1. Slight change 2. Major change
		a. Type of activities in which resident is currently involved
		b. Extent of resident involvement in activities

SECTION O. MEDICATIONS

1.	NUMBER OF MEDICATIONS	*(Record the number of different medications used in the last 7 days; enter "0" if none used)*
2.	NEW MEDICATIONS	*(Resident currently receiving medications that were initiated during the last 90 days)* 0. No 1. Yes
3.	INJECTIONS	*(Record the number of DAYS injections of any type received during the last 7 days; enter "0" if none used)*
4.	DAYS RECEIVED THE FOLLOWING MEDICATION	*(Record the number of DAYS during last 7 days; enter "0" if not used. Note—enter "1" for long-acting meds used less than weekly)*

a. Antipsychotic			d. Hypnotic	
b. Antianxiety			e. Diuretic	
c. Antidepressant				

SECTION P. SPECIAL TREATMENTS AND PROCEDURES

1.	SPECIAL TREATMENTS, PROCEDURES, AND PROGRAMS	a. SPECIAL CARE—*Check treatments or programs received during the last 14 days*

TREATMENTS			
a.	Chemotherapy	l.	Ventilator or respirator
b.	Dialysis		**PROGRAMS**
c.	IV medication	m.	Alcohol/drug treatment program
d.	Intake/output	n.	Alzheimer's/dementia special care unit
e.	Monitoring acute medical condition	o.	Hospice care
f.	Ostomy care	p.	Pediatric unit
g.	Oxygen therapy	q.	Respite care
h.	Radiation	r.	Training in skills required to return to the community (e.g., taking medications, house work, shopping, transportation, ADLs)
i.	Suctioning		
j.	Tracheostomy care	s.	NONE OF ABOVE
k.	Transfusions		

4.	DEVICES AND RESTRAINTS	*(Use the following codes for last 7 days:)* 0. Not used 1. Used less than daily 2. Used daily
		Bed rails
		a. — Full bed rails on all open sides of bed
		b. — Other types of side rails used (e.g., half rail, one side)
		c. Trunk restraint
		d. Limb restraint
		e. Chair prevents rising
5.	HOSPITAL STAY(S)	Record number of times resident was admitted to hospital with an overnight stay in last 90 days (or since last assessment if less than 90 days). *(Enter 0 if no hospital admissions)*
6.	EMERGENCY ROOM (ER) VISIT(S)	Record number of times resident visited ER without an overnight stay in last 90 days (or since last assessment if less than 90 days). *(Enter 0 if no ER visits)*
7.	PHYSICIAN VISITS	In the LAST 14 DAYS (or since admission if less than 14 days in facility) how many days has the physician (or authorized assistant or practitioner) examined the resident? *(Enter 0 if none)*
8.	PHYSICIAN ORDERS	In the LAST 14 DAYS (or since admission if less than 14 days in facility) how many days has the physician (or authorized assistant or practitioner) changed the resident's orders? *Do not include order renewals without change. (Enter 0 if none)*
9.	ABNORMAL LAB VALUES	Has the resident had any abnormal lab values during the last 90 days (or since admission)? 0. No 1. Yes

SECTION Q. DISCHARGE POTENTIAL AND OVERALL STATUS

1.	DISCHARGE POTENTIAL	a. Resident expresses/indicates preference to return to the community
		0. No 1. Yes
		b. Resident has a support person who is positive towards discharge
		0. No 1. Yes
		c. Stay projected to be of a short duration— discharge projected within 90 days (do not include expected discharge due to death)
		0. No 2. Within 31-90 days
		1. Within 30 days 3. Discharge status uncertain

b. THERAPIES

b. **THERAPIES** - Record the number of days and total minutes each of the following therapies was administered *(for at least 15 minutes a day)* in the last 7 calendar days *(Enter 0 if none or less than 15 min. daily)*

[Note—count only post admission therapies]

(A) = # of days administered for 15 minutes or more

(B) = total # of minutes provided in last 7 days

	DAYS (A)	MIN (B)
a. Speech - language pathology and audiology services		
b. Occupational therapy		
c. Physical therapy		
d. Respiratory therapy		
e. Psychological therapy (by any licensed mental health professional)		

2. INTERVEN-TION PROGRAMS FOR MOOD, BEHAVIOR, COGNITIVE LOSS	(Check all interventions or strategies used in last 7 days—no matter where received)	
	Special behavior symptom evaluation program	a.
	Evaluation by a licensed mental health specialist in last 90 days	b.
	Group therapy	c.
	Resident-specific deliberate changes in the environment to address mood/behavior patterns—e.g., providing bureau in which to rummage	d.
	Reorientation—e.g., cueing	e.
	NONE OF ABOVE	f.

3. NURSING REHABILITA-TION RESTOR-ATIVE CARE	Record the *NUMBER OF DAYS* each of the following rehabilitation or restorative techniques or practices was provided to the resident for *more than or equal to 15 minutes per day in the last 7 days* *(Enter 0 if none or less than 15 min. daily.)*	
	a. Range of motion (passive)	f. Walking
	b. Range of motion (active)	g. Dressing or grooming
	c. Splint or brace assistance	h. Eating or swallowing
	TRAINING AND SKILL PRACTICE IN:	i. Amputation/prosthesis care
	d. Bed mobility	j. Communication
	e. Transfer	k. Other

2.	**OVERALL CHANGE IN CARE NEEDS**	Resident's overall self sufficiency has changed significantly as compared to status of **90 days ago** (or since last assessment if less than 90 days)

0. No change   1. Improved—receives fewer   2. Deteriorated—receives
                     supports, needs less   more support
                     restrictive level of care

SECTION R. ASSESSMENT INFORMATION

1. PARTICIPA-TION IN ASSESS-MENT	a. Resident:	0. No	1. Yes	
	b. Family:	0. No	1. Yes	2. No family
	c. Significant other:	0. No	1. Yes	2. None

2. SIGNATURES OF PERSONS COMPLETING THE ASSESSMENT:

a. Signature of RN Assessment Coordinator (sign on above line)

b. Date RN Assessment Coordinator signed as complete

	Month	Day	Year

c. Other Signatures	Title	Sections	Date
d.			Date
e.			Date
f.			Date
g.			Date
h.			Date

MDS 2.0 01/30/98

549

Resident _____

SECTION T. THERAPY SUPPLEMENT FOR MEDICARE PPS

	SPECIAL TREAT-MENTS AND PROCE-DURES			

1. | **SPECIAL TREAT-MENTS AND PROCE-DURES**

a. RECREATION THERAPY—*Enter number of days and total minutes of recreation therapy administered (for at least 15 minutes a day) in the last 7 days (Enter 0 if none)*

	DAYS	MIN
	(A)	(B)

(A) = # of days administered for 15 minutes or more
(B) = total # of minutes provided in last 7 days

Skip unless this is a Medicare 5 day or Medicare readmission/return assessment.

b. ORDERED THERAPIES—*Has physician ordered any of following therapies to begin in FIRST 14 days of stay—physical therapy, occupational therapy, or speech pathology service?*
0. No   1. Yes

If not ordered, skip to item 2

c. Through day 15, provide an estimate of the number of days when at least 1 therapy service can be expected to have been delivered.

d. Through day 15, provide an estimate of the number of therapy minutes (across the therapies) that can be expected to be delivered?

2. | **WALKING WHEN MOST SELF SUFFICIENT**

Complete item 2 if ADL self-performance score for TRANSFER (G.1.b.A) is 0,1,2, or 3 AND at least one of the following are present:
- Resident received physical therapy involving gait training (P1.b.c)
- Physical therapy was ordered for the resident involving gait training (T.1.b)
- Resident received nursing rehabilitation for walking (P3.f)
- Physical therapy involving walking has been discontinued within the past 180 days

Skip to item 3 if resident did not walk in last 7 days

(FOR FOLLOWING FIVE ITEMS, BASE CODING ON THE EPISODE WHEN THE RESIDENT WALKED THE FARTHEST WITHOUT SITTING DOWN. INCLUDE WALKING DURING REHABILITATION SESSIONS)

a. Furthest distance walked without sitting down during this episode.

0. 150+ feet	3. 10-25 feet
1. 51-149 feet	4. Less than 10 feet
2. 26-50 feet	

b. Time walked without sitting down during this episode.

0. 1-2 minutes   3. 11-15 minutes
1. 3-4 minutes   4. 16-30 minutes
2. 5-10 minutes   5. 31+ minutes

c. Self-Performance in walking during this episode.

0. *INDEPENDENT*—No help or oversight

1. *SUPERVISION*—Oversight, encouragement or cueing provided

2. *LIMITED ASSISTANCE*—Resident highly involved in walking; received physical help in guided maneuvering of limbs or other nonweight bearing assistance

3. *EXTENSIVE ASSISTANCE*—Resident received weight bearing assistance while walking

d. Walking support provided associated with this episode (code regardless of resident's self-performance classification).

0. No setup or physical help from staff
1. Setup help only
2. One person physical assist
3. Two+ persons physical assist

e. Parallel bars used by resident in association with this episode.

0. No   1. Yes

Medicare			State	

3.	CASE MIX GROUP			

SECTION V. RESIDENT ASSESSMENT PROTOCOL SUMMARY

Resident's Name:	Medical Record No.:

1. Check if RAP is triggered.

2. For each triggered RAP, use the RAP guidelines to identify areas needing further assessment. Document relevant assessment information regarding the resident's status.

   • Describe:
   — Nature of the condition (may include presence or lack of objective data and subjective complaints).
   — Complications and risk factors that affect your decision to proceed to care planning.
   — Factors that must be considered in developing individualized care plan interventions.
   — Need for referrals/further evaluation by appropriate health professionals.

   • Documentation should support your decision-making regarding whether to proceed with a care plan for a triggered RAP and the type(s) of care plan interventions that are appropriate for a particular resident.

   • Documentation may appear anywhere in the clinical record (e.g., progress notes, consults, flowsheets, etc.).

3. Indicate under the Location of RAP Assessment Documentation column where information related to the RAP assessment can be found.

4. For each triggered RAP, indicate whether a new care plan, care plan revision, or continuation of current care plan is necessary to address the problem(s) identified in your assessment. The Care Planning Decision column must be completed within 7 days of completing the RAI (MDS and RAPs).

A. RAP PROBLEM AREA	(a) Check if triggered	Location and Date of RAP Assessment Documentation	(b) Care Planning Decision—check if addressed in care plan
1. DELIRIUM	☐		☐
2. COGNITIVE LOSS	☐		☐
3. VISUAL FUNCTION	☐		☐
4. COMMUNICATION	☐		☐

5. ADL FUNCTIONAL/ REHABILITATION POTENTIAL	☐	☐
6. URINARY INCONTINENCE AND INDWELLING CATHETER	☐	☐
7. PSYCHOSOCIAL WELL-BEING	☐	☐
8. MOOD STATE	☐	☐
9. BEHAVIORAL SYMPTOMS	☐	☐
10. ACTIVITIES	☐	☐
11. FALLS	☐	☐
12. NUTRITIONAL STATUS	☐	☐
13. FEEDING TUBES	☐	☐
14. DEHYDRATION/FLUID MAINTENANCE	☐	☐
15. DENTAL CARE	☐	☐
16. PRESSURE ULCERS	☐	☐
17. PSYCHOTROPIC DRUG USE	☐	☐
18. PHYSICAL RESTRAINTS	☐	☐

B.

1. Signature of RN Coordinator for RAP Assessment Process

2. ☐☐ — ☐☐ — ☐☐☐☐
   Month   Day   Year

3. Signature of Person Completing Care Planning Decision

4. ☐☐ — ☐☐ — ☐☐☐☐
   Month   Day   Year

MDS 2.0 01/30/98

553

RESIDENT ASSESSMENT PROTOCOL TRIGGER LEGEND FOR REVISED RAPS (FOR MDS VERSION 2.0)

Key:
- ● = One item required to trigger
- ❷ = Two items required to trigger
- ✱ = One of these three items, plus at least one other item required to trigger
- @ = When both ADL triggers present, maintenance takes precedence

Proceed to RAP Review once triggered

RAP problem areas (column headers):
Delirium · Cognitive Loss/Dementia · Visual Function · Communication · ADL-Rehabilitation Trigger A @ · ADL-Maintenance Trigger B @ · Urinary Incontinence and Indwelling Catheter · Psychosocial Well-Being · Mood State · Behavioral Symptoms · Activities Trigger A · Activities Trigger B · Falls · Nutritional Status · Feeding Tubes · Dehydration/Fluid Maintenance · Dental Care · Pressure Ulcers · Psychotropic Drug Use · Physical Restraints

Code	MDS ITEM	CODE
B2a	Short term memory	1
B2b	Long term memory	
B4	Decision making	1,2,3
B4	Change in decision making	3
B5a to B5f	Indicators of delirium	2
B6	Change in cognitive status	2
C1	Hearing	1,2,3
C4	Expression by others	1,2,3
C6	Understand others	1,2,3
C7	Change in communication	2
D1	Vision	1,2,3
D2a	Side vision problem	1
E1a to E1p	Indicators of depression, anxiety, sad mood	1,2
E1o	Repetitive movement	1,2
E1o	Withdrawal from activities	1,2
E2	Mood persistency	1,2
E3	Change in Mood	2
E4aA	Wandering	1,2,3
E4aA - E4eA	Behavioral symptoms	1,2,3
E5	Change in behavioral symptoms	1
E5	Change in behavioral symptoms	2

Code	Item			
F1d	Establishes own goals			
F2a to F2d	Unsettled relationships	✓		
F3a	Strong ... past roles	✓		
F3b	Lost roles	✓		
F3c	Deterioration in ...			
G1aA - G1jA	ADL self-performance	1,2,3,4		
G1aA	Bed mobility			●
G2A	Bathing	1,2,3,4		
G5b	Reduce while sitting	✓		●
G6a	Balance			●
G5f	Resident ... ... capable	✓		●
H1a	Bowel incontinence	1,2,3,4		●
H1b	Bladder	✓		
H2b	Constipation	✓		
H2d	Fecal impaction	✓		
H3c,d,e	Catheter use	✓		
H5g	Use of	✓		
I1i	Hypotension	✓		
	Peripheral vascular disease	✓		
I1ee	Depression	✓		
	... ...	✓		
I1l	Glaucoma	✓		
	...	✓		
I3	Dehydration diagnosis	276.5		
J1a	Weight fluctuation	✓		
J1c	Dehydrated	✓		
J1d	Insufficient fluid	✓		
J1f	Dizziness	✓		
	...	✓		
J1i	Hallucinations	✓		
	... ...	✓		
J1k	Lung aspirations	✓		
	... ...	✓		

555

RESIDENT ASSESSMENT PROTOCOL TRIGGER LEGEND FOR REVISED RAPS (FOR MDS VERSION 2.0)

Key:
● = One item required to trigger
❷ = Two items required to trigger
* = One of these three items, plus at least one other item required to trigger
ⓐ = When both ADL triggers present, maintenance takes precedence

Proceed to RAP Review once triggered

MDS ITEM		CODE	Delirium	Cognitive Loss/Dementia	Visual Function	Communication	ADL-Rehabilitation Trigger A ⓐ	ADL-Maintenance Trigger B ⓐ	Urinary Incontinence and Indwelling Catheter	Psychosocial Well-Being	Mood State	Behavioral Symptoms	Activities Trigger A	Activities Trigger B	Falls	Nutritional Status	Feeding Tubes	Dehydration/Fluid Maintenance	Dental Care	Pressure Ulcers	Psychotropic Drug Use	Physical Restraints
J4a,b	Fell	✓												●						●		
J4c	Hip fracture	✓																		●		
K1b	Swallowing problem	✓																		●		
K1c	Mouth pain																			●		
K3a	Weight loss	1													●			●				
K4a	Hunger/dehydration														●							
K4c	Leave 25% food	✓													●	●	●					
K5a	Parenteral/IV feeding														●	●	●					
K5b	Feeding tube	✓													●							
K5c	Mechanically altered	✓													●							
K5d	Syringe feeding	✓													●							
K5e	Therapeutic diet	✓													●							
L1a,c,d,e	Dental	✓													●			●				
M2a	Pressure ulcer	2,3,4																●				
M2d	Pressure ulcer	1,2,3,4																	●			
M3	Previous pressure ulcer	1																	●			
M3c	Impaired tactile sense	✓																	●			
N1a	Awake morning													❷								
N2	Involved in activities	0												❶								

556

N2																						N2
	Involved in activities	2,3						●														N2
05a,b	Makes change in daily routine	1,2		●																		05a,b
04a	Antipsychotics	1,7								*												04a
04b	Antianxiety	1,2								*												04b
04c	Antidepressants	1,7		●		●				*												04c
04d	Diuretic	1,2																				04d
P4c	Trunk restraint	1,2				●		●														P4c
P4c	Hypnotic/sedative	1,2		●				●														P4c
P4d	Limb restraint	1,2							●													P4d
P4e	Chair prevents rising	1,2							●													P4e

Numeric Identifier: _____

MDS QUARTERLY ASSESSMENT FORM

A1.	RESIDENT NAME	a. (First)	b. (Middle Initial)	c. (Last)	d. (Jr/Sr)
A2.	ROOM NUMBER				
A3.	ASSESSMENT REFERENCE DATE	a. Last day of MDS observation period — Month / Day / Year			
		b. Original (0) or corrected copy of form (enter number of correction)			
A4a	DATE OF REENTRY	Date of reentry from most recent temporary discharge to a hospital in last 90 days (or since last assessment or admission if less than 90 days) — Month / Day / Year			
A6.	MEDICAL RECORD NO.				
B1.	COMATOSE	(Persistent vegetative state/no discernible consciousness) 0. No 1. Yes (Skip to Section G)			
B2.	MEMORY	(Recall of what was learned or known) a. Short-term memory OK—seems/appears to recall after 5 minutes 0. Memory OK 1. Memory problem b. Long-term memory OK—seems/appears to recall long past 0. Memory OK 1. Memory problem			
B4.	COGNITIVE SKILLS FOR DAILY DECISION-MAKING	(Made decisions regarding tasks of daily life) 0. INDEPENDENT—decisions consistent/reasonable 1. MODIFIED INDEPENDENCE—some difficulty in new situations only 2. MODERATELY IMPAIRED—decisions poor; cues/supervision required 3. SEVERELY IMPAIRED—never/rarely made decisions			
B5.	INDICATORS OF DELIRIUM—PERIODIC DISORDERED THINKING/AWARENESS	(Code for behavior in the last 7 days.) [Note: Accurate assessment requires conversations with staff and family who have direct knowledge of resident's behavior over this time]. 0. Behavior not present 1. Behavior present, not of recent onset 2. Behavior present, over last 7 days appears different from resident's usual functioning (e.g., new onset or worsening) a. EASILY DISTRACTED—(e.g., difficulty paying attention; gets sidetracked)			

E1.	INDICATORS OF DEPRESSION, ANXIETY, SAD MOOD (cont.)	VERBAL EXPRESSIONS OF DISTRESS	SLEEP-CYCLE ISSUES
		f. Expressions of what appear to be unrealistic fears—e.g., fear of being abandoned, left alone, being with others	j. Unpleasant mood in morning
			k. Insomnia/change in usual sleep pattern
		g. Recurrent statements that something terrible is about to happen—e.g., believes he or she is about to die, have a heart attack	SAD, APATHETIC, ANXIOUS APPEARANCE
			l. Sad, pained, worried facial expressions—e.g., furrowed brows
			m. Crying, tearfulness
		h. Repetitive health complaints—e.g., persistently seeks medical attention, obsessive concern with body functions	n. Repetitive physical movements—e.g., pacing, hand wringing, restlessness, fidgeting, picking
			LOSS OF INTEREST
		i. Repetitive anxious complaints/concerns (non-health related) e.g., persistently seeks attention/reassurance regarding schedules, meals, laundry, clothing, relationship issues	o. Withdrawal from activities of interest—e.g., no interest in long standing activities or being with family/friends
			p. Reduced social interaction
E2.	MOOD PERSISTENCE	One or more indicators of depressed, sad or anxious mood were not easily altered by attempts to "cheer up", console, or reassure the resident over last 7 days 0. No mood indicators 1. Indicators present, easily altered 2. Indicators present, not easily altered	
E4.	BEHAVIORAL SYMPTOMS	(A) Behavioral symptom frequency in last 7 days 0. Behavior not exhibited in last 7 days 1. Behavior of this type occurred 1 to 3 days in last 7 days 2. Behavior of this type occurred 4 to 6 days, but less than daily 3. Behavior of this type occurred daily (B) Behavioral symptom alterability in last 7 days 0. Behavior not present OR behavior was easily altered 1. Behavior was not easily altered	(A) (B)
		a. WANDERING (moved with no rational purpose, seemingly oblivious to needs or safety)	
		b. VERBALLY ABUSIVE BEHAVIORAL SYMPTOMS (others were threatened, screamed at, cursed at)	
		c. PHYSICALLY ABUSIVE BEHAVIORAL SYMPTOMS (others were hit, shoved, scratched, sexually abused)	

558

d. SOCIALLY INAPPROPRIATE/DISRUPTIVE BEHAVIORAL SYMPTOMS (made disruptive sounds, noisiness, screaming, self-abusive acts, sexual behavior or disrobing in public, smeared/threw food/feces, hoarding, rummaged through others' belongings)

e. RESISTS CARE (resisted taking medications/injections, ADL assistance, or eating)

G1. (A) ADL SELF-PERFORMANCE—(Code for resident's *PERFORMANCE OVER ALL SHIFTS during last 7 days—Not including setup*)

0. INDEPENDENT—No help or oversight —OR— Help/oversight provided only 1 or 2 times during last 7 days

1. SUPERVISION—Oversight, encouragement or cueing provided 3 or more times during last 7 days —OR— Supervision (3 or more times) plus physical assistance provided only 1 or 2 times during last 7 days

2. LIMITED ASSISTANCE—Resident highly involved in activity; received physical help in guided maneuvering of limbs or other nonweight bearing assistance 3 or more times —OR—More help provided only 1 or 2 times during last 7 days

3. EXTENSIVE ASSISTANCE—While resident performed part of activity, over last 7-day period, help of following type(s) provided 3 or more times:
 —Weight-bearing support
 —Full staff performance during part (but not all) of last 7 days

4. TOTAL DEPENDENCE—Full staff performance of activity during entire 7 days

8. ACTIVITY DID NOT OCCUR during entire 7 days

(A)

a.	BED MOBILITY	How resident moves to and from lying position, turns side to side, and positions body while in bed
b.	TRANSFER	How resident moves between surfaces—to/from: bed, chair, wheelchair, standing position (EXCLUDE to/from bath/toilet)
c.	WALK IN ROOM	How resident walks between locations in his/her room.
d.	WALK IN CORRIDOR	How resident walks in corridor on unit.
e.	LOCOMOTION ON UNIT	How resident moves between locations in his/her room and adjacent corridor on same floor. If in wheelchair, self-sufficiency once in chair
f.	LOCOMOTION OFF UNIT	How resident moves to and returns from off unit locations (e.g., areas set aside for dining, activities, or treatments). If facility has only one floor, how resident moves to and from distant areas on the floor. If in wheelchair, self-sufficiency once in chair
g.	DRESSING	How resident puts on, fastens, and takes off all items of street clothing, including donning/removing prosthesis
h.	EATING	How resident eats and drinks (regardless of skill). Includes intake of nourishment by other means (e.g., tube feeding, total parenteral nutrition).

MDS 2.0 01/30/98

---

b. PERIODS OF ALTERED PERCEPTION OR AWARENESS OF SURROUNDINGS—(e.g., moves lips or talks to someone not present; believes he/she is somewhere else; confuses night and day)

c. EPISODES OF DISORGANIZED SPEECH—(e.g., speech is incoherent, nonsensical, irrelevant, or rambling from subject to subject; loses train of thought)

d. PERIODS OF RESTLESSNESS—(e.g., fidgeting or picking at skin, clothing, napkins, etc; frequent position changes; repetitive physical movements or calling out)

e. PERIODS OF LETHARGY—(e.g., sluggishness; staring into space; difficult to arouse; little body movement)

f. MENTAL FUNCTION VARIES OVER THE COURSE OF THE DAY—(e.g., sometimes better, sometimes worse; behaviors sometimes present, sometimes not)

C4. MAKING SELF UNDERSTOOD
(Expressing information content—however able)
0. UNDERSTOOD
1. USUALLY UNDERSTOOD—difficulty finding words or finishing thoughts
2. SOMETIMES UNDERSTOOD—ability is limited to making concrete requests
3. RARELY/NEVER UNDERSTOOD

C6. ABILITY TO UNDERSTAND OTHERS
(Understanding verbal information content—however able)
0. UNDERSTANDS
1. USUALLY UNDERSTANDS—may miss some part/intent of message
2. SOMETIMES UNDERSTANDS—responds adequately to simple, direct communication
3. RARELY/NEVER UNDERSTANDS

E1. INDICATORS OF DEPRESSION, ANXIETY, SAD MOOD
(Code for indicators observed in last 30 days, irrespective of the assumed cause)
0. Indicator not exhibited in last 30 days
1. Indicator of this type exhibited up to five days a week
2. Indicator of this type exhibited daily or almost daily (6, 7 days a week)

VERBAL EXPRESSIONS OF DISTRESS

a. Resident made negative statements—e.g., "Nothing matters; Would rather be dead; What's the use; Regrets having lived so long; Let me die"

b. Repetitive questions—e.g., "Where do I go; What do I do?"

c. Repetitive verbalizations—e.g., calling out for help, ("God help me")

d. Persistent anger with self or others—e.g., easily annoyed, anger at placement in nursing home; anger at care received

e. Self deprecation—e.g., "I am nothing; I am of no use to anyone"

J5.	**STABILITY OF CONDITIONS**	Conditions/diseases make resident's cognitive, ADL, mood or behavior status unstable—(fluctuating, precarious, or deteriorating)	a.
		Resident experiencing an acute episode or a flare-up of a recurrent or chronic problem	b.
		End-stage disease, 6 or fewer months to live	c.
		NONE OF ABOVE	d.
K3.	**WEIGHT CHANGE**	a. Weight loss—5 % or more in last 30 days; or 10 % or more in last 180 days 0. No 1. Yes	
		b. Weight gain—5 % or more in last 30 days; or 10 % or more in last 180 days 0. No 1. Yes	
K5.	**NUTRITIONAL APPROACHES**	Feeding tube	b.
		On a planned weight change program	h.
		NONE OF ABOVE	i.
M1.	**ULCERS** (Due to any cause)	*(Record the number of ulcers at each ulcer stage—regardless of cause. If none present at a stage, record "0" (zero). Code all that apply during last 7 days. Code 9 = 9 or more.)* **[Requires full body exam.]**	**Number at Stage**
		a. Stage 1. A persistent area of skin redness (without a break in the skin) that does not disappear when pressure is relieved.	
		b. Stage 2. A partial thickness loss of skin layers that presents clinically as an abrasion, blister, or shallow crater.	
		c. Stage 3. A full thickness of skin is lost, exposing the subcutaneous tissues - presents as a deep crater with or without undermining adjacent tissue.	
		d. Stage 4. A full thickness of skin and subcutaneous tissue is lost, exposing muscle or bone.	
M2.	**TYPE OF ULCER**	*(For each type of ulcer, code for the highest stage in the last 7 days using scale in item M1—i.e., 0=none; stages 1, 2, 3, 4)*	
		a. Pressure ulcer—any lesion caused by pressure resulting in damage of underlying tissue	
		b. Stasis ulcer—open lesion caused by poor circulation in the lower extremities	
N1.	**TIME AWAKE**	*(Check appropriate time periods over last 7 days)* Resident awake all or most of time (i.e., naps no more than one hour per time period) in the:	
		Morning a. ☐ Evening c.	
		Afternoon b. ☐ NONE OF ABOVE d.	
		(If resident is comatose, skip to Section O)	

i.	**TOILET USE**	How resident uses the toilet room (or commode, bedpan, urinal); transfer on/off toilet, cleanses, changes pad, manages ostomy or catheter, adjusts clothes	
j.	**PERSONAL HYGIENE**	How resident maintains personal hygiene, including combing hair, brushing teeth, shaving, applying makeup, washing/drying face, hands, and perineum (EXCLUDE baths and showers)	
G2.	**BATHING**	How resident takes full-body bath/shower, sponge bath, and transfers in/out of tub/shower (EXCLUDE washing of back and hair.) *Code for most dependent in self-performance.* (A) BATHING SELF-PERFORMANCE codes appear below	**(A)**
		0. Independent—No help provided	
		1. Supervision—Oversight help only	
		2. Physical help limited to transfer only	
		3. Physical help in part of bathing activity	
		4. Total dependence	
		8. Activity itself did not occur during entire 7 days	
G4.	**FUNCTIONAL LIMITATION IN RANGE OF MOTION**	*(Code for limitations during last 7 days that interfered with daily functions or placed residents at risk of injury)* (A) RANGE OF MOTION 0. No limitation 1. Limitation on one side 2. Limitation on both sides	(B) VOLUNTARY MOVEMENT 0. No loss 1. Partial loss 2. Full loss
			(A) (B)
		a. Neck	
		b. Arm—Including shoulder or elbow	
		c. Hand—Including wrist or fingers	
		d. Leg—Including hip or knee	
		e. Foot—Including ankle or toes	
		f. Other limitation or loss	
G6.	**MODES OF TRANSFER**	*(Check all that apply during last 7 days)*	
		Bedfast all or most of time a.	
		Bed rails used for bed mobility or transfer b.	
		NONE OF ABOVE f.	
H1.	**CONTINENCE SELF-CONTROL CATEGORIES** *(Code for resident's PERFORMANCE OVER ALL SHIFTS)*	0. CONTINENT—Complete control *[includes use of indwelling urinary catheter or ostomy device that does not leak urine or stool]*	
		1. USUALLY CONTINENT—BLADDER, incontinent episodes once a week or less; BOWEL, less than weekly	
		2. OCCASIONALLY INCONTINENT—BLADDER, 2 or more times a week but not daily; BOWEL, once a week	

	3.	**FREQUENTLY INCONTINENT**—BLADDER, tended to be incontinent daily, but some control present (e.g., on day shift); BOWEL, 2-3 times a week
	4.	**INCONTINENT**—Had inadequate control BLADDER, multiple daily episodes; BOWEL, all (or almost all) of the time
H2.	BOWEL CONTINENCE	
a.		Control of bowel movement, with appliance or bowel continence programs, if employed
b.	BLADDER CONTINENCE	Control of urinary bladder function, if dribbles, volume insufficient to soak through underpants), with appliances (e.g., foley) or continence programs, if employed
H2.	BOWEL ELIMINATION PATTERN	Fecal impaction d. NONE OF ABOVE e.
H3.	APPLIANCES AND PROGRAMS	Any scheduled toileting plan a. Indwelling catheter d. Bladder retraining program b. Ostomy present i. External (condom) catheter c. NONE OF ABOVE j.
I2.	INFECTIONS	Urinary tract infection in last 30 days m. NONE OF ABOVE
I3.	OTHER CURRENT DIAGNOSES AND ICD-9 CODES	*(Include only those diseases diagnosed in the last 90 days that have a relationship to current ADL status, cognitive status, mood or behavior status, medical treatments, nursing monitoring, or risk of death)* a. ___ . ___ b. ___ . ___
J1.	PROBLEM CONDITIONS	*(Check all problems present in last 7 days)* Dehydrated; output exceeds input a. Hallucinations c. NONE OF ABOVE i. / p.
J2.	PAIN SYMPTOMS	*(Code the highest level of pain present in the last 7 days)* **a. FREQUENCY** with which resident complains or shows evidence of pain 0. No pain *(skip to J4)* 1. Pain less than daily 2. Pain daily **b. INTENSITY of pain** 1. Mild pain 2. Moderate pain 3. Times when pain is horrible or excruciating
J4.	ACCIDENTS	*(Check all that apply)* Fell in past 30 days a. Hip fracture in last 180 days c. Fell in past 31-180 days b. Other fracture in last 180 days d. NONE OF ABOVE e.

MDS 2.0 01/30/98

N2.	AVERAGE TIME INVOLVED IN ACTIVITIES	(When awake and not receiving treatments or ADL care) 0. Most—more than 2/3 of time 2. Little—less than 1/3 of time 1. Some—from 1/3 to 2/3 of time 3. None
O1.	NUMBER OF MEDICATIONS	*(Record the number of different medications used in the last 7 days; enter "0" if none used)*
O4.	DAYS RECEIVED THE FOLLOWING MEDICATION	*(Record the number of DAYS during last 7 days; enter "0" if not used. Note—enter "1" for long-acting meds used less than weekly)* a. Antipsychotic d. Hypnotic b. Antianxiety e. Diuretic c. Antidepressant
P4.	DEVICES AND RESTRAINTS	Use the following codes for last 7 days: 0. Not used 1. Used less than daily 2. Used daily Bed rails a. — Full bed rails on all open sides of bed b. — Other types of side rails used (e.g., half rail, one side) c. Trunk restraint d. Limb restraint e. Chair prevents rising
Q2.	OVERALL CHANGE IN CARE NEEDS	Resident's overall level of self sufficiency has changed significantly as compared to status of 90 days ago (or since last assessment if less than 90 days) 0. No change 1. Improved—receives fewer 2. Deteriorated—receives supports, needs less more support restrictive level of care
R2.	SIGNATURES OF PERSONS COMPLETING THE ASSESSMENT:	
	a. Signature of RN Assessment Coordinator (sign on above line)	
	b. Date RN Assessment Coordinator signed as complete	Month Day Year
	c. Other Signatures Title Sections Date	
	d. Date	
	e. Date	
	f. Date	
	g. Date	

Numeric Identifier _____

MDS QUARTERLY ASSESSMENT FORM
(OPTIONAL VERSION FOR RUG III)

A1.	RESIDENT NAME	a. (First)	b. (Middle Initial)	c. (Last)	d. (Jr/Sr)
A2.	ROOM NUMBER				
A3.	ASSESSMENT REFERENCE DATE	a. Last day of MDS observation period Month — Day — Year b. Original (0) or corrected copy of form (enter number of correction)			
A4.	DATE OF REENTRY	Date of reentry from most recent temporary discharge to a hospital in last 90 days (or since last assessment or admission if less than 90 days) Month — Day — Year			
A6.	MEDICAL RECORD NO.				
B1.	COMATOSE	(Persistent vegetative state/no discernible consciousness) 0. No 1. Yes (Skip to Section G)			

B2.	MEMORY	(Recall of what was learned or known)
		a. Short-term memory OK—seems/appears to recall after 5 minutes
		  0. Memory OK 1. Memory problem
		b. Long-term memory OK—seems/appears to recall long past
		  0. Memory OK 1. Memory problem			

B3.	MEMORY/ RECALL ABILITY	(Check all that resident was normally able to recall during last 7 days) Current season — a. Location of own room — b. Staff names/faces — c. That he/she is in a nursing home — d. NONE OF ABOVE are recalled — e.			
B4.	COGNITIVE SKILLS FOR DAILY DECISION-MAKING	(Made decisions regarding tasks of daily life) 0. INDEPENDENT—decisions consistent/reasonable 1. MODIFIED INDEPENDENCE—some difficulty in new situations only 2. MODERATELY IMPAIRED—decisions poor; cues/supervision required 3. SEVERELY IMPAIRED—never/rarely made decisions			

E1.	INDICATORS OF DEPRESSION, ANXIETY, SAD MOOD	**VERBAL EXPRESSIONS OF DISTRESS** a. Resident made negative statements—e.g., *"Nothing matters; Would rather be dead; What's the use; Regrets having lived so long; Let me die"* b. Repetitive questions—e.g., *"Where do I go; What do I do?"* c. Repetitive verbalizations—e.g., calling out for help, (*"God help me"*) d. Persistent anger with self or others—e.g., easily annoyed, anger at placement in nursing home; anger at care received e. Self deprecation—e.g., *"I am nothing; I am of no use to anyone"* f. Expressions of what appear to be unrealistic fears—e.g., fear of being abandoned, left alone, being with others g. Recurrent statements that something terrible is about to happen—e.g., believes he or she is about to die, have a heart attack	**h.** Repetitive health complaints—e.g., persistently seeks medical attention, obsessive concern with body functions **i.** Repetitive anxious complaints/concerns (non-health related) e.g., persistently seeks attention/ reassurance regarding schedules, meals, laundry, clothing, relationship issues **SLEEP-CYCLE ISSUES** **j.** Unpleasant mood in morning **k.** Insomnia/change in usual sleep pattern **SAD, APATHETIC, ANXIOUS APPEARANCE** **l.** Sad, pained, worried facial expressions—e.g., furrowed brows **m.** Crying, tearfulness **REPETITIVE PHYSICAL MOVEMENTS** **n.** Repetitive physical movements—e.g., pacing, hand wringing, restlessness, fidgeting, picking **LOSS OF INTEREST** **o.** Withdrawal from activities of interest—e.g., no interest in long standing activities or being with family/friends **p.** Reduced social interaction
E2.	MOOD PERSISTENCE	One or more indicators of depressed, sad or anxious mood were not easily altered by attempts to "cheer up", console, or reassure the resident over last 7 days 0. No mood 1. Indicators present, 2. Indicators present, indicators easily altered not easily altered	
E4.	BEHAVIORAL SYMPTOMS	(A) *Behavioral symptom frequency in last 7 days* 0. Behavior not exhibited in last 7 days 1. Behavior of this type occurred 1 to 3 days in last 7 days 2. Behavior of this type occurred 4 to 6 days, but less than daily 3. Behavior of this type occurred daily	

(B) Behavioral symptom alterability in last 7 days
0. Behavior not present OR behavior was easily altered
1. Behavior was not easily altered

	(A)	(B)
a. WANDERING (moved with no rational purpose, seemingly oblivious to needs or safety)		
b. VERBALLY ABUSIVE BEHAVIORAL SYMPTOMS (others were threatened, screamed at, cursed at)		
c. PHYSICALLY ABUSIVE BEHAVIORAL SYMPTOMS (others were hit, shoved, scratched, sexually abused)		
d. SOCIALLY INAPPROPRIATE/DISRUPTIVE BEHAVIORAL SYMPTOMS (made disruptive sounds, noisiness, screaming, self-abusive acts, sexual behavior or disrobing in public, smeared/threw food/feces, hoarding, rummaged through others' belongings)		
e. RESISTS CARE (resisted taking medications/injections, ADL assistance, or eating)		

G1. (A) ADL SELF-PERFORMANCE—*(Code for resident's PERFORMANCE OVER ALL SHIFTS during last 7 days—Not including setup)*

0. INDEPENDENT—No help or oversight —OR— Help/oversight provided only 1 or 2 times during last 7 days

1. SUPERVISION—Oversight, encouragement or cueing provided 3 or more times during last 7 days —OR— Supervision (3 or more times) plus physical assistance provided only 1 or 2 times during last 7 days

2. LIMITED ASSISTANCE—Resident highly involved in activity; received physical help in guided maneuvering of limbs or other nonweight bearing assistance 3 or more times —OR—More help provided only 1 or 2 times during last 7 days

3. EXTENSIVE ASSISTANCE—While resident performed part of activity, over last 7-day period, help of following type(s) provided 3 or more times:
— Weight-bearing support
— Full staff performance during part (but not all) of last 7 days

4. TOTAL DEPENDENCE—Full staff performance of activity during entire 7 days

8. ACTIVITY DID NOT OCCUR during entire 7 days

(B) ADL SUPPORT PROVIDED—*(Code for MOST SUPPORT PROVIDED OVER ALL SHIFTS during last 7 days; code regardless of resident's self-performance classification)*

0. No setup or physical help from staff
1. Setup help only
2. One person physical assist
3. Two+ persons physical assist

8. ADL activity itself did not occur during entire 7 days

		(A) SELF-PERF	(B) SUPPORT
a.	BED MOBILITY	How resident moves to and from lying position, turns side to side, and positions body while in bed	
b.	TRANSFER	How resident moves between surfaces—to/from: bed, chair, wheelchair, standing position (EXCLUDE to/from bath/toilet)	

MDS 2.0 01/30/98

B5.	INDICATORS OF DELIRIUM— PERIODIC DISORDERED THINKING/ AWARENESS	*(Code for behavior in the last 7 days.) [Note: Accurate assessment requires conversations with staff and family who have direct knowledge of resident's behavior over this time].*

0. Behavior not present
1. Behavior present, not of recent onset
2. Behavior present, over last 7 days appears different from resident's usual functioning (e.g., new onset or worsening)

a. EASILY DISTRACTED—(e.g., difficulty paying attention; gets sidetracked)
b. PERIODS OF ALTERED PERCEPTION OR AWARENESS OF SURROUNDINGS—(e.g., moves lips or talks to someone not present; believes he/she is somewhere else; confuses night and day)
c. EPISODES OF DISORGANIZED SPEECH—(e.g., speech is incoherent, nonsensical, irrelevant, or rambling from subject to subject; loses train of thought)
d. PERIODS OF RESTLESSNESS—(e.g., fidgeting or picking at skin, clothing, napkins, etc; frequent position changes; repetitive physical movements or calling out)
e. PERIODS OF LETHARGY—(e.g., sluggishness; staring into space; difficult to arouse; little body movement)
f. MENTAL FUNCTION VARIES OVER THE COURSE OF THE DAY—(e.g., sometimes better, sometimes worse; behaviors sometimes present, sometimes not)

C4.	MAKING SELF UNDERSTOOD	*(Expressing information content—however able)*

0. UNDERSTOOD
1. USUALLY UNDERSTOOD—difficulty finding words or finishing thoughts
2. SOMETIMES UNDERSTOOD—ability is limited to making concrete requests
3. RARELY/NEVER UNDERSTOOD

C6.	ABILITY TO UNDER- STAND OTHERS	*(Understanding verbal information content—however able)*

0. UNDERSTANDS
1. USUALLY UNDERSTANDS—may miss some part/intent of message
2. SOMETIMES UNDERSTANDS—responds adequately to simple, direct communication
3. RARELY/NEVER UNDERSTANDS

E1.	INDICATORS OF DEPRES- SION, ANXIETY, SAD MOOD	*(Code for indicators observed in last 30 days, irrespective of the assumed cause)*

0. Indicator not exhibited in last 30 days
1. Indicator of this type exhibited up to five days a week
2. Indicator of this type exhibited daily or almost daily (6, 7 days a week)

563

Resident ______________________

G1.			(A)	(B)
c.	WALK IN ROOM	How resident walks between locations in his/her room		
d.	WALK IN CORRIDOR	How resident walks in corridor on unit		
e.	LOCOMOTION ON UNIT	How resident moves between locations in his/her room and adjacent corridor on same floor. If in wheelchair, self-sufficiency once in chair		
f.	LOCOMOTION OFF UNIT	How resident moves to and returns from off unit locations (e.g., areas set aside for dining, activities, or treatments). **If facility has only one floor,** how resident moves to and from distant areas on the floor. If in wheelchair, self-sufficiency once in chair		
g.	DRESSING	How resident puts on, fastens, and takes off all items of **street clothing**, including donning/removing prosthesis		
h.	EATING	How resident eats and drinks (regardless of skill). Includes intake of nourishment by other means (e.g., tube feeding, total parenteral nutrition)		
i.	TOILET USE	How resident uses the toilet room (or commode, bedpan, urinal); transfer on/off toilet, cleanses, changes pad, manages ostomy or catheter, adjusts clothes		
j.	PERSONAL HYGIENE	How resident maintains personal hygiene, including combing hair, brushing teeth, shaving, applying makeup, washing/drying face, hands, and perineum (EXCLUDE baths and showers)		

G2.	BATHING	How resident takes full-body bath/shower, sponge bath, and transfers in/out of tub/shower (EXCLUDE washing of back and hair.) ***Code for most dependent** in self-performance.* (A) BATHING SELF PERFORMANCE codes appear below	(A)
		0. Independent—No help provided	
		1. Supervision—Oversight help only	
		2. Physical help limited to transfer only	
		3. Physical help in part of bathing activity	
		4. Total dependence	
		8. Activity itself did not occur during entire 7 days	
G3.	TEST FOR BALANCE (see training manual)	(*Code for ability during test in the **last 7 days***) 0. Maintained position as required in test 1. Unsteady, but able to rebalance self without physical support 2. Partial physical support during test; or stands (sits) but does not follow directions for test 3. Not able to attempt test without physical help	
		a. Balance while standing	
		b. Balance while sitting—position, trunk control	

Numeric Identifier ______________________

H3.	APPLIANCES AND PROGRAMS	Any scheduled toileting plan	a.	Indwelling catheter	d.
		Bladder retraining program	b.	Ostomy present	i.
		External (condom) catheter	c.	*NONE OF ABOVE*	j.

Check only those diseases that have a relationship to current ADL status, cognitive status, mood and behavior status, medical treatments, nursing monitoring, or risk of death. (Do not list inactive diagnoses)

I1.	DISEASES	*(If none apply, CHECK the NONE OF ABOVE box)*			
		MUSCULOSKELETAL		Multiple sclerosis	w.
		Hip fracture	m.	Quadriplegia	z.
		NEUROLOGICAL		**PSYCHIATRIC/MOOD**	
		Aphasia	r.	Depression	ee.
		Cerebral palsy	s.	Manic depressive (bipolar disease)	ff.
		Cerebrovascular accident (stroke)	t.	**OTHER**	
		Hemiplegia/Hemiparesis	v.	*NONE OF ABOVE*	rr.
I2.	INFECTIONS	*(If none apply, CHECK the NONE OF ABOVE box)*			
		Antibiotic resistant infection (e.g., Methicillin resistant staph)	a.	Septicemia	g.
				Sexually transmitted diseases	h.
		Clostridium difficile (c. diff.)	b.	Tuberculosis	i.
		Conjunctivitis	c.	Urinary tract infection **in last 30 days**	j.
		HIV infection	d.	Viral hepatitis	k.
		Pneumonia	e.	Wound infection	l.
		Respiratory infection	f.	NONE OF ABOVE	m.
I3.	OTHER CURRENT DIAGNOSES AND ICD-9 CODES	(*Include **only those diseases diagnosed in the last 90 days that have a relationship** to current ADL status, cognitive status, mood or behavior status, medical treatments, nursing monitoring, or risk of death*)			
		a. ______________		| | | |•| |	
		b. ______________		| | | |•| |	
J1.	PROBLEM CONDITIONS	(***Check all problems present** in **last 7 days** unless other time frame is indicated*)			
		INDICATORS OF FLUID STATUS		**OTHER**	
				Delusions	e.
		Weight gain or loss of 3 or more pounds within a 7 day period	a.	Edema	g.
				Fever	h.
				Hallucinations	i.

G4.	FUNCTIONAL LIMITATION IN RANGE OF MOTION	(Code for limitations during last 7 days that interfered with daily functions or placed residents at risk of injury)		
		(A) RANGE OF MOTION	(A)	(B)
		0. No limitation		
		1. Limitation on one side		
		2. Limitation on both sides		
		a. Neck		
		b. Arm—Including shoulder or elbow		
		c. Hand—Including wrist or fingers		
		d. Leg—Including hip or knee		
		e. Foot—Including ankle or toes		
		f. Other limitation or loss		
G6.	MODES OF TRANSFER	(Check all that apply during last 7 days)		
		Bedfast all or most of time	a.	
		Bed rails used for bed mobility or transfer	b.	
		NONE OF ABOVE	f.	
G7.	TASK SEGMENTA-TION	Some or all of ADL activities were broken into subtasks during last 7 days so that resident could perform them 0. No 1. Yes		

H1.	CONTINENCE SELF-CONTROL CATEGORIES (Code for resident's PERFORMANCE OVER ALL SHIFTS)	
	0. CONTINENT—Complete control [includes use of indwelling urinary catheter or ostomy device that does not leak urine or stool]	
	1. USUALLY CONTINENT—BLADDER, incontinent episodes once a week or less; BOWEL, less than weekly	
	2. OCCASIONALLY INCONTINENT—BLADDER, 2 or more times a week but not daily; BOWEL, once a week	
	3. FREQUENTLY INCONTINENT—BLADDER, tended to be incontinent daily, but some control present (e.g., on day shift); BOWEL, 2-3 times a week	
	4. INCONTINENT—Had inadequate control BLADDER, multiple daily episodes; BOWEL, all (or almost all) of the time	
a.	BOWEL CONTI-NENCE	Control of bowel movement, with appliance or bowel continence programs, if employed
b.	BLADDER CONTI-NENCE	Control of urinary bladder function (if dribbles, volume insufficient to soak through underpants), with appliances (e.g., foley) or continence programs, if employed
H2.	BOWEL ELIMINATION PATTERN	Diarrhea	c.	NONE OF ABOVE	e.
		Fecal impaction	d.		

		Inability to lie flat due to shortness of breath	b.	Internal bleeding	j.
		Dehydrated; output exceeds input	c.	Recurrent lung aspirations in last 90 days	k.
		Insufficient fluid; did NOT consume all/almost all liquids provided during last 3 days	d.	Shortness of breath	l.
				Unsteady gait	n.
				Vomiting	o.
				NONE OF ABOVE	p.

J2.	PAIN SYMPTOMS	(Code the highest level of pain present in the last 7 days)			
		a. FREQUENCY with which resident complains or shows evidence of pain		b. INTENSITY of pain	
		0. No pain (skip to J4)		1. Mild pain	
		1. Pain less than daily		2. Moderate pain	
		2. Pain daily		3. Times when pain is horrible or excruciating	
J4.	ACCIDENTS	(Check all that apply)			
		Fell in past 30 days	a.	Hip fracture in last 180 days	c.
		Fell in past 31-180 days	b.	Other fracture in last 180 days	d.
				NONE OF ABOVE	e.
J5.	STABILITY OF CONDITIONS	Conditions/diseases make resident's cognitive, ADL, mood or behavior status unstable—(fluctuating, precarious, or deteriorating)			a.
		Resident experiencing an acute episode or a flare-up of a recurrent or chronic problem				b.
		End-stage disease, 6 or fewer months to live				c.
		NONE OF ABOVE				d.
K1.	ORAL PROBLEMS	Chewing problem			a.
		Swallowing problem				b.
		NONE OF ABOVE				d.

K2.	HEIGHT AND WEIGHT	Record (a.) height in inches and (b.) weight in pounds. Base weight on most recent measure in last 30 days; measure weight consistently in accord with standard facility practice—e.g., in a.m. after voiding, before meal, with shoes off, and in nightclothes	a. HT (in.)	b. WT (lb.)

K3.	WEIGHT CHANGE	a. Weight loss—5 % or more in last 30 days; or 10 % or more in last 180 days 0. No 1. Yes
		b. Weight gain—5 % or more in last 30 days; or 10 % or more in last 180 days 0. No 1. Yes

MDS 2.0 01/30/98

565

Resident ____

Numeric Identifier ____

K5.	NUTRITIONAL APPROACHES	(Check all that apply in last 7 days)	
		Parenteral/IV	a. On a planned weight change program
		Feeding tube	b. NONE OF ABOVE

M1.	ULCERS (Due to any cause)	(Record the number of ulcers at each ulcer stage—regardless of cause. If none present at a stage, record "0" (zero). Code all that apply during last 7 days. Code 9 = 9 or more.) [Requires full body exam.]	Number at Stage
		a. Stage 1. A persistent area of skin redness (without a break in the skin) that does not disappear when pressure is relieved.	
		b. Stage 2. A partial thickness loss of skin layers that presents clinically as an abrasion, blister, or shallow crater.	
		c. Stage 3. A full thickness of skin is lost, exposing the subcutaneous tissues - presents as a deep crater with or without undermining adjacent tissue.	
		d. Stage 4. A full thickness of skin and subcutaneous tissue is lost, exposing muscle or bone.	

M2.	TYPE OF ULCER	(For each type of ulcer, code for the highest stage in the last 7 days using scale in item M1—i.e., stages 1, 2, 3, 4) 0=none;	
		a. Pressure ulcer—any lesion caused by pressure resulting in damage of underlying tissue	
		b. Stasis ulcer—open lesion caused by poor circulation in the lower extremities	

M4.	OTHER SKIN PROBLEMS OR LESIONS PRESENT	(Check all that apply during last 7 days)	
		Abrasions, bruises	a.
		Burns (second or third degree)	b.
		Open lesions other than ulcers, rashes, cuts (e.g., cancer lesions)	c.
		Rashes—e.g., intertrigo, eczema, drug rash, heat rash, herpes zoster	d.
		Skin desensitized to pain or pressure	e.
		Skin tears or cuts (other than surgery)	f.
		Surgical wounds	g.
		NONE OF ABOVE	h.

M5.	SKIN TREATMENTS	(Check all that apply during last 7 days)	
		Pressure relieving device(s) for chair	a.
		Pressure relieving device(s) for bed	b.
		Turning/repositioning program	c.
		Nutrition or hydration intervention to manage skin problems	d.
		Ulcer care	e.
		Surgical wound care	f.

P1.	SPECIAL TREATMENTS, PROCEDURES, AND PROGRAMS	a. SPECIAL CARE—Check treatments or programs received during the last 14 days		
		TREATMENTS		PROGRAMS
		Chemotherapy	a.	Ventilator or respirator	l.
		Dialysis	b.	Alcohol/drug treatment program	m.
		IV medication	c.	Alzheimer's/dementia special care unit	n.
		Intake/output	d.	Hospice care	o.
		Monitoring acute medical condition	e.	Pediatric unit	p.
		Ostomy care	f.	Respite care	q.
		Oxygen therapy	g.	Training in skills required to return to the community (e.g., taking medications, house work, shopping, transportation, ADLs)	
		Radiation	h.		
		Suctioning	i.		r.
		Tracheostomy care	j.		
		Transfusions	k.	NONE OF ABOVE	s.

b. THERAPIES - Record the number of days and total minutes each of the following therapies was administered (for at least 15 minutes a day) in the last 7 calendar days (Enter 0 if none or less than 15 min. daily)

[Note—count only post admission therapies]

(A) = # of days administered for 15 minutes or more

(B) = total # of minutes provided in last 7 days

	DAYS (A)	MIN (B)
a. Speech - language pathology and audiology services		
b. Occupational therapy		
c. Physical therapy		
d. Respiratory therapy		
e. Psychological therapy (by any licensed mental health professional)		

P3.	NURSING REHABILITATION/ RESTORATIVE CARE	Record the NUMBER OF DAYS each of the following rehabilitation or restorative techniques or practices was provided to the resident for more than or equal to 15 minutes per day in the last 7 days (Enter 0 if none or less than 15 min. daily)			
		a. Range of motion (passive)		f. Walking	
		b. Range of motion (active)		g. Dressing or grooming	
		c. Splint or brace assistance		h. Eating or swallowing	
		TRAINING AND SKILL PRACTICE IN:		i. Amputation/prosthesis care	
		d. Bed mobility		j. Communication	
		e. Transfer		k. Other	

	Surgical wound care	f.
	Application of dressings (with or without topical medications) other than to feet	g.
	Application of ointments/medications (other than to feet)	h.
	Other preventative or protective skin care (other than to feet)	i.
	NONE OF ABOVE	j.
M6. FOOT PROBLEMS AND CARE	*(Check all that apply during last 7 days)*	
	Resident has one or more foot problems—e.g., corns, calluses, bunions, hammer toes, overlapping toes, pain, structural problems	a.
	Infection of the foot—e.g., cellulitis, purulent drainage	b.
	Open lesions on the foot	c.
	Nails/calluses trimmed during last 90 days	d.
	Received preventative or protective foot care (e.g., used special shoes, inserts, pads, toe separators)	e.
	Application of dressings (with or without topical medications)	f.
	NONE OF ABOVE	g.

N1. TIME AWAKE	*(Check appropriate time periods over last 7 days)* Resident awake all or most of time (i.e., naps no more than one hour per time period) in the:		
	Morning	a.	Evening	c.
	Afternoon	b.	NONE OF ABOVE	d.

(If resident is comatose, skip to Section O)

N2. AVERAGE TIME INVOLVED IN ACTIVITIES	*(When awake and not receiving treatments or ADL care)* 0. Most—more than 2/3 of time 2. Little—less than 1/3 of time 1. Some—from 1/3 to 2/3 of time 3. None	
O1. NUMBER OF MEDICATIONS	*(Record the number of different medications used in the last 7 days; enter "0" if none used)*	
O3. INJECTIONS	*(Record the number of DAYS injections of any type received during the last 7 days; enter "0" if none used)*	

O4. DAYS RECEIVED THE FOLLOWING MEDICATION	*(Record the number of DAYS during last 7 days; enter "0" if not used. Note—enter "1" for long-acting meds used less than weekly)*		
	a. Antipsychotic	d. Hypnotic	
	b. Antianxiety	e. Diuretic	
	c. Antidepressant		

MDS 2.0 01/30/98

P4. DEVICES AND RESTRAINTS	*Use the following codes for last 7 days:* 0. Not used 1. Used less than daily 2. Used daily	
	Bed rails	
	a. — Full bed rails on all open sides of bed	
	b. — Other types of side rails used (e.g., half rail, one side)	
	c. Trunk restraint	
	d. Limb restraint	
	e. Chair prevents rising	
P7. PHYSICIAN VISITS	In the LAST 14 DAYS (or since admission if less than 14 days in facility) how many days has the physician (or authorized assistant or practitioner) examined the resident? *(Enter 0 if none)*	
P8. PHYSICIAN ORDERS	In the LAST 14 DAYS (or since admission if less than 14 days in facility) how many days has the physician (or authorized assistant or practitioner) changed the resident's orders? *Do not include order renewals without change. (Enter 0 if none)*	
Q2. OVERALL CHANGE IN CARE NEEDS	Resident's overall level of self sufficiency has changed significantly as compared to status of 90 days ago (or since last assessment if less than 90 days) 0. No change 1. Improved—receives fewer 2. Deteriorated—receives supports, needs less more support restrictive level of care	

R2. SIGNATURES OF PERSONS COMPLETING THE ASSESSMENT:

a. Signature of RN Assessment Coordinator (sign on above line)

b. Date RN Assessment Coordinator signed as complete

	Month	Day	Year

c. Other Signatures	Title	Sections	Date
d.			Date
e.			Date
f.			Date
g.			Date
h.			Date

MDS QUARTERLY ASSESSMENT FORM
(OPTIONAL VERSION FOR RUG-III 1997 Update)

A1.	**RESIDENT NAME**	a. (First) b. (Middle Initial) c. (Last) d. (Jr/Sr)
A2.	**ROOM NUMBER**	
A3.	**ASSESSMENT REFERENCE DATE**	a. Last day of MDS observation period Month — Day — Year b. Original (0) or corrected copy of form (enter number of correction)
A4a.	**DATE OF REENTRY**	Date of reentry from most recent temporary discharge to a hospital in last 90 days (or since last assessment or admission if less than 90 days) Month — Day — Year
A6.	**MEDICAL RECORD NO.**	
B1.	**COMATOSE**	(Persistent vegetative state/no discernible consciousness) 0. No 1. Yes (Skip to Section G)
B2.	**MEMORY**	(Recall of what was learned or known) a. Short-term memory OK—seems/appears to recall after 5 minutes 0. Memory OK 1. Memory problem b. Long-term memory OK—seems/appears to recall long past 0. Memory OK 1. Memory problem
B3.	**MEMORY/ RECALL ABILITY**	(Check all that resident was normally able to recall during last 7 days) Current season [a] Location of own room [b] That he/she is in a nursing home [d] Staff names/faces [c] NONE OF ABOVE are recalled [e]
B4.	**COGNITIVE SKILLS FOR DAILY DECISION-MAKING**	(Made decisions regarding tasks of daily life) 0. INDEPENDENT—decisions consistent/reasonable 1. MODIFIED INDEPENDENCE—some difficulty in new situations only 2. MODERATELY IMPAIRED—decisions poor; cues/supervision required 3. SEVERELY IMPAIRED—never/rarely made decisions

E1.	**INDICATORS OF DEPRESSION, ANXIETY, SAD MOOD**	**VERBAL EXPRESSIONS OF DISTRESS** a. Resident made negative statements—e.g., "Nothing matters; Would rather be dead; What's the use; Regrets having lived so long; Let me die" b. Repetitive questions—e.g., "Where do I go; What do I do?" c. Repetitive verbalizations—e.g., calling out for help, ("God help me") d. Persistent anger with self or others—e.g., easily annoyed, anger at placement in nursing home; anger at care received e. Self deprecation—e.g., "I am nothing; I am of no use to anyone" f. Expressions of what appear to be unrealistic fears—e.g., fear of being abandoned, left alone, being with others g. Recurrent statements that something terrible is about to happen—e.g., believes he or she is about to die, have a heart attack	h. Repetitive health complaints—e.g., persistently seeks medical attention, obsessive concern with body functions i. Repetitive anxious complaints/concerns (non-health related) e.g., persistently seeks attention/reassurance regarding schedules, meals, laundry, clothing, relationship issues **SLEEP-CYCLE ISSUES** j. Unpleasant mood in morning k. Insomnia/change in usual sleep pattern **SAD, APATHETIC, ANXIOUS APPEARANCE** l. Sad, pained, worried facial expressions—e.g., furrowed brows m. Crying, tearfulness n. Repetitive physical movements—e.g., pacing, hand wringing, restlessness, fidgeting, picking **LOSS OF INTEREST** o. Withdrawal from activities of interest—e.g., no interest in long standing activities or being with family/friends p. Reduced social interaction
E2.	**MOOD PERSISTENCE**	One or more indicators of depressed, sad or anxious mood were not easily altered by attempts to "cheer up", console, or reassure the resident over last 7 days 0. No mood 1. Indicators present, 2. Indicators present, indicators easily altered not easily altered	
E4.	**BEHAVIORAL SYMPTOMS**	(A) *Behavioral symptom frequency in last 7 days* 0. Behavior not exhibited in last 7 days 1. Behavior of this type occurred 1 to 3 days in last 7 days 2. Behavior of this type occurred 4 to 6 days, but less than daily 3. Behavior of this type occurred daily	

B5. INDICATORS OF DELIRIUM—PERIODIC DISORDERED THINKING/AWARENESS

(Code for behavior in the last 7 days.) [Note: Accurate assessment requires conversations with staff and family who have direct knowledge of resident's behavior over this time].

0. Behavior not present
1. Behavior present, not of recent onset
2. Behavior present, over last 7 days appears different from resident's usual functioning (e.g., new onset or worsening)

a. EASILY DISTRACTED—(e.g., difficulty paying attention; gets sidetracked)

b. PERIODS OF ALTERED PERCEPTION OR AWARENESS OF SURROUNDINGS—(e.g., moves lips or talks to someone not present; believes he/she is somewhere else; confuses night and day)

c. EPISODES OF DISORGANIZED SPEECH—(e.g., speech is incoherent, nonsensical, irrelevant, or rambling from subject to subject; loses train of thought)

d. PERIODS OF RESTLESSNESS—(e.g., fidgeting or picking at skin, clothing, napkins, etc; frequent position changes; repetitive physical movements or calling out)

e. PERIODS OF LETHARGY—(e.g., sluggishness; staring into space; difficult to arouse; little body movement)

f. MENTAL FUNCTION VARIES OVER THE COURSE OF THE DAY—(e.g., sometimes better, sometimes worse; behaviors sometimes present, sometimes not)

C4. MAKING SELF UNDERSTOOD

(Expressing information content—however able)

0. UNDERSTOOD
1. USUALLY UNDERSTOOD—difficulty finding words or finishing thoughts
2. SOMETIMES UNDERSTOOD—ability is limited to making concrete requests
3. RARELY/NEVER UNDERSTOOD

C6. ABILITY TO UNDERSTAND OTHERS

(Understanding verbal information content—however able)

0. UNDERSTANDS
1. USUALLY UNDERSTANDS—may miss some part/intent of message
2. SOMETIMES UNDERSTANDS—responds adequately to simple, direct communication
3. RARELY/NEVER UNDERSTANDS

E1. INDICATORS OF DEPRESSION, ANXIETY, SAD MOOD

(Code for indicators observed in last 30 days, irrespective of the assumed cause)

0. Indicator not exhibited in last 30 days
1. Indicator of this type exhibited up to five days a week
2. Indicator of this type exhibited daily or almost daily (6, 7 days a week)

(B) Behavioral symptom alterability in last 7 days

0. Behavior not present OR behavior was easily altered
1. Behavior was not easily altered

	(A)	(B)
a. WANDERING (moved with no rational purpose, seemingly oblivious to needs or safety)		
b. VERBALLY ABUSIVE BEHAVIORAL SYMPTOMS (others were threatened, screamed at, cursed at)		
c. PHYSICALLY ABUSIVE BEHAVIORAL SYMPTOMS (others were hit, shoved, scratched, sexually abused)		
d. SOCIALLY INAPPROPRIATE/DISRUPTIVE BEHAVIORAL SYMPTOMS (made disruptive sounds, noisiness, screaming, self-abusive acts, sexual behavior or disrobing in public, smeared/threw food/feces, hoarding, rummaged through others' belongings)		
e. RESISTS CARE (resisted taking medications/ injections, ADL assistance, or eating)		

G1. (A) ADL SELF-PERFORMANCE—(Code for resident's PERFORMANCE OVER ALL SHIFTS during last 7 days—Not including setup)

0. INDEPENDENT—No help or oversight —OR— Help/oversight provided only 1 or 2 times during last 7 days

1. SUPERVISION—Oversight, encouragement or cueing provided 3 or more times during last 7 days —OR— Supervision (3 or more times) plus physical assistance provided only 1 or 2 times during last 7 days

2. LIMITED ASSISTANCE—Resident highly involved in activity; received physical help in guided maneuvering of limbs or other nonweight bearing assistance 3 or more times —OR—More help provided only 1 or 2 times during last 7 days

3. EXTENSIVE ASSISTANCE—While resident performed part of activity, over last 7-day period, help of following type(s) provided 3 or more times:
— Weight-bearing support
— Full staff performance during part (but not all) of last 7 days

4. TOTAL DEPENDENCE—Full staff performance of activity during entire 7 days

8. ACTIVITY DID NOT OCCUR during entire 7 days

(B) ADL SUPPORT PROVIDED—(Code for MOST SUPPORT PROVIDED OVER ALL SHIFTS during last 7 days; code regardless of resident's self-performance classification)

0. No setup or physical help from staff
1. Setup help only
2. One person physical assist
3. Two+ persons physical assist

8. ADL activity itself did not occur during entire 7 days

		(A) SELF-PERF	(B) SUPPORT
a.	BED MOBILITY	How resident moves to and from lying position, turns side to side, and positions body while in bed		
b.	TRANSFER	How resident moves between surfaces—to/from: bed, chair, wheelchair, standing position (EXCLUDE to/from bath/toilet)		

MDS 2.0 01/30/98

G1.		(A)	(B)
c.	**WALK IN ROOM** — How resident walks between locations in his/her room		
d.	**WALK IN CORRIDOR** — How resident walks in corridor on unit		
e.	**LOCOMOTION ON UNIT** — How resident moves between locations in his/her room and adjacent corridor on same floor. If in wheelchair, self-sufficiency once in chair		
f.	**LOCOMOTION OFF UNIT** — How resident moves to and returns from off unit locations (e.g., areas set aside for dining, activities, or treatments). If facility has only one floor, how resident moves to and from distant areas on the floor. If in wheelchair, self-sufficiency once in chair		
g.	**DRESSING** — How resident puts on, fastens, and takes off all items of **street** clothing, including donning/removing prosthesis		
h.	**EATING** — How resident eats and drinks (regardless of skill). Includes intake of nourishment by other means (e.g., tube feeding, total parenteral nutrition)		
i.	**TOILET USE** — How resident uses the toilet room (or commode, bedpan, urinal); transfer on/off toilet, cleanses, changes pad, manages ostomy or catheter, adjusts clothes		
j.	**PERSONAL HYGIENE** — How resident maintains personal hygiene, including combing hair, brushing teeth, shaving, applying makeup, washing/drying face, hands, and perineum (EXCLUDE baths and showers)		

G2.	**BATHING** — How resident takes full-body bath/shower, sponge bath, and transfers in/out of tub/shower (EXCLUDE washing of back and hair.) Code for most dependent in self-performance. (A) BATHING SELF-PERFORMANCE codes appear below	(A)
	0. Independent—No help provided	
	1. Supervision—Oversight help only	
	2. Physical help limited to transfer only	
	3. Physical help in part of bathing activity	
	4. Total dependence	
	8. Activity itself did not occur during entire 7 days	

G3.	**TEST FOR BALANCE** (see training manual)	
	(Code for ability during test in the last 7 days)	
	0. Maintained position as required in test	
	1. Unsteady, but able to rebalance self without physical support	
	2. Partial physical support during test; or stands (sits) but does not follow directions for test	
	3. Not able to attempt test without physical help	
	a. Balance while standing	
	b. Balance while sitting—position, trunk control	

H3.	**APPLIANCES AND PROGRAMS**	Any scheduled toileting plan	a.	Indwelling catheter	d.
		Bladder retraining program	b.	Ostomy present	i.
		External (condom) catheter	c.	NONE OF ABOVE	j.

I1.	**DISEASES**	**Check only those diseases that have a relationship to current ADL status, cognitive status, mood and behavior status, medical treatments, nursing monitoring, or risk of death. (Do not list inactive diagnoses)**	
		(*If none apply, CHECK the NONE OF ABOVE box*)	
		ENDOCRINE/METABOLIC/NUTRITIONAL	Hemiplegia/Hemiparesis — v.
		Diabetes mellitus — a.	Multiple sclerosis — w.
		MUSCULOSKELETAL	Quadriplegia — z.
		Hip fracture — m.	PSYCHIATRIC/MOOD
		NEUROLOGICAL	Depression — ee.
		Aphasia — r.	Manic depressive (bipolar disease) — ff.
		Cerebral palsy — s.	OTHER
		Cerebrovascular accident (stroke) — t.	NONE OF ABOVE — rr.

I2.	**INFECTIONS**	(*If none apply, CHECK the NONE OF ABOVE box*)	
		Antibiotic resistant infection (e.g., Methicillin resistant staph) — a.	Septicemia — g.
		Clostridium difficile (c. diff.) — b.	Sexually transmitted diseases — h.
		Conjunctivitis — c.	Tuberculosis — i.
		HIV infection — d.	Urinary tract infection in last 30 days — j.
		Pneumonia — e.	Viral hepatitis — k.
		Respiratory infection — f.	Wound infection — l.
			NONE OF ABOVE — m.

I3.	**OTHER CURRENT DIAGNOSES AND ICD-9 CODES**	(*Include only those diseases diagnosed in the last 90 days that have a relationship to current ADL status, cognitive status, mood or behavior status, medical treatments, nursing monitoring, or risk of death*)	
		a.	· ·
		b.	· ·

J1.	**PROBLEM CONDITIONS**	(*Check all problems present in last 7 days unless other time frame is indicated*)	
		INDICATORS OF FLUID STATUS	OTHER
		a.	Delusions — e.
		b.	

G4.	FUNCTIONAL LIMITATION IN RANGE OF MOTION	(Code for limitations during last 7 days that interfered with daily functions or placed residents at risk of injury) (A) RANGE OF MOTION 0. No limitation 1. Limitation on one side 2. Limitation on both sides	(B) VOLUNTARY MOVEMENT 0. No loss 1. Partial loss 2. Full loss	(A)	(B)
		a. Neck			
		b. Arm—Including shoulder or elbow			
		c. Hand—Including wrist or fingers			
		d. Leg—Including hip or knee			
		e. Foot—Including ankle or toes			
		f. Other limitation or loss			

G6.	MODES OF TRANSFER	(Check all that apply during last 7 days)	
		Bedfast all or most of time	a.
		Bed rails used for bed mobility or transfer	b.
		NONE OF ABOVE	

G7.	TASK SEGMENTATION	Some or all of ADL activities were broken into subtasks during last 7 days so that resident could perform them 0. No 1. Yes	

H1.	CONTINENCE SELF-CONTROL CATEGORIES (Code for resident's PERFORMANCE OVER ALL SHIFTS)
	0. CONTINENT—Complete control [includes use of indwelling urinary catheter or ostomy device that does not leak urine or stool]
	1. USUALLY CONTINENT—BLADDER, incontinent episodes once a week or less; BOWEL, less than weekly
	2. OCCASIONALLY INCONTINENT—BLADDER, 2 or more times a week but not daily; BOWEL, once a week
	3. FREQUENTLY INCONTINENT—BLADDER, tended to be incontinent daily, but some control present (e.g., on day shift); BOWEL, 2-3 times a week
	4. INCONTINENT—Had inadequate control BLADDER, multiple daily episodes; BOWEL, all (or almost all) of the time

a.	BOWEL CONTINENCE	Control of bowel movement, with appliance or bowel continence programs, if employed	
b.	BLADDER CONTINENCE	Control of urinary bladder function (if dribbles, volume insufficient to soak through underpants), with appliances (e.g., foley) or continence programs, if employed	

H2.	BOWEL ELIMINATION PATTERN	Diarrhea	c.	NONE OF ABOVE	e.
		Fecal impaction	d.		

		Weight gain or loss of 3 or more pounds within a 7 day period	Edema	g.
	a.	Inability to lie flat due to shortness of breath	Fever	h.
			Hallucinations	i.
	b.	Dehydrated; output exceeds input	Internal bleeding	j.
			Recurrent lung aspirations in last 90 days	k.
	c.		Shortness of breath	l.
		Insufficient fluid; did NOT consume all/almost all liquids provided during last 3 days	Unsteady gait	n.
	d.		Vomiting	o.
			NONE OF ABOVE	p.

J2.	PAIN SYMPTOMS	(Code the highest level of pain present in the last 7 days)	
		a. FREQUENCY with which resident complains or shows evidence of pain 0. No pain (skip to J4) 1. Pain less than daily 2. Pain daily	b. INTENSITY of pain 1. Mild pain 2. Moderate pain 3. Times when pain is horrible or excruciating

J4.	ACCIDENTS	(Check all that apply)	
		Fell in past 30 days	a.
		Fell in past 31-180 days	b.
		Hip fracture in last 180 days	c.
		Other fracture in last 180 days	d.
		NONE OF ABOVE	e.

J5.	STABILITY OF CONDITIONS	Conditions/diseases make resident's cognitive, ADL, mood or behavior status unstable—(fluctuating, precarious, or deteriorating)	a.
		Resident experiencing an acute episode or a flare-up of a recurrent or chronic problem	b.
		End-stage disease, 6 or fewer months to live	c.
		NONE OF ABOVE	d.

K1.	ORAL PROBLEMS	Chewing problem	a.
		Swallowing problem	b.
		NONE OF ABOVE	d.

K2.	HEIGHT AND WEIGHT	Record (a.) height in inches and (b.) weight in pounds. Base weight on most recent measure in last 30 days; measure weight consistently in accord with standard facility practice—e.g., in a.m. after voiding, before meal, with shoes off, and in nightclothes	a. HT (in.)	b. WT (lb.)

K3.	WEIGHT CHANGE	a. Weight loss—5 % or more in last 30 days; or 10 % or more in last 180 days 0. No 1. Yes	a.
		b. Weight gain—5 % or more in last 30 days; or 10 % or more in last 180 days 0. No 1. Yes	b.

MDS 2.0 01/30/98

K5. NUTRITIONAL APPROACHES

(Check all that apply in last 7 days)

- a. Parenteral/IV
- b. Feeding tube
- On a planned weight change program ... h.
- NONE OF ABOVE ... i.

K6. PARENTERAL OR ENTERAL INTAKE

(Skip to Section M if neither 5a nor 5b is checked)

a. Code the proportion of total calories the resident received through parenteral or tube feedings in the **last 7 days**

0. None	3. 51% to 75%
1. 1% to 25%	4. 76% to 100%
2. 26% to 50%	

b. Code the average fluid intake per day by IV or tube in **last 7 days**

0. None	3. 1001 to 1500 cc/day
1. 1 to 500 cc/day	4. 1501 to 2000 cc/day
2. 501 to 1000 cc/day	5. 2001 or more cc/day

M1. ULCERS (Due to any cause)

(Record the number of ulcers at each ulcer stage—regardless of cause. If none present at a stage, record "0" (zero). Code all that apply during last 7 days. Code 9 = 9 or more.) [Requires full body exam.]

Number at Stage

- a. **Stage 1.** A persistent area of skin redness (without a break in the skin) that does not disappear when pressure is relieved.
- b. **Stage 2.** A partial thickness loss of skin layers that presents clinically as an abrasion, blister, or shallow crater.
- c. **Stage 3.** A full thickness of skin is lost, exposing the subcutaneous tissues - presents as a deep crater with or without undermining adjacent tissue.
- d. **Stage 4.** A full thickness of skin and subcutaneous tissue is lost, exposing muscle or bone.

M2. TYPE OF ULCER

(For each type of ulcer, code for the highest stage in the last 7 days using scale in item M1—i.e., 0=none; stages 1, 2, 3, 4)

- a. Pressure ulcer—any lesion caused by pressure resulting in damage of underlying tissue
- b. Stasis ulcer—open lesion caused by poor circulation in the lower extremities

M4. OTHER SKIN PROBLEMS OR LESIONS PRESENT

(Check all that apply during last 7 days)

- a. Abrasions, bruises
- b. Burns (second or third degree)
- c. Open lesions other than ulcers, rashes, cuts (e.g. cancer lesions)
- d. Rashes—e.g., intertrigo, eczema, drug rash, heat rash, herpes zoster
- e. Skin desensitized to pain or pressure
- f. Skin tears or cuts (other than surgery)
- g. Surgical wounds
- h. NONE OF ABOVE

P1. SPECIAL TREATMENTS, PROCEDURES, AND PROGRAMS

a. SPECIAL CARE—*Check treatments or programs received during the last 14 days*

TREATMENTS

- a. Chemotherapy
- b. Dialysis
- c. IV medication
- d. Intake/output
- e. Monitoring acute medical condition
- f. Ostomy care
- g. Oxygen therapy
- h. Radiation
- i. Suctioning
- j. Tracheostomy care
- k. Transfusions
- l. Ventilator or respirator

PROGRAMS

- m. Alcohol/drug treatment program
- n. Alzheimer's/dementia special care unit
- o. Hospice care
- p. Pediatric unit
- q. Respite care
- r. Training in skills required to return to the community (e.g., taking medications, house work, shopping, transportation, ADLs)
- s. NONE OF ABOVE

b. THERAPIES - Record the number of days and total minutes each of the following therapies was administered (for at least 15 minutes a day) in the **last 7 calendar days** (Enter 0 if none or less than 15 min. daily)

[Note—count only post admission therapies]

(A) = # of days administered for 15 minutes or more
(B) = total # of minutes provided in last 7 days

	DAYS	MIN
	(A)	(B)
a. Speech - language pathology and audiology services		
b. Occupational therapy		
c. Physical therapy		
d. Respiratory therapy		
e. Psychological therapy (by any licensed mental health professional)		

P3. NURSING REHABILITATION/RESTORATIVE CARE

Record the NUMBER OF DAYS each of the following rehabilitation or restorative techniques or practices was provided to the resident for more than or equal to 15 minutes per day in the last 7 days (Enter 0 if none or less than 15 min. daily.)

- a. Range of motion (passive)
- b. Range of motion (active)
- c. Splint or brace assistance

TRAINING AND SKILL PRACTICE IN:

- d. Bed mobility
- e. Transfer
- f. Walking
- g. Dressing or grooming
- h. Eating or swallowing
- i. Amputation/prosthesis care
- j. Communication
- k. Other

M5.	SKIN TREAT-MENTS	Pressure relieving device(s) for chair	a.
		Pressure relieving device(s) for bed	b.
	(Check all that apply during last 7 days)	Turning/repositioning program	c.
		Nutrition or hydration intervention to manage skin problems	d.
		Ulcer care	e.
		Surgical wound care	f.
		Application of dressings (with or without topical medications) other than to feet	g.
		Application of ointments/medications (other than to feet)	h.
		Other preventative or protective skin care (other than to feet)	i.
		NONE OF ABOVE	j.
M6.	FOOT PROBLEMS AND CARE	Resident has one or more foot problems—e.g., corns, calluses, bunions, hammer toes, overlapping toes, pain, structural problems	a.
		Infection of the foot—e.g., cellulitis, purulent drainage	b.
	(Check all that apply during last 7 days)	Open lesions on the foot	c.
		Nails/calluses trimmed during last 90 days	d.
		Received preventative or protective foot care (e.g., used special shoes, inserts, pads, toe separators)	e.
		Application of dressings (with or without topical medications)	f.
		NONE OF ABOVE	g.

N1.	TIME AWAKE	(Check appropriate time periods over last 7 days) Resident awake all or most of time (i.e., naps no more than one hour per time period) in the:	
		Morning	a.	Evening	c.
		Afternoon	b.	NONE OF ABOVE	d.

(If resident is comatose, skip to Section O)

| N2. | AVERAGE TIME INVOLVED IN ACTIVITIES | (When awake and not receiving treatments or ADL care) 0. Most—more than 2/3 of time 2. Little—less than 1/3 of time 1. Some—from 1/3 to 2/3 of time 3. None | |

O1.	NUMBER OF MEDICA-TIONS	(Record the number of different medications used in the last 7 days; enter "0" if none used)	
O3.	INJECTIONS	(Record the number of DAYS injections of any type received during the last 7 days; enter "0" if none used)	
O4.	DAYS RECEIVED THE FOLLOWING MEDICATION	(Record the number of DAYS during last 7 days; enter "0" if not used. Note—enter "1" for long-acting meds used less than weekly)	
		a. Antipsychotic		d. Hypnotic	
		b. Antianxiety		e. Diuretic	
		c. Antidepressant			

P4.	DEVICES AND RESTRAINTS	Use the following codes for last 7 days: 0. Not used 1. Used less than daily 2. Used daily	
		Bed rails	
		a. — Full bed rails on all open sides of bed	a.
		b. — Other types of side rails used (e.g., half rail, one side)	b.
		c. Trunk restraint	c.
		d. Limb restraint	d.
		e. Chair prevents rising	e.
P7.	PHYSICIAN VISITS	In the LAST 14 DAYS (or since admission if less than 14 days in facility) how many days has the physician (or authorized assistant or practitioner) examined the resident?? (Enter 0 if none)	a.
P8.	PHYSICIAN ORDERS	In the LAST 14 DAYS (or since admission if less than 14 days in facility) how many days has the physician (or authorized assistant or practitioner) changed the resident's orders? Do not include order renewals without change. (Enter 0 if none)	b.
Q2.	OVERALL CHANGE IN CARE NEEDS	Resident's overall level of self sufficiency has changed significantly as compared to status of 90 days ago (or since last assessment if less than 90 days) 0. No change 1. Improved—receives fewer 2. Deteriorated—receives supports, needs less more support restrictive level of care	
R2.	SIGNATURES OF PERSONS COMPLETING THE ASSESSMENT:		

a. Signature of RN Assessment Coordinator (sign on above line)

b. Date RN Assessment Coordinator signed as complete

	Month	Day	Year

c. Other Signatures	Title	Sections	Date
d.			Date
e.			Date
f.			Date
g.			Date
h.			Date

MDS 2.0 01/30/98

573

MINIMUM DATA SET (MDS) — *VERSION 2.0*

FOR NURSING HOME RESIDENT ASSESSMENT AND CARE SCREENING

DISCHARGE TRACKING FORM [do not use for temporary visits home]

SECTION AA. IDENTIFICATION INFORMATION

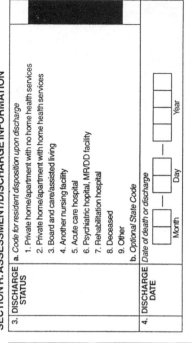

1.	RESIDENT NAME③	a. (First)	b. (Middle Initial)	c. (Last)	d. (Jr/Sr)
2.	GENDER③	1. Male	2. Female		
3.	BIRTHDATE③	Month — Day — Year			
4.	RACE/ ETHNICITY③	1. American Indian/Alaskan Native 2. Asian/Pacific Islander 3. Black, not of Hispanic origin	4. Hispanic 5. White, not of Hispanic origin		
5.	SOCIAL SECURITY③ AND MEDICARE NUMBERS ⓑ [C in 1ˢᵗ box if non med. no.]	a. Social Security Number b. Medicare number (or comparable railroad insurance number)			
6.	FACILITY PROVIDER NO.ⓒ	a. State No. b. Federal No.			
7.	MEDICAID NO. ["+" if pending, "N" if not a Medicaid recipient] ⓕ				
8.	REASONS FOR ASSESS-MENT	[Note—Other codes do not apply to this form] a. Primary reason for assessment 6. Discharged—return not anticipated 7. Discharged—return anticipated 8. Discharged prior to completing initial assessment			

SECTION R. ASSESSMENT/DISCHARGE INFORMATION

3.	DISCHARGE STATUS	a. Code for resident disposition upon discharge 1. Private home/apartment with no home health services 2. Private home/apartment with home health services 3. Board and care/assisted living 4. Another nursing facility 5. Acute care hospital 6. Psychiatric hopital, MR/DD facility 7. Rehabilitation hospital 8. Deceased 9. Other b. Optional State Code
4.	DISCHARGE DATE	Date of death or discharge Month — Day — Year

9. SIGNATURES OF STAFF COMPLETING FORM			
	Title	Sections	Date
a. Signatures			Date
b.			Date
c.			Date

SECTION AB. DEMOGRAPHIC INFORMATION
[Complete only for stays less than 14 days] (AA8a=8)

1.	DATE OF ENTRY	*Date the stay began. Note — Does not include readmission if record was closed at time of temporary discharge to hospital, etc. In such cases, use prior admission date*
		[ ][ ] — [ ][ ] — [ ][ ][ ][ ]
		Month Day Year
2.	ADMITTED FROM (AT ENTRY)	1. Private home/apt. with no home health services 2. Private home/apt. with home health services 3. Board and care/assisted living/group home 4. Nursing home 5. Acute care hospital 6. Psychiatric hospital, MR/DD facility 7. Rehabilitation hospital 8. Other

SECTION A. IDENTIFICATION AND BACKGROUND INFORMATION

6.	MEDICAL RECORD NO.	

⊙ = Key items for computerized resident tracking

☐ = When box blank, must enter number or letter   [a.] = When letter in box, check if condition applies

MDS 2.0 01/30/98

MINIMUM DATA SET (MDS) — *VERSION 2.0*
FOR NURSING HOME RESIDENT ASSESSMENT AND CARE SCREENING

REENTRY TRACKING FORM

SECTION AA. IDENTIFICATION INFORMATION

1.	RESIDENT NAME⓪	a. (First)	b. (Middle Initial)	c. (Last)	d. (Jr/Sr)

2.	GENDER⓪	1. Male	2. Female

3.	BIRTHDATE⓪	Month — Day — Year

4.	RACE/ ETHNICITY⓪	1. American Indian/Alaskan Native 4. Hispanic 2. Asian/Pacific Islander 5. White, not of 3. Black, not of Hispanic origin Hispanic origin

5.	SOCIAL SECURITY⓪ AND MEDICARE NUMBERS ⓪ [C in 1st box if non med. no.]	a. Social Security Number __ __ __ — __ __ — __ __ __ __ b. Medicare number (or comparable railroad insurance number)

6.	FACILITY PROVIDER NO.⓪	a. State No. b. Federal No.

7.	MEDICAID NO. ["+" if pending, "N" if not a Medicaid recipient] ⓪	

8.	REASONS FOR ASSESS-MENT	[Note—Other codes do not apply to this form] a. Primary reason for assessment 9. Reentry

9. SIGNATURES OF PERSONS COMPLETING FORM

	Title	Sections	Date
a. Signatures			Date
b.			Date
c.			Date

SECTION A. IDENTIFICATION AND BACKGROUND INFORMATION

4a.	DATE OF REENTRY	Date of reentry		
		Month	Day	Year
4b.	ADMITTED FROM (AT REENTRY)	1. Private home/apt. with no home health services 2. Private home/apt. with home health services 3. Board and care/assisted living/group home 4. Nursing home 5. Acute care hospital 6. Psychiatric hospital, MR/DD facility 7. Rehabilitation hospital 8. Other		
6.	MEDICAL RECORD NO.			

⊙ = Key items for computerized resident tracking

☐ = When box blank, must enter number or letter   a. = When letter in box, check if condition applies

577

INDEX

.

ISBN 0-07-034458-2

90000

9 780070 344587